POINTERS TO CANCER PROGNOSIS

DEVELOPMENTS IN ONCOLOGY

Recent volumes

M.P. Hacker, E.B. Double and I. Krakoff, eds., Platinum Coordination Complexes in Cancer Chemotherapy. ISBN 0-89838-619-5

M.J. van Zwieten, The Rat as Animal Model in Breast Cancer Research: A Histopathological Study of Radiation- and Hormone-Induced Rat Mammary Tumors. ISBN 0-89838-624-1

B. Löwenberg and A. Hagenbeek, eds., Minimal Residual Disease in Acute Leukemia. ISBN 0-89838-630-6

I. van der Waal and G.B. Snow, eds., Oral Oncology. ISBN 0-89838-631-4

B.W. Hancock and A.H. Ward, eds., Immunological Aspects of Cancer. ISBN 0-89838-664-0

K.V. Honn and B.F. Sloane, Hemostatic Mechanisms and Metastasis. ISBN 0-89838-667-5

K.R. Harrap, W. Davis and A.H. Calvert, eds., Cancer Chemotherapy and Selective Drug Development. ISBN 0-89838-673-X

C.J.H. van de Velde and P.H. Sugarbaker, eds., Liver Metastasis. ISBN 0-89838-648-5

D.J. Ruiter, K. Welvaart and S. Ferrone, eds., Cutaneous Melanoma and Precursor Lesions. ISBN 0-89838-689-6

S.B. Howell, ed., Intra-arterial and Intracavitary Cancer Chemotherapy. ISBN 0-89838-691-8

D.L. Kisner and J.F. Smyth, eds., Interferon Alpha-2: Pre-Clinical and Clinical Evaluation. ISBN 0-89838-701-9

P. Furmanski, J.C. Hager and M.A. Rich, eds., RNA Tumor Viruses, Oncogenes, Human Cancer and Aids: On the Frontiers of Understanding. ISBN 0-89838-703-5

J. Talmadge, I.J. Fidler and R.K. Oldham, Screening for Biological Response Modifiers: Methods and Rationale. ISBN 0-89838-712-4

J.C. Bottino, R.W. Opfell and F.M. Muggia, eds., Liver Cancer. ISBN 0-89838-713-2

P.K. Pattengale, R.J. Lukes and C.R. Taylor, Lymphoproliferative Diseases: Pathogenesis, Diagnosis, Therapy. ISBN 0-89838-725-6

F. Cavalli, G. Bonadonna and M. Rozencweig, eds., Malignant Lymphomas and Hodgkin's Disease: Experimental and Therapeutic Advances. ISBN 0-89838-727-2

L. Baker, F. Valeriote and V. Ratanatharathorn, eds., Biology and Therapy of Acute Leukemia. .ISBN 0-89838-728-0

J. Russo, ed., Immunocytochemistry in Tumor Diagnosis. ISBN 0-89838-737-X

R.L. Ceriani, ed., Monoclonal Antibodies and Breast Cancer. ISBN 0-89838-739-6

D.E. Peterson, G.E. Elias and S.T. Sonis, eds., Head and Neck Management of the Cancer Patient. ISBN 0-89838-747-7

D.M. Green, Diagnosis and Management of Malignant Solid Tumors in Infants and Children. ISBN 0-89838-750-7

K.A. Foon and A.C. Morgan, Jr., eds., Monoclonal Antibody Therapy of Human Cancer. ISBN 0-89838-754-X

J.G. McVie, W. Bakker, Sj.Sc. Wagenaar and D. Carney, eds., Clinical and Experimental Pathology of Lung Cancer. ISBN 0-89838-764-7

K.V. Honn, W.E. Powers and B.F. Sloane, eds., Mechanisms of Cancer Metastasis. ISBN 0-89838-765-5

K. Lapis, L.A. Liotta and A.S. Rabson, eds., Biochemistry and Molecular Genetics of Cancer Metastasis. ISBN 0-89838-785-X

A.J. Mastromarino, ed., Biology and Treatment of Colorectal Cancer Metastasis. ISBN 0-89838-786-8

M.A. Rich, J.C. Hager and J. Taylor-Papadimitriou, eds., Breast Cancer: Origins, Detection and Treatment. ISBN 0-89838-792-2

D.G. Poplack, L. Massimo and P. Cornaglia-Ferraris, eds., The Role of Pharmacology in Pediatric Oncology. ISBN 0-89838-795-7

A. Hagenbeek and B. Löwenberg, eds., Minimal Residual Disease in Acute Leukemia 1986. ISBN 0-89838-799-X

F.M. Muggia and M. Rozencweig, eds., Clinical Evaluations of Anti-Tumor Therapy. ISBN 0-89838-803-1

F.A. Valeriote and F.A. Baker, eds., Biochemical Modulation of Anticancer Agents: Experimental and Clinical Approaches. ISBN 0-89838-827-9

B.A. Stoll, ed., Pointers to Cancer Prognosis. ISBN 0-89838-841-4

K.H. Hollmann and J.M. Verley, eds., New Frontiers in Mammary Pathology 1986. ISBN 0-89838-852-X

POINTERS TO CANCER PROGNOSIS

edited by

Basil A. Stoll
Honorary consultant physician to Oncology Departments
St. Thomas' Hospital and Royal Free Hospital, London, U.K.

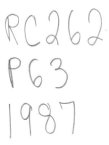

RC262
P63
1987

1987 **MARTINUS NIJHOFF PUBLISHERS**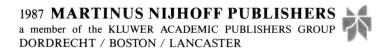
a member of the KLUWER ACADEMIC PUBLISHERS GROUP
DORDRECHT / BOSTON / LANCASTER

Distributors

for the United States and Canada: Kluwer Academic Publishers, P.O. Box 358, Accord Station, Hingham, MA 02018-0358, USA
for the UK and Ireland: Kluwer Academic Publishers, MTP Press Limited, Falcon House, Queen Square, Lancaster LA1 1RN, UK
for all other countries: Kluwer Academic Publishers Group, Distribution Center, P.O. Box 322, 3300 AH Dordrecht, The Netherlands

Library of Congress Cataloging in Publication Data

```
Pointers to cancer prognosis.

   (Developments in oncology ; 48)
   Includes index.
   1. Cancer--Prognosis.  I. Stoll, Basil A. (Basil
Arnold)  II. Series.  [DNLM: 1. Neoplasms.  2. Prognosis.
W1 DE998N v.48 / QZ 200 P752]
RC262.P63  1987      616.99'4075      86-23673
ISBN 0-89838-841-4
```

ISBN 0-89838-841-4

PRINTED IN THE NETHERLANDS

Contents

Contributors

S.J. Arnott, F.R.C.S. (Ed), F.R.C.R.
Consultant, Department of Radiotherapy, St. Bartholomew's Hospital, London, UK

N.F. Boyd, M.D., F.R.C.P. (C)
Associate Professor of Medicine, Princess Margaret Hospital; Clinical Epidemiologist, Ludwig Institute, Toronto, Ontario, Canada

A. Philippe Chahinian, M.D.
Associate Professor, Department of Neoplastic Diseases, Mount Sinai School of Medicine, New York, USA

Ann F. Chambers, Ph.D.
Assistant Professor, Department of Radiation Oncology, University of Western Ontario, London, Ontario, Canada

Philip R. Clingan, M.B., B.S., F.R.A.C.P.
Terry Fox Fellow, Ontario Cancer Institute; Research Fellow, Ludwig Institute, Toronto, Ontario, Canada

John Craven, M.D., F.R.C.S.
Consultant Surgeon, York District Hospital, York, UK

John D. Crissman, M.D.
Professor of Pathology, Wayne State University; Director of Anatomic Pathology, Harper Hospital, Detroit, Michigan, USA

Alon J. Dembo, M.D., F.R.C.P. (C)
Associate Professor, Department of Radiology, University of Toronto; Radiation Oncologist, Princess Margaret Hospital, Toronto, Ontario, Canada

Robert O. Dillman, M.D., F.A.C.P.
Assistant Professor of Medicine, University of California, San Diego, School of Medicine and Cancer Center; Chief, Hematology/Oncology, San Diego VA Medical Center, USA

Michael L. Friedlander, M.B., Ch.B., Ph.D., M.R.C.P., F.R.A.C.P.
Staff Specialist in Oncology, Royal Prince Alfred Hospital; Honorary Consultant, Ludwig Institute, Sydney, Australia

W.M. Gregory, B.Sc.
Department of Medical Oncology, St. Bartholomew's Hospital, London, UK

M. Harding, Ph.D., M.R.C.P.
Senior Registrar, C.R.C. Department of Medical Oncology, University of Glasgow, UK

John Harris, Ph.D.
Assistant Professor, Department of Radiation Oncology, University of Western Ontario, London, Ontario, Canada

Ian R. Hart, B.V.Sc., Ph.D.
Staff Scientist, Imperial Cancer Research Fund, London, UK

Andrew M. Hoy, M.R.C.P., F.R.C.R.
Medical Director, The Princess Alice Hospice, Esher, Surrey; Honorary Consultant in Radiotherapy and Oncology, St. Thomas' Hospital, London, UK

S.B. Kaye, M.D., M.R.C.P.
Professor, C.R.C. Department of Medical Oncology, University of Glasgow, UK

Leslie Levin, M.D., M.R.C.P., F.R.C.P. (C)
Associate Professor and Acting Chairman, Department of Radiation Oncology, University of Western Ontario; Chief, Medical Oncology, Ontario Cancer Foundation, London, Ontario, Canada

T.A. Lister, M.D., F.R.C.P.
Reader and Consultant in Medical Oncology, Department of Medical Oncology, St. Bartholomew's Hospital, London, UK

E. Jane Ormerod, Ph.D.
Postdoctoral Research Fellow, Imperial Cancer Research Fund, London, UK

Walter B. Panko, Ph.D.
Associate Professor of Pathology, Assistant Professor of Cell Biology, The Methodist Hospital; Baylor College of Medicine, Houston, Texas, USA

Santilal P. Parbhoo, Ph. D., F.R.C.S.
Senior Lecturer and Consultant Surgeon, Academic Department of Surgery, Royal Free Hospital and School of Medicine, London UK

A.H.G. Paterson, M.D., F.R.C.P. (Ed), F.A.C.P.
Associate Professor of Medicine, University of Alberta; Senior Specialist in Medical Oncology, Cross Cancer Institute, Edmonton, Alberta, Canada

M.A. Richards, M.A., M.R.C.P.
I.C.R.F. Research Fellow and Honorary Senior Registrar, Department of Medical Oncology, St. Bartholomew's Hospital, London, UK

Michael H. Rosen, M.D.
Edith Rafton Fellow, Department of Neoplastic Diseases, Mount Sinai School of Medicine, New York, USA

Julian Rosenman, Ph.D., M.D.
Assistant Professor, Division of Radiation Therapy, University of North Carolina, Chapel Hill, North Carolina, USA

Kevin P. Ryan, M.D.
Division of Hematology/Oncology, University of California, San Diego, School of Medicine and Cancer Center, San Diego, California, USA

Mary R. Schwartz, M.D.
Assistant Professor of Pathology, Pathologist, The Methodist Hospital; Baylor College of Medicine, Houston, Texas, USA

Basil A. Stoll, F.F.R., F.R.C.R.
Honorary Consulting Physician, Departments of Oncology, St. Thomas' Hospital and Royal Free Hospital, London, UK

Gillian M. Thomas, B.Sc., M.D., F.R.C.P. (C)
Assistant Professor, Department of Radiology, University of Toronto; Radiation Oncologist, Princess Margaret Hospital, Toronto, Ontario, Canada

M. Tubiana, M.D.
Professor and Director, Institut Gustave Roussy, Villejuif, France

Mahesh Varia, M.D.
Associate Professor, Division of Radiation Therapy, University of North Carolina, Chapel Hill, North Carolina, USA

Gordon Williams, M.B., F.R.C.S.
Consultant Urologist and Honorary Senior Lecturer, Royal Postgraduate Medical School, Hammersmith Hospital, London, UK

Richard J. Zarbo, M.D.
Assistant Professor of Pathology, Wayne State University; Direction of Immunocytochemistry, Harper Hospital, Detroit, Michigan, USA

Preface

The last 30 years have seen little improvement in the age-adjusted mortality rates for most common types of cancer, and until we develop more effective and less damaging treatment modalities for these tumours, selection of each patient's treatment must depend on prognostic pointers. These lead to a calculated trade-off between our estimate of likely benefit to the patient, as against cost in terms of quality of life.

But changes have occurred recently in our understanding of the traditional prognostic pointers used for selecting such individualised treatment. First, it is increasingly recognised that the stage at which a tumour presents is more related to the chromological age of the tumour (how far it has progressed before diagnosis) than to its biological characteristics. While advanced chronological age of the tumour may predict a greater likelihood of early death, only biological criteria can predict the tumour growth rate, the likelihood of prolonged survival, the likely course of the disease after the first recurrence or the likehood of response to systemic therapy.

Second, there is increasing use of failure analysis in relating the clinical and biological characteristics of tumours to their response to standard treatments. In the past, the relationship was interpreted mainly in terms of survival rate, but the site and timing of first recurrence and the pattern and timing of subsequent spread provide a better assessment of the control possible from local or systemic therapy.

Third, the unifactorial statistical analysis of prognostic factors in cancer has recently given way to multivariate analysis. In the latter approach, the various factors found to be related to prognosis are compared both for their relative importance and also for how they act independently of other factors.

Fourth, for many years it has been widely assumed that the growth rate of a tumour runs parallel to its metastatic potential, but now that it is possible to measure the tumour replication rate, there is increasing evidence to the contrary. Recent reports suggest that specific metastasis genes regulate the cancer cell's ability to express enzymes which facilitate invasion of the stroma, and favour implantation and establishment of distant metastases. Invasiveness, not replicating activity, is the major factor determining a cancer's lethality.

Finally, there is increasing evidence that tumours undergo 'progression', implying that most tumour populations are clonally heterogeneous by the time they present clinically, and that their biological aggressiveness may change still further by the time the first recurrence manifests. Even subsequently, tumours are capable of evolving a new variant which can outflank any systemic therapy being given. Only by recognising such progression can we plan appropriate treatment when the biology of a tumour changes.

The above considerations have implications for research but also affect the selection of treatment for our next cancer patient. Thus, there is a serious danger of 'overkill' unless we distinguish cases offering a likelihood of prolonged survival with minimal treatment (as in slowly growing prostatic or breast cancer), from those with biologically aggressive tumours for which aggressive therapy is imperative. Again, the selection of high-risk patients for adjuvant systemic therapy must be based on indices shown to have an independent effect on prognosis in multivariate analysis. Finally, in cases where alternative treatments are possible (as in lymphoma or breast cancer), we must attempt to identify patients at risk of failure to a specific treatment in order to permit early application of alternative treatment.

The book sets out to satisfy two distinct needs: the first sections aim to estimate the relative strengths of standard prognostic pointers in different types of cancer; the final section provides an up-to-the-minute guide to the use of multifactorial indices of prognosis and responsiveness for selecting individualised treatment for each common type of cancer. In these aims, I acknowledge my gratitude to the contributors who responded so magnificently to the demanding challenge issued to them. To make each chapter complete in itself, some minor points of overlap have been permitted.

London, 1987   Basil A. Stoll

I. Clinical pointers to prognosis

1. Clinical pointers to rapid growth

S.P. PARBHOO

The growth tempo of tumours has, until recently, received little attention in relation to the clinical management of cancer, yet, when it can be recognised (as in the case of inflammatory cancer), the dynamic biological characterisation of a tumour may provide a much better clue to its clinical behaviour than does its histopathological picture. Even now, information on the growth rate and kinetics of tumours is scanty and based on studies of a small number of tumours. This chapter will examine clinical behaviour of rapidly growing malignant tumours in relation to underlying biological phenomena, under the following headings:
– Inflammatory cancer and other rapidly growing tumours
– Clinical demonstration of rapid growth
– Relationship of rapid growth to biological indices
– Changes in tumour growth rate
– Relationship of rapid growth to immune deficiency states
– Prospects for clinical detection of rapidly growing tumours

Inflammatory cancer and other rapidly growing tumours

There is a clinical impression that sarcomas, embryonal tumours and lymphomas are the fastest growing tumours whereas most breast cancers and adenocarcinomas are relatively slow growing. This is supported by Fig. 1 which compares the rate of growth of various malignancies from one cell to 10^9 cells, when the tumour becomes clinically manifest. The figure is based on a small number of studies. There are however, subsets of tumours within all groups which grow rapidly, and some are listed in Table 1.

The traditional clinical terms applied to rapidly growing tumours are inflammatory or hurricane tumours. The former term is usually applied to the loco-regional features of a tumour visible to the clinician, whereas the term hurricane is more commonly applied to rapidly growing tumours with early and widespread metastatic deposits in the bones and viscera. Inflammatory cancers demonstrate the

4

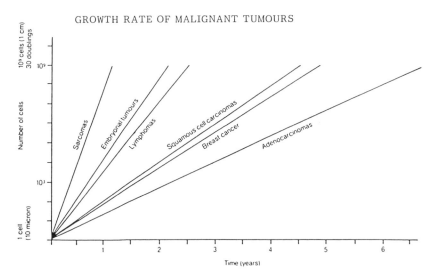

Figure 1. Comparative growth rates of cancer.

clinical features of bacterial inflammation namely, swelling, redness, heat and tenderness. In addition, their size increases rapidly, vascular markings are prominent and necrosis and ulceration of the overlying skin are common. Subcutaneous inflammatory tumours invade the skin and cause lymphoedema with peau d'orange. Widespread lymphatic permeation will cause nodularity, thickening and induration over large areas (e.g. carcinoma en-cuirasse over the chest wall).

There may be a field change such as that seen with extensive recurrence after mastectomy, when multiple nodules appear rapidly and extend rapidly to cover a wide area of the chest wall, or when multiple basal cell or squamous carcinomata appear over a wide area of skin. In the case of malignant melanoma, rapid growth

---

Table 1. Examples of rapidly growing cancers

Sarcoma
  Sarcoma in immunocompromised host
Embryonal tumours
  'Hurricane' testicular tumour
  Testicular teratoma
  Chorio carcinoma
Neuroblastoma
Nephroblastoma
Hepatoblastoma
Spindle and giant cell thyroid cancer
Inflammatory cancer
  Breast, thyroid, melanoma
Aggressive/subterranean basal cell carcinoma
Anaplastic carcinoma

---

may cause multiple pigmented nodules to appear on the skin or on the surface of organs such as the liver or bowel.

Although inflammatory carcinomas have been recognised in patients with carcinoma of the breast for over a century [1], it was the classical report by Lee and Tannenbaum [2] which established inflammatory carcinoma of the breast as a clinical entity. An inflammatory appearance has also been reported in some cases of bronchial, gynaecological and pancreatic cancers and in malignant melanoma. Inflammatory cancer probably represents the most active end of the spectrum of any rapidly growing tumour and whereas inflammatory cancers of the breast are diagnosed in 1.5–4% of all patients presenting with breast cancer, fast growing tumours probably represent between 10 and 20% of all breast cancers [3, 4]. In Tunisia, more than half the women presenting with breast cancer have rapidly progressing cancer but the reason for this exceptional incidence is unclear [5].

Rapidly growing breast cancers are, in general, not easily identified clinically. Denoix [6] introduced the concept of a fast growing phase (FGP) and described three types of rapidly progressive breast cancer:

FGP 3 (inflammatory breast cancer) which usually presents no diagnostic problems. The breast is red, tender, warm and with prominent vascular markings, and the cutaneous lymphangitis and oedema give rise to the peau d'orange appearance. The axillary nodes may be enlarged and matted.

FGP 2 shows peritumoural or skin oedema, pinkish colour of the skin, tenderness on palpation and enlarged axillary nodes.

FGP 1 is based on the growth rate of the tumour as shown by its having doubled its volume within the previous two months. This category is thus largely based on the clinical history and lacks objectivity, unless the patient is a good observer or the cancer has been monitored without treatment for more than two months.

Clinical recognition of rapid growth depends on the site of the primary or metastatic cancer. While small tumours may be lost in a large breast, one may get a false impression of rapid growth in a female patient with small breasts or in men with carcinoma. The change in size of the tumour may be obvious even to the patient [7, 8, 9]. A useful index of rate of growth can be obtained from the patient's history in a variety of malignancies including cancers of the lung, colon, rectum, larynx and Hodgkins lymphoma [7, 10]. Rapid enlargement of the tumour usually leads to a short delay in reporting symptoms [11].

Other manifestations of rapidly growing tumour are the appearance of rapidly enlarging regional nodes sometimes complicated by limb oedema. Also the appearance of cerebral oedema, rupture of the capsule of a solid organ (such as haemoperitoneum from ruptured primary liver cell cancer), ulceration or fungation through the skin or perforation or fistulation of the bowel. Rapid enlargement of lytic bone lesions may lead to pathological fractures and may be associated with hypercalcaemia. In addition, rapid development of complications may point to rapid growth of tumour. Thus, superior vena-caval obstruction is most commonly seen in association with bronchogenic or breast cancer or lymphoma, but may also be seen with rapidly growing thyroid cancer of the spindle and giant cell type [12].

Rapidly growing tumours tend to show multiple sites of metastatic disease, with extensive lesions in the lungs, liver of bones rather than localised lesions. While solitary lesions in bone, liver or lung may progress slowly or remain stable over long periods of time, multiple deposits tend to grow much more rapidly. In addition, multiple deposits may show different generations of sizes, suggesting repeated showers of tumour emboli.

Rapidly growing tumours have a predilection for growing into blood vessels and this is especially seen with sarcoma, renal cell carcinoma and primary liver cell cancer. Thus, sarcomata have a high incidence of pulmonary secondaries. Inferior vena-caval and hepatic vein obstruction is sometimes seen in patients with renal cell carcinoma, giving rise to the Budd-Chiari syndrome [13].

The rate of growth of large well-defined metastatic deposits is easier to follow than that of the diffusely infiltrating type. The growth rate of a metastasis declines progressively with increasing size of the lesion and this is accompanied by a greater tendency to necrosis. It has therefore been suggested that it may be more accurate to judge advancing growth on the basis of the appearance of new lesions, rather than by change in size of existing lesions.

Slowly growing multiple nodules may cause massive enlargement of the liver without associated jaundice, liver failure or ascites. In contrast, diffuse infiltration of the liver is often associated with features of liver failure. Rapidly growing tumour is suggested by the appearance of jaundice when the liver is not grossly enlarged, contrasting with a likelihood of slowly growing tumour in a non-jaundiced patient with a liver full of discrete metastatic deposits.

The clinical and metabolic consequences of rapidly growing cancers are relate both to the tumour and to the concomitant necrosis which is common in these tumours. Thus, pyrexia and hyperuricaemia are common. Large sarcomata, or primary liver cell cancers with high metabolic rate, may also produce a clinical picture of hypoglycaemia.

Clinical demonstration of rapid growth

Radiological evidence

Rapidly growing metastases in bone tend to produce progressive lytic lesions in plain radiographs of the skeleton (Fig. 2), as opposed to more slowly growing lesions which cause blastic or mixed lytic and blastic lesions. In the case of lung metastases, rapidly growing tumours usually have characteristic features on radiology. Some patients demonstrate several crops of lung metastases at different stages in development, while a miliary pattern indicates extensive embolisation

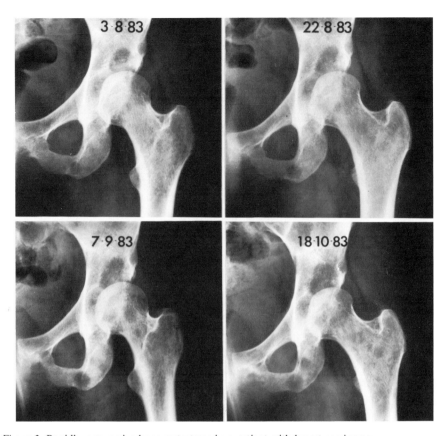

Figure 2. Rapidly progressive bone metastases in a patient with breast carcinoma.

of a tumour to the lungs. Extensive interstitial infiltration of the lungs gives the radiological appearance of lymphangitis carcinomatosa. 'Cannonball' metastases are usually associated with sarcomata, renal cell carcinoma and embryonal tumours of childhood.

The doubling time (Dt) of a tumour is the time taken for it to double its clinical volume. Those tumours where it is 7 days or less are predominantly rapidly growing in nature [14]. In the case of colorectal cancer, it is reported that the doubling time of pulmonary metastases is 5–6 times longer than that of the primary tumour [15, 16], but in the case of Ewing's sarcoma and osteogenic sarcoma, the Dt of the primary bone tumour is said to be longer than that of the pulmonary metastases [17]. Kusuma *et al.* [18] compared 163 primary breast cancer with 49 metastases in various sites and found no difference between their mean doubling times, but others [19, 20] have found that the Dt of metastases was shorter than that of the primary cancer. No firm conclusions are possible.

Mammography has been used to measure the growth rate of primary breast cancer. Discrete lesions seen on mammography generally have a slower rate of growth and are dense due to a greater content of fibrous tissue and calcium. This type of tumour is usually seen in the elderly patient with a history of a lump for several years. On the other hand, inflammatory or necrotic rapidly growing tumours may be only faintly visible, reflecting diffuse infiltration and a lesser content of fibrous tissue.

Fournier *et al.* [21] carried out serial mammography in 53 patients with primary breast cancer and found no correlation between histological characteristics and doubling times. Previously, Gershon-Cohen [22] described 16 patients in whom they were able to measure untreated carcinoma in the breast on at least two separate occasions, and calculated the doubling time of the tumours to vary between 81–834 days. Galante *et al.* [23] studied 196 non-selected patients with breast cancer by two mammographic examination with an interval of about 30 days. They found that 15.8% of their patients had fast growing cancers but there was no statistical correlation with age or menopausal status.

In a series of 32 primary breast cancers whose growth was measured by serial mammography, Spratt [24] found no association between the doubling time and the mammary parenchymal patterns as defined by Wolfe [25]. This suggests that the subset of rapidly growing breast cancers are unlikely to be identified early on the basis of mammographic patterns.

Mammographic studes have the deficiency that a number of rapidly growing cancers, especially of the inflammatory type, are not easily visualised. However, when changes such as blurring of the tumour outline, skin thickening, dilatation of the adjacent veins and microcalcification are present, the prognosis is poor [26]. Mammography is also less useful in assessing the regrowth of tumour in the irradiated breast because of the increased density and skin oedema.

Temperature change

An inflammatory appearance or increased temperature of the skin overlying a tumour may signify rapid growth of the tumour. The increase in temperature may be obvious on palpation if more than 2°C, and may be associated with gross inflammatory changes or only slight erythema. Often there is associated skin oedema. In the absence of obvious inflammatory change, there may be dilated veins coursing over the tumour or in the overlying skin. Most clinicians are familiar with the large vessels coursing over sarcomata and rapidly growing metastatic deposits, but it is seen more commonly in breast cancer. The temperature of the skin may be objectively measured either by infra-red thermography or liquid crystal thermography while that of the tumour is measured by implanted electrodes. By these techniques, dynamic studies have been carried out on the diurnal temperature variation in the tumour [22].

Intra-tumoural temperature measurements of fast growing breast cancers indicate that the metabolic activity of the tumour generates the heat measured at the surface of the breast. Gautherie [28] found a positive correlation between the metabolic heat production and the tumour volume doubling time (Dt). Other studies [see 3] report that fast growing hot breast cancers show a further rise in the temperature of 1–1.5°C over the tumour area after intravenous or peroral bolus of glucose. This response to glucose was not seen in benign breast conditions.

Spitalier *et al.* [29] and Pietra [30] used infra-red thermography to study the extent of the area with increased temperature, in relation to clinical findings. They claim that the increase in temperture was never less than 4°C in patients with fast growing tumours. The grading system used by these authors and their findings are shown in Table 2. This clearly shows that in patients with inflammatory stages 2 and 3, the temperature increase is highest and the area in which this occurs is also the most extensive. The use of this classification would also allow us to identify those patients without obvious inflammatory cancer but whose tumours may be growing rapidly.

Using liquid crystal thermography, Ratz *et al.* [31] examined the lateral extent of basal cell carcinomas and found the greatest temperature difference in highly cellular tumours and no difference in low cellularity morphea basal cell cancers. Thermography has also been used in malignant melanomas as an advance on infra-red photography. Tapernoux and Hesslar [32] reported a correlation between temperature and degree of malignancy in two thirds of the cases examined. Apart from metabolic activity, other causes for the temperature rise in the vicinity of tumours may be increased vascularity, increased flow rate or in increased heat conduction between the tumour and the skin. The last may be due to oedema and lymphatic obstruction, so that thermo-conductivity may be much greater than when the tumour is surrounded by fat.

Increased vascularity of a tumour, seen either on the surface or by angiography, is believed by the clinician to be evidence of high malignant activity. Such an abnormal tumour circulation, with or without a blush and late venous pooling,

Table 2. Clinical apprearance and extent of temperature change in breast cancer

Clinical grade	Increase °C	Area of temperature change
FGP* (signs of fast growth)		
1	4–10	S_1^{**} S_2
2	4–12	S_2 S_4
3 (obvious inflammatory cancer)	5–15	S_4

FGP*	Fast growing phase
S_1^{**}	Not more than 1 quadrant
S_2	Not more than 2 quadrants
S_3	Area greater than 2 quadrants but not beyond the breast
S_4	Area extending beyond breast

is seen only in a minority of tumours. However, in experimental animal tumours, no significant increase in blood flow is seen and there is no correlation between the rate of growth and blood supply of breast or liver cancers [33].

Operative findings

At operation, the tissues around rapidly growing tumours are often oedematous, almost gelatinous, facilitating dissection around the tumour. Large draining vessels, up to a centimeter in diameter are common and because of the danger of heavy blood loss, sufficient blood should be crossed matched and hypotensive anaesthesia used. In addition, the use of pre-operative angiography will help localise some of the larger feeding arteries which can be ligated early in the operation to minimise blood loss. In the case of large, highly vascular tumours it may be possible to embolise the main feeder vessels but, if these are numerous, arterial embolisation is unlikely to effective in decreasing tumour vascularity. Tumour excision should be carried out within 48–72 hours of embolisation, otherwise the collateral circulation adapts rapidly.

Large tumours often show haemorrhagic and necrotic areas. Necrosis is generally thought to be related to the tumour outgrowing its blood supply, but in addition, increased intratumoural pressure may interfere with tissue blood flow [34]. Experiments by Tveit *et al*. [35] indicate that increased tumour pressure may obstruct capillary blood flow and the resultant necrosis of cancer cells will result in an further increase in interstitial fluid pressure.

Relationship of rapid growth to biological indices

This will be discussed in relation to histopathology, cytology, hormone receptor status and tumour markers.

Histopathology

A variety of grading schemes have been used to identify rapidly growing breast cancers but there have been few attempts to correlate the grading of breast cancer with clinical or mammographic growth rate. In a serial mammographic study of 18 patients, Gershon-Cohen *et al*. [36] found no correlation between the doubling time and histological type of breast cancer. Spratt *et al*. [24] noted similar overall findings in 32 patients with breast cancer but reported that rapidly growing cancers had a border exhibiting increased fibrous tissue reaction and a higher nuclear grade.

Jackson and Adams [31] reviewed the histology in 33 patients with clinically aggressive basal cell carcinoma, and concluded that it was indistinguishable from the ordinary non-aggressive variety studied in 435 patients. A WHO report indicated that the morphoea type of lesion showed a typically histological pattern but had a greater tendency to recur and progress than other forms [38]. In a clinico/pathological review of 100 unselected consecutive cases of basal cell cancer, Jacobs et al. [39] found 10% of histologically aggressive lesions which they considered more likely to recur.

Cytological grading

Mouriquand et al. [40] correlated cytological grading with tumour growth rate as reflected by the FGP classification. Using their own criteria, they proposed grading into well differentiated tumours (I) intermediate groups (II) and anaplastic tumours (III). In a consecutive series of 91 breast cancers they found 18 to be clinically FGP3, and all of these showed a marked local or diffuse increase in temperature over 3°C by thermography. Of these 18 tumours, 15 proved to be cytological grade III, the others being grade II; none was grade I. They suggest that it may be possible to establish an estimate of tumour growth rate merely by analysis of cytological criteria.

Hormone receptor status

Low levels of oestrogen and progesterone receptors (ER, PR) have been found in inflammatory breast cancers [41–44] and in most cases with early local recurrence [45, 46]. The reported correlation depends on the cut-off points used for ER/PR positivity. In Tunisia, where fast growing breast cancers are frequent, ER levels are said to be low, whether or not inflammatory changes are seen [44].

Tumour marker levels

CEA (carcinoembryonic antigen) is the most widely used biological marker of cancer, but it is non-specific for cancer and its usefulness varies markedly from one type of cancer to another. Apart from colorectal cancers, CEA has been most extensively used in breast cancer assessment and the highest levels of plasma CEA have been noted with visceral (especially liver) metastases [47, 48].

Serial studies have show an exponential rate of increase in CEA levels similar to gross growth rates of metastatic cancer, while Mughal et al. [48] have reported rapid increase in CEA levels related to progression, and rapid falls following response to cytoxic chemotherapy. Others have noted marked rise in CEA levels following cytotoxic chemotherapy in lung and breast cancer, possibly a result of increased release of cytosol CEA following chemotherapeutic tumour necrosis [49, 50]. In a propective study of 628 patients with node-positive early breast cancer, Wang *et al.* [51] noted that those with a preoperative level higher than 10ng/ml had earlier recurrence as compared with those with levels less than 2.5ng/ml. The high levels (found in 5 per cent of the patients) were also associated with a reduced survival rate suggesting a subset of fast growing aggressive cancers.

Changes in tumour growth rate

The growth curve of cancers is not constant but may vary at different periods in the natural evolution of the tumour [52]. The exponential curve observed by measuring the growth rate of human cancers in skin nodules, metastatic deposits, primary lung or breast cancers, is based on a very limited part of the life history of the cancer [53].

Studies of the growth pattern of individual metastases indicates that the growth rate declines progressively as the size of a lesion increases so that the size of large lesions tends to plateau while smaller tumours continue to grow rapidly [54, 55]. There also appears to be an upper limit of the size to which the metastases grow, and Brennan *et al.* [55] have shown that for pulmonary lesions, a diameter of 4 cm is the upper limit for more than 90% of metastases. It is possible therefore to find that large measurable lesions do not change perceptibly while multiple microscopic foci are rapidly adding to the patient's tumour burden.

Rapid growth during pregnancy and lactation

Cancers developing during pregnancy or lactation are thought to have a poor prognosis. Increased hormone production, alteration in the hormone status or production of growth factors may play a part if a deleterious effect of pregnancy or lactation is shown. Contrary to popular belief, it is now accepted that the prognosis for breast cancer is no different in pregnant and non-pregnant women and that termination of pregnancy does not improve survival [56, 57].

However, some malignant melanomas are hormonally influenced and it is claimed that pregnancy and delivery may produce variable effects such as exacerbation, recurrence or regression in some cases [58, 59]. The finding of oestrogen receptor protein in approximately 20% of melanomas adds further weight to the possibility of hormonal influence, and may explain more rapid growth during pregnancy [60].

Shiu *et al.* [61] showed that pregnant women were more likely to have aggressive melanoma with itching, ulceration, bleeding and a higher incidence of lymph node involvement. The five year survival rate was no different in Stage 1 melanoma, but marked differences were seen in the 5 year survival rates for Stage

2 cases (melanoma during pregnancy 29%, parous patient with activation of melanoma during pregnancy 22%, non-parous patient 55%, other parous women 51%).

Lymphomas seen during pregnancy do not appear to have a more aggressive pattern and the prognosis is no different from that seen in non-pregnant patients [62]. In general, therefore, no general conclusions can be drawn regarding increased growth rate of cancer during pregnancy, although some tumours may show sub-sets of patients with more rapidly growing tumours.

Tumour flare

This term is usually applied to apparent clinical exacerbation in soft tissue deposits of breast cancer shortly after commencing hormone therapy [63]. Intradermal and subcutaneous metastases swell and become painful while the overlying skin may become erythematous. Rarely 'flare' of lung metastases has been reported [64, 65]. These inflammatory phenomena may be due either to sudden acceleration of growth, local stromal reaction to tumour products, or necrosis. Serial measurements of tumour area in lesions that showed a flare phenomenon, have failed to show any increase in growth rate after starting Tamoxifen therapy [65].

A similar phenomenon is seen in breast or prostate cancer patients with bone metastases, in whom treatment may cause increase in existing pain and appearance of pain at *new* sites. This increase in bone pain may occur immediately after hormone injection (as in prostatic cancer) or during the first three weeks after starting oral treatment in breast cancer. Use of a high dose loading schedule of Tamoxifen in breast cancer patients appears to hasten the onset of pain [66] but it usually resolves spontaneously despite continued use of the drug. Similar observations have been made on the flare following the start of oestrogen or androgen therapy in breast cancer [67].

Powles [68] has suggested that the exacerbation of bone pain in association with hypercalcaemia may be related to prostaglandin released by the tumour and this may apply also to soft tissue flare. The inflammatory changes associated with soft tissue flare are likely to be response to tumour necrosis rather than to a rapid increase in tumour growth rate. A dramatic example of this has been reported [69] where localised pain, erythema and tenderness occurred over a primary breast cancer in a 70 year old woman treated with Tamoxifen. The patient stopped the treatment because of the symptoms, and at mastectomy, the tumour was found to be an infiltrating duct cancer with almost total tumour necrosis.

Hypercalcaemia is sometimes found to be associated with increased bone pain shortly after the start of therapy. This third manifestation of flare may occur after either oestrogen, Tamoxifen or progestogen therapy [66, 70–73]. Mechanisms of the three manifestations of flare are poorly understood, but it has been suggested that if flare represents acceleration of tumour growth, it may be due to stimulation by lower levels of circulating hormone as the dose builds up to a therapeutic level [74].

Relationship of rapid growth to immune deficiency states

There is evidence that the incidence of cancer is higher and its growth more rapid in patients who have immune deficiency states. However, the observation applies especially to particular types of cancer and to particular subsets of patients. The incidence of such cancers is small but this may be because many patients die much earlier and may not have the time to develop the cancer. The immune deficiency states may be due to: (a) Genetic immuno deficiencies; (b) Auto-immune states e.g. primary biliary cirrhosis, Hashimoto's thyroiditis, rheumatoid arthritis, vitiligo; (c) Immunosuppression e.g. transplant anti-rejection therapy, immuno-suppressive drugs; (c) Acquired immune deficiency syndrome (AIDS).

Patients with auto-immune conditions such as Sjögren's Syndrome, scleroderma or primary biliary cirrhosis have been noted to have an increased incidence of malignancy [75, 76]. Kinlen *et al.* [77] amongst others, have reported an increased incidence of non-Hodgkins lymphoma in patients on chronic renal dialysis, and the immunosuppressive factor of uraemia has been postulated as a contributory cause. The malignancies found in immunosuppressed patients were predominantly lymphomas and epithelial tumours of the skin, lip, cervix and uterus [78].

Kaposi's sarcoma is seen in 25% of patients with AIDS. Beta cell lymphomas are also part of the spectrum of neoplastic complications of HTLV III infection. Other carcinomas, such as those of the anus and anorectum, have been described in homosexual men but their relationship to HTLV III infection is uncertain. In patients with AIDS, Kaposi's lymphoma and sarcoma grow rapidly and contribute to the demise of the patient [79], but because of simultaneous bacterial, viral and fungal infections, it is difficult to assess the mortality related to rapidly growing tumours in this group of patients.

Certain ethnic groups such as Africans in Zaire and Mozambique, Hong Kong-Chinese and South Vietnamese have a high incidence of primary liver cell cancer (PLCC) producing alpha foetoprotein. Some of these liver cancers are rapidly growing, as demonstrated by the development of interval cancers between annual screens of serum alpha foetoprotein [80]. Rapidly growing aggresive cancers of the breast and anorectum have also been reported in West Africans amongst a young population. While inherited genetic susceptibility is possible, it is more likely that environmental factors affecting the immune system, such as malaria, viral hepatitis and other viral infections may play the major role. The demography of a number of cancers in Africa appears to be related to areas where the population has a high incidence of relative immunodeficiency as a result of

malnutrition and recurrent stressing of the reticulo-endothelial system by infection.

Prospects for clinical detection of rapidly growing cancers

Measurement of temperature in a tumour may provide a pointer to its biological
behaviour and help in the selection of appropriate management for the patient.
The temperature of tumours can be assessed by thermography [27], and rapidly
growing cancers show the greatest rise in surface temperature as detected by
contact liquid crystal or infra-red thermography. Indolent and deeper cancers
cannot be detected using these techniques. Microwave thermography – a new
technique of measuring thermal radiation from the tissues of the body in the
microwave region – may obtain a measure of the temperature of tumours at a
depth of several centimetres [82]. Prototype equipment using this technique is
being used and may help to distinguish temperature increase due to increased
vascularity from that due to metabolic activity [82]. Refinements of microwave
thermography may allow dynamic studies of deep tumours without invasive
probes.

Dynamic studies of breast temperature to assess the change in circadian rhythm
may provide further information about the metabolism of individual breast
cancers [27, 83]. In addition, the change in temperature of the tumour and the
overlying breast may be used as a marker of response to hormone therapy early
in the course of treatment [84]. Because of the circadian rhythm of breast
temperature, serial measurements need to be taken at the same time of the day
and single readings may be misleading.

Chronobiological studies involving repeated measurements over a 24 hour
period, should prove more accurate and may also provide more useful information. Rapidly growing tumours with short doubling time tend to shift from
circadian to ultradian (<20 hours) rhythm, while tumours with a long doubling
time showed a 24 hour rhythm, but the acrophase in the tumourous breast
preceded the acrophase in the contralateral normal breast [85].

There is some evidence that animal and human breast tumour cells show a
circadian mitotic cell cycle [86, 87] and studies of P32 uptake in untreated human
breast cancer showed a circadian shythm [88]. Stoll and Burch [89] confirmed the
circadian rhythmicity of P32 uptake in some breast cancers using surface Geiger
counters and observed parallel changes in surface temperature. This suggests that
surface temperature may reflect metabolism of the underlying tumour and may
indicate the time of maximum tumour sensitivity to therapy. It may therefore have
implications for the timing of radiotherapy or cytotoxic chemotherapy.

Gautherie and Gros [27] have recorded surface tumour temperatures by radio-
telethermometry. One sensor was sited over the tumour 'hot spot' (as defined by
infra-red thermography) and the other sensor on a matched site on the other

breast. They confirmed that the shift from circadian to ultradian rhythm was associated with anaplastic tumours, a short doubling time, and a greater elevation of skin temperature.

Conclusion

The tempo of tumour growth is often overlooked by the clinician in his management decision, except in obvious cases such as inflammatory cancer. The latter is merely one extreme of a wide spectrum of growth rates. Clinical features of rapid growth as described in this chapter can help to identify tumours with a highly malignant potential and can supplement information derived from imaging and laboratory investigations. Newly developing techniques of dynamic thermography involving measurement of circadian rhythms may help to recognise rapidly growing tumours. They may also help to plan specific timing of therapy.

References

1. Bell CA: *A System of Operative Surgery*. Vol. 2, Longman, London, 1814, p. 136
2. Lee BJ, Tannenbaum NE: Inflammatory carcinoma of the breast. *Surg Gynec Obstet* 39: 580–595, 1924
3. Pluygers E, Beauduin M: Assessing growth activity in the primary tumour. In: *Secondary Spread in Breast Cancer*, BA Stoll (Ed), 1977, p. 15–30, William Heinemann, London
4. Lloyd Williams K: Unpublished, 1985
5. Levine PH, Mourali N, Tabbane F, Costa J, Mesa-Tejada R, Spiegelman S, Munez LR, Bekesi JC: Immunopathologic features of rapidly progressing breast cancer (RPBC) in Tunisia. *Proc AM Assoc Cancer Res* 21: 170, 1980
6. Denoix P: In: *La Maladie Cancereuse*. JB Bailliere & Fils Paris, 1968, p. 135
7. Feinstein AR: Symptoms as an index of biologic behaviour and prognosis in human cancer. *Nature* 209: 241–245, 1966
8. Charlson ME, Feinstein AR: The Auxometric Dimension. A new method for using rate of growth in prognostic staging of breast cancer. *JAMA* 288: 180–185, 1974
9. Boyd NF, Meakin JW, Hayward JL, Brown TC: Clinical estimation of the growth rate of breast cancer. *Cancer* 48: 1037–1042, 1981
10. Axtell LM, Myers MH, Thomas LH: Prognostic indicators in Hodgkin's disease. *Cancer* 29: 1481–1488, 1972
11. Clack NH, Blumenson LE, Bross ID: Therapeutic implications from a mathematical model characterizing the course of breast cancer. *Cancer* 24: 960–971, 1969
12. Aldinger KA, Samaan NA, Ibanez M, Hill CS: Anaplastic carcinoma of the thyroid. *Cancer* 41: 2267–2275, 1978
13. Sherlock S: In: *Disease of the Liver and Biliary System*. 1968, p. 246, Blackwell, Oxford
14. Nathan NH, Collins VP, Adams RA: Differentiation of benign and malignant pulmonary nodules by growth rate. *Radiology* 79: 221–232, 1962
15. Welin S, Youker J, Spratt SS: The rates and patterns of growth of 375 tumours of the large intestine and rectum observed serially by double contrast enema study. *Am J Roentgenol* 90: 673–681, 1963

16. Spratt JS, Spratt TL: Rates of growth of pulmonary metastases and host survival. *Ann Surg* 159: 161–171, 1974

17. Spratt JS: The rates of growth of skeletal sarcomas. *Cancer* 18: 14–24, 1965

18. Kusuma S, Spratt JS, Donegan WL, Watson FR, Cunningham C: The gross rates of growth of human mammary carcinoma. *Cancer* 30: 594–599, 1972

19. Charbit A, Malaise EP, Tubiana M: Relationship between the pathological nature and the growth rate of human tumours. *Eur J Cancer* 7: 307–315, 1971

20. Steel G: Cell population kinetics in relation to the growth and treatment of cancer. In: *Growth Kinetics of Tumours*. Clarendon Press, Oxford, 1977

21. Fournier VD, Kuttig H, Kubli F: Wachstumsgeschwindigkeit des mammakarzinomas und roentgenologische fruhdiagnosen. *Strahlentherapie* 151: 318–332, 1926

22. Ingleby H, Gershon-Cohen J: In: *Comparative Anatomy, Pathology and Roentgenology of the Breast*. University of Pennsylvania Press, Philadelphia, 1960, p. 359

23. Galante E, Gallus G, Guzzon A, Settoni I, Bertuccelli M, Di Pietro S: Growth rate in the interpretation of the natural history of breast cancer. *Review on Endocrine-related Cancer* (Suppl) 14: 41–44, 1984

24. Spratt JS, Heuser L, Kuhns JG, Reiman HM, Buchanan JB, Polk HC, Sandoz J: Association between the actual doubling times of primary breast cancer with histopathologic characteristics and Wolfe's parenchymal mammographic patterns. *Cancer* 47: 2265–2268, 1981

25. Wolfe JN: Breast pattern classification and observation. *Radiology* 127: 343–344, 1978

26. Stewart HJ, Songhorabadi S, Gravelle IH, Apsimon HT: Mammographic tumour contour and prognosis in breast cancer. *Reviews on Endocrine-related Cancer* Suppl. 14: 183–187, 1984

27. Gautherie M, Gros C: Circadian rhythm alterations of skin temperature in breast cancer. *Chronobiologia* 4: 1–17, 1977

28. Gautherie M, Thermobiological assessment of benign and malignant breast disease. *Am J Obstet Gynaecol* 147: 861–869, 1983

29. Spitalier JM, Clerc S, Giraud D, Ayme Y, Pietra JC, Almaric R: La notion thermovisuelle de croissance rapide dans les cancers du sein. *Mediterranee Medicale* 76, 1, 1974

30. Pietra JC: La telethermographie dynamique dans les cancers du sein en phase evolutive. *Thesis, Marseille* (cited by Plugyers and Beauduin 1977), 1974

31. Ratz JL, Bailin PL: Liquid-crystal thermography in determining the lateral extents of basal cell carcinomas. *J Dermatol Surg Oncol* 7: 27–31, 1981

32. Tapernoux B, Hessler C: Thermography of malignant melanomas. *J Dermatol Surg Oncol* 3: 299–30, 1977

33. Gullino PM, Grantham FH: Studies on the exchange of fluids between host and tumour. 1. A method for growing 'tissue isolated tumours in laboratory animals'. *J Natl Cancer Inst* 27: 679–693, 1961

34. Falk P: Differences in vascular pattern between the spontaneous and the transplanted C3H mouse mammary carcinoma. *Eur J Cancer and Clin Oncol* 18: 155–165, 1982

35. Tveit E, Hultborn R, Weiss L: Pathogenesis of tumour necrosis in induced rat mammary tumours. *Reviews on Endocrine-related Cancer* (Suppl) 14: 107–109, 1984

36. Gershon-Cohen J, Berger SM, Klickstein HS: Roentgengraphy of breast cancer moderating concept of 'Biologic predeterminism'. *Cancer* 16: 961–964, 1963

37. Jackson R, Adams BH: Horrifying basal cell carcinoma. *J Surg Oncol* 5: 431–433, 1973

38. Ten-Seldam REJ, Helwig EB: Histological typing of skin tumours. *World Health Organisation*. Geneva 1974, 48–49

39. Jacobs GH, Rippley JJ, Altini K: Prediction of aggressive behaviour in basal cell carcinoma. *Cancer* 49: 533–537, 1982

40. Mouriquand J, Vrousos C, Vincent F, Aguettaz G: L'aspect cytologique des tumeurs du sein en poussee evolutive (cited by Plugyers and Beauduin 1977) In: *Explorations Fonctionnelles en Senologie*, R Lambotte and GF Leroux (Eds), 1975

18

41. Harvey HA, Lipton A, Lusch CJ: Estrogen receptor status in inflammatory breast carcinoma. *Proc Am Soc Clin Oncol* 20: 431, 1979

42. De la Rue JC, May-Lewin F, Mouriesse H, Contesso G, Sancho-Garnier H: Oestrogen and progesterone cytosolic receptors in clinically inflammatory tumours of the human breast. *Br J Cancer* 44: 911–916, 1981

43. Antoniades K, Spector H: Quantitative oestrogen receptor values and growth of carcinoma of the breast before surgical intervention. *Cancer* 50: 793–796, 1982

44. Levine PH, Tabbane F, Muenz LR, Kamaraju LS, Das S, Polivy S, Belhassen S, Scholl SM, Bekes JG, Mourali N: Hormone receptors in rapidly progressing breast cancer. *Cancer* 54: 3012–3016, 1984

45. Hahnel R: Oestrogen receptor status, breast cancer growth and prognosis. *Reviews on Endocrine-Related Cancer* 8: 5–11, 1981

46. Nicholson RI, Wilson DW, Richards G, Griffiths K, Williams M, Elston CW, Blamey RW: Biological and clinical aspects of oestrogen receptor measurements in rapidly progressing breast cancer. *Proc 9th Int Cong Pharmacol* 3, 75–79, 1984

47. Lee YTN: Serial tests of carcinoembryonic antigen in patients with breast cancer. *Am J Clin Oncol* 6: 287–293, 1983

48. Mughal AW, Hortobagyi GN, Fritsche HA, Buzdar AU, Yap HW, Blumenschein GR: Serial Plasma carcinoembryonic antigen measurements during treatment of metastatic breast cancer. *JAMA* 249: 1881–1886, 1983

49. Waalkes TP, Abeloff MD, Woo KB, Ettinger DS, Ruddon RW, Aldenderfer P: Carcinoembryonic antigen for monitoring patients with small cell carcinoma of the lung during treatment. *Cancer* 40: 4420–4427, 1980

50. Krieger G, Wander HE, Prangen M, Bandlow G, Beyer JH, Nagel GA: Bestimmung des carcinoembryonalen antigens (CEA) zur voraussage des therapieerfolges beim metastasierenden mammakarzinom. *Dtsch med Wschr* 108: 610–614, 1983

51. Wang DY, Knyba RE, Bulbrook RD, Millis RR, Hayward JL: Serum carcinoembryonic antigen in the diagnosis and prognosis of women with breast cancer. *Eur J Cancer Clin Oncol* 20: 25–31, 1984

52. Foulds L: Neoplastic Development. In: *Neoplastic Development*. Academic Press, New York, 1977, p. 2

53. Spratt JS Jr: Growth kinetics in mammary cancer. In: *Secondary Spread in Breast Cancer*. A Stoll (Ed) Heinemann, London, 1977, p. 3

54. Brindley CO, Markoff E and Schneiderman MA: Direct observation of lesion size and number as a method of following the growth of human tumors. *Cancer* 12: 139–146, 1959

55. Brennan MJ, Prychodko W and Horeglad S: In: *Biological Interactions in Normal and Neoplastic Growth*. MJ Brennan and WL Simpson (Ed) Little Brown & Co. Boston, 1962, p. 739

56. Peters MV: The effect of pregnancy on breast cancer. In: *Prognostic Factors in Breast Carcinoma*. Forrest APM, Kunkler PB (Eds) William and Wilkins, Baltimore, 1968, p. 65

57. Anderson JM: Mammary cancers and pregnancy. *Brit Med J* 1: 1124–1127, 1979

58. Pack GT, Scharnagel IM: The prognosis for malignant melanoma in the pregnant woman. *Cancer* 4: 324–334, 1951

59. George PA, Fortner JG, Pack GT: Melanoma with pregnancy. A report of 115 cases. *Cancer* 13: 854–859, 1960

60. Fisher RI, Neifeld JP, Lippman NE: Oestrogen receptors in human malignant melanoma. *Lancet* 2: 337–338, 1976

61. Shiu MH, Schottenfeld D, MacLean B, Fortner JG: Adverse effect of pregnancy. *Cancer* 37: 181–187, 1976

62. Boesen E: Unpublished, 1986

63. Stoll BA: The significance of tumour 'stimulation' by Tamoxifen. *Recent Results in Cancer Research* 71: 149–15, 1980

64. Tanaka M, Adachi I, Kimura S, Yamaguchi K, Kikuchi K, Abe K: *Jap J Clin Oncol* 11: 545, 1981

65. Tormey DC, Simon R.M., Lippmann ME, Bull JM, Myers CE: Evaluation of Tamoxifen dose in advanced breast cancer. *Cancer Treat Rep* 60: 1451–1459, 1976

66. Parbhoo SP: Serial monitoring in management of bone metastases. In: *Screening and Monitoring of Cancer*. BA Stoll (Ed), Wiley, Chichester, 1985, p. 355–406

67. Stoll BA: Hormonal management in breast cancer. In: *Hormonal Management in Breast Cancer*. Pitman Medical, London, 1964, p. 59

68. Powles TJ: Factors influencing metastasis in bone. In: *Secondary Spread in Breast Cancer*. BA Stoll (Ed), Heinemann, London, 1977, p. 89

69. Britton JP and Sagar PM: Tamoxifen and breast pain. *Brit Med J* 291:1172, 1985

70. Hall TC, Dederick MM, Nevinny HB: Prognostic value of hormonally induced hypercalcaemia in breast cancer. *Cancer Chemotherapy Reports* 30: 21–24, 1963

71. Plotkin D, Lechner J, Jung WE, Rposen PJ: Tamoxifen flare in advanced breast cancer. *JAMA* 240: 2644–2646, 1978

72. Otteman LA, Long HJ: Hypercalcaemic flare with megestrol acetate. *Cancer Treat Reports*: 1420–1421, 1980

73. Matelski H, Green R, Huberman M, Lokich J, Zipoli T: Randomized trial of oestrogen vs tamoxifen therapy for advanced breast cancer. *Am J Clin Oncol* 8: 128–133, 1985

74. Alexieva-Figusch J, van Gilse HA: Flare and rebound regression in the hormone therapy of breast cancer. *Rev Endoc Related Cancer* 21: 5–10, 1985

75. Talbot JH, Barrocas M: Carcinoma of the lung in systemic sclerosis. *Semin Arthritis Rheum* 9: 191–217, 1980

77. Mills PR, Boyle P, Quigley EMM: Primary biliary cirrhosis: an increased incidence of extrahepatic malignancies. *J Clin Path* 35: 541–543, 1982

78. Kinlen LJ, Eastwood JB, Kerr DNS: Cancer in patients receiving dialysis. *Br Med J* I: 1401–1403, 1980

78. Penn I: Malignancies associated with immunosoppresive or cytotoxic therapy. *Surgery* 83: 492–502, 1978

79. MacDonald Burns DC: Unpublished, 1985

80. Purves LR: Alpha fetoprotein and the diagnosis of liver cell carcinoma. In: *Liver cell cancer*. Cameron HM, Warwick GP, Linsell CA (Eds). Elsevier Amsterdam, 1976, p. 61

81. Meyers PC, Barrett AH: Microwave thermography of normal and cancerous breast tissue. *Proc NY Acad Sci* 335–340, 1980

82. Love TJ: Thermography as an indicator of blood perfusion. *Proc NY Acad Sci* 335: 67–85, 1980

83. Phillips MJ, Wilson DW, Simpson HW, Fahmy DR, Groom GV, Phillips MEA, Pierrepoint CG, Blamey RW, Kalberg F, Griffiths K: Characterisation of breast skin temperature rhythms of women in relation to menstrual status. *Acta Endocrinologica* 96: 350–360, 1981

84. Mansfield CM, Carabasi RA, Wells W and Borman K: Circadian rhythm in the skin temperture of normal and cancerous breasts. *Int J Chronobiol* 1: 235–243, 1973

85. Simpson HW: An outline of mammary chronophysiology and pathology: A new tumour marker. In: *Tumour Markers*. Griffiths K, Neville AM, Pierrepoint CG (Ed): 317–339, Alpha Omega Publishers, Cardiff, 1977

86. Badran AF, Echave Lanos JM: Persistence of metabolic circadian rhythm in mammary carcinoma after 35 generations. *J Natl Can Inst* 35: 285–290, 1965

87. Rosene G, Halberg F: Circadian rhythms. *Bull All India Inst Med* Sci 4: 77–94, 1970

88. Bleehan NM, Bryant THE: In vivo studies of radioactive phosphorus in malignant tumours. *Clin Radiology* 18: 237–244, 1967

89. Stoll BA, Burch WM: Surface detection of circadian rhythm in P32 content of cancer of the breast. *Cancer* 21: 193–197, 1968

2. Clinical history as a guide to prognosis

P.R. CLINGAN and N.F. BOYD

Clinical trials in cancer show that treatment may have different results in patients with different prognostic characteristics (1–3). This chapter reviews the scientific evidence that the patient's clinical history can provide pointers to the outcome of cancer. After setting out the principles of classifying such information, it shows how it can be used to define prognostically distinctive groups of patients. It then decribes how in studies meeting scientific requirements, these methods of classification have been used to study the prognosis in cancers of the lung, rectum and breast, Hodgkin's disease and acute lymphoblastic leukemia.

Patients with cancer are presently classified according to the site, histology, and anatomical extent of the tumour. Despite the undoubted relevance of these features to the prognosis of cancer, they are a static classification of a process that is dynamic. Patients who are found to have tumours of the same size at the time of diagnosis, will be assigned to the same anatomical stage of disease, but their prognosis will differ if their tumours differ in rate of growth or metastatic potential [4, 5].

Classifying the symptoms of patients with cancer

Patients found to have cancer may be asymptomatic, but if symptoms are present, their type and duration may, with suitable methods of classification, be used to estimate prognosis. Initially, symptoms are classified according to whether they arise from the tumour at its site of origin (primary symptoms), arise remote from the tumour but do not denote metastatic spread of the tumour (systematic symptoms), or arise remote from the tumour and do denote metastatic spread of the tumour (metastatic symptoms) [6, 7].

Primary symptoms

Primary symptoms arise from the general region of the primary tumour e.g. a lump in breast cancer, cough in lung cancer or rectal bleeding in rectal cancer. Primary symptoms can also arise from the effects of a primary tumour on adjacent organs, e.g. frequency of micturition due to bladder irritation by a pelvic mass. Primary symptoms thus arise at the site of origin of the tumour but provide no information as to whether the tumour has spread beyond its anatomical site of origin.

Systemic symptoms

Systemic symptoms include the general effects of a tumour on the host, such as fatigue, weight loss, or fever, or the effects of tumour products such as hormones. They manifest in sites remote from the primary tumour, or in the body as a whole, but again do not necessarily indicate that the tumour has spread beyond its site of origin.

Metastatic symptoms

Metastatic symptoms, by contrast, imply that the cancer has physically disseminated from its site of origin. They arise as a result of the invasion by cancer of tissue remote from the primary site of the tumour, and include symptoms such as bone pain, brachial plexus involvement by axillary nodes or seizures from brain metastasis. Metastatic symptoms can also arise when a primary tumour spreads contiguously to regional organs, for example, when rectal cancer invades the bladder.

Patients with cancer may of course have other, unrelated disease that can cause symptoms [7, 8] and a method is required for assessing them when they arise. In general, symptoms fall into one of three mutually exclusive categories – those that are clearly attributable to cancer and could definitely not have been caused by any other co-existing disease, those that are definitely not caused by cancer, and those that are of equivocal attribution [7]. Each of the studies of specific diseases that are described below has developed explicit criteria for the classification of symptoms of uncertain attribution. The purpose of these criteria is not to provide an unequivocally 'correct' attribution of symptoms but to ensure that uncertainties of this kind are handled in a consistent way.

Estimating the prognosis using the classification of symptoms

Feinstein [5, 7] has formally set out a classification of symptoms in a way that allows inferences to be made about rate of growth un tumours, but their rationale will be intuitively recognized by most clinicians. Examples include patients in whom a large breast cancer is found within a few months of a completely normal breast examination, or in whom a large lung tumour appears shortly after a normal chest radiograph. Rapid growth of the tumour is shown by its rapid progression from being undetectable to a large size.

On the other hand, the circumstances in which a tumour is detected may indicate that it is slowly growing. Cancers that are detected in asymptomatic patients as the result of routine examination are likely to be slowly growing. Slowly growing tumours (by definition) have a longer interval between inception and detection than do rapidly growing tumours. Because the probability of detecting asymptomatic disease at routine examination is proportional to the length of time that disease is present, routine examinations are more likely to find slowly growing varieties of cancer. This phenomenon is the same as the problem of 'length bias' that may complicate the interpretation of screening programmes for cancer.

A slowly growing tumour may also be presumed if known to have been present for a long time without having undergone dissemination. (Cancers may be known to have been present for a long time either because of their symptoms or because they have been observed directly as abnormalities on examination.) On the other hand, cancers that have caused symptoms for only a short time but have undergone discernible change within that time, or those with metastatic symptoms as their first manifestation, are likely to be rapidly growing. Rate of growth is undeterminate in cancers that have caused symptoms for only a short time and that have not changed or given rise to metastatic symptoms, and also in cancers that have been present for long periods and have changed [4, 6, 7].

Study of the clinical course of a particular group of patients requires selection of a specified time in their disease history (called zero time), at which the patients will be characterized, and from which their subsequent survival will be measured. Thus, in a study of the correlation between oestrogen receptor assay and survival in patients with breast cancer, zero time might be specified as the time of diagnosis; oestrogen receptor status would be characterized at that time, and survival time would be recorded for patients with different receptor values.

A group of such patients is referred to as an 'inception cohort' [8]. This term refers to any group of patients assembled at a common point in their clinical course and while this time point is often the time of diagnosis, it could be some other suitable point in time. For example, in the sudy of prognosis of patients with metastatic breast cancer, zero time might be the date at which metastases were first identified.

Evaluation of the influence of a prognostic variable also requires examination of the influence of other known variables on its association with survival. A factor in the clinical history which influences survival should not do so because of its association with some other prognostic factor. Significant factors should be independent [4].

Complete follow-up is essential in prognostic studies because patients who are lost to follow-up are unlikely to have experienced the same outcome as those who remain. Patients are lost to follow-up either because they die or because they are well enough to move away from the environment of the investigator. Attempts to presume outcome in such cases may be influenced by knowledge of the patients initial prognostic characteristics. To avoid such possible sources of bias, all patients in the inception cohort should be assessed with the same frequency and using the same set of tests.

Finally, the replication of experimental results is essential, and before we can accept a report that a variable influences prognosis in cancer, the observation needs to be confirmed in a further population of patients [10, 11]. The sections that follow will give examples of the application of these principles to specific malignant diseases.

Lung cancer

The symptomatic classification of patients with lung cancer was first developed in a study of 596 patients [12]. In this scheme, the patient may have primary symptoms only, systemic symptoms only, metastatic symptoms only, or a combination of primary, systemic and metastatic symptoms. The presence of metastatic symptoms implies an unfavourable growth pattern and a poor prognosis. As described above, analysis of the length of time for which primary symptoms are present allows conclusions to be drawn about the growth rate of the tumour.

If symptoms are of short duration, the growth rate of the tumour is indeterminate. Symptoms may be of short duration because the tumour has grown rapidly, or because symptoms have occurred late in the course of a slowly growing tumour. If, however, primary symptoms have been present for a long time, and no systemic or metastatic symptoms have developed, then the tumour is likely to be slowly growing. In asymptomatic patients, the length of time for which disease has been present cannot be assessed, but as discussed above, disease that is detected in asymptomatic patients is likely to be slowly growing.

The classification of symptoms according to their origin and duration resulted in the formation of 5 clinical stages: Stage 1 contained asymptomatic patients; Stage 2 contained patients with primary symptoms only which were of long duration (greater than or equal to 6 months); Stage 3 contained patients with primary symptoms of less than 6 months duration; Stage 4 contained patients with systemic symptoms; Stage 5 contained patients with metastatic symptoms. It was found that 32% of those in clinical Stage 1 survived for 5 years, compared to 18% in Stage 2, 10% in Stage 3, 8% in Stage 4 and 0% in Stage 5. That these prognostic variables were independent was shown by taking into account the anatomical stage and histological features of the tumour. It showed that the survival gradient associated with the symptomatic categories persisted when these factors were taken into account.

In a further study of 678 patients [13], the 5 stage clinical system was condensed to create 3 new categories indolent, obtrusive and deleterious. The indolent group included patients who were asymptomatic or who had primary symptoms for longer than 6 months (that is, stages 1 and 2 in the earlier classification). The obtrusive group contained patients with primary symptoms that were less than 6 months duration, with or without the systemic symptoms of weight loss, fatigue, and anorexia, but without evidence of metastases (stages 3 and 4 in the earlier classification). The deleterious group contained patients who had metastatic symptoms (earlier called stage 5).

In this new 3 stage grouping, the 5 year survival was 17% for the indolent group, 7% for the obtrusive group, and 0% for the deleterious group. When anatomical features were taken into consideration, these clinical prognostic groups were again able to predict survival within each stage, as shown in Table 1. Within each anatomical group the three symptom stages were associated with differences in 5 year survival rate. Also, the extent of anatomical spread of the tumour influenced prognosis within each symptom stage.

Other investigators have shown a direct relationship between these categories of indolent, obtrusive and deleterious disease, and the growth rate of lung cancers as measured on serial chest x-rays [14].

Rectal cancer

Symptom stages were formed and named in a manner similar to that used in lung cancer, in order to analyze the effects of symptomatic staging in rectal cancer [13]. Stage 1, named indolent, contained patients who were asymptomatic at the time rectal cancer was detected, or those who had had primary symptoms (such as rectal bleeding) for longer than 6 months but without systemic or metastatic symptoms. Clinical Stage 2, called obtrusive, comprised patients with primary symptoms that had been present for less than 6 months, or those who had systemic symptoms such as weight loss, anorexia or fatigue, but without metastatic

Table 1. Five-year survival rates in lung cancer according to symptom stage and anatomic group

Symptom stage	Anatomic group			Total
	Localized	Regional	Distant	
'Indolent'	17/71 (24%)	3/31 (10%)	1/23 (4%)	21/125 (17%)
'Obtrusive'	18/118 (15%)	5/100 (5%)	1/116 (1%)	24/334 (7%)
'Deleterious'	9/29 (0%)	0/49 (0%)	0/141 (0%)	0/219 (0%)
Total	35/218 (16%)	8/180 (4%)	2/280 (1%)	45/678 (7%)

(Adapted from Ref. 13).

symptoms. Stage 3, named deleterious, contained patients with metastatic symptoms.

The 5 year survival rates for these symptomatic groupings in patients who had surgical resection (shown in Table 2) were 52% for Stage 1, 33% for Stage 2 and 0% for Stage 3. These gradients and survival rates were comparable to those created by anatomical methods of staging rectal cancer according to the extent of the spread of the tumour in the excised rectum. Five year survival rates obtained in the same population with anatomical methods of classification were 57% for patients with disease confined to the bowel wall, 26% for patients with localized spread beyond the bowal wall, and 6% for patients with distant spread. When survival by symptom stages was compared with that by anatomical staging, there was a gradient within each anatomical stage according to clinical stage, and also within each clinical stage according to anatomical stage, indicating that the two methods of assessing prognosis were independent of each other.

An attempt to replicate such symptomatic staging of carcinoma of the rectum was unable to confirm that it was independently related to prognosis [15]. The medical records on which this study was based, however, often did not provide the detailed information required to assign patients to a symptom stage. This study, however, did show that several clinical features identified in patients with rectal cancer were associated with prognostic distinctions. These features included the presence or absence of metastatic disease, fixation of the tumour, the presence of absence of an annular tumour, and the presence or absence of the systemic symptoms of weight loss, anorexia, weakness and anemia.

Using these clinical features, the patients were divided into 4 clinical classes. Class 4 had metastatic disease, Class 3 has a fixed rectal tumour, but no metastases, Class 2 had an annular rectal tumour or the presence of systemic symptoms, and Class 1 had none of the previously mentioned features (i.e. no metastases, no fixation of rectal tumour, a tumour that was not annular, and no systemic symptoms.) Five year survival in these classes was 72% for Class 1, 40% for Class 2, 20% for Class 3 and 2% for Class 4. It was again possible to show

Table 2. Five-year survival rates after surgical resection of rectal cancer according to symptom stage and anatomical group

Symptom stage	Anatomic group			Total
	Localized	Regional	Distant	
'Indolent'	36/50 (72%)	6/15 (40%)	1/18 (6%)	43/83 (52%)
'Obtrusive'	34/70 (49%)	6/31 (19%)	2/28 (7%)	42/129 (33%)
'Deleterious'	0/2 (0%)	—	0/7 (0%)	0/9 (0%)
Total	70/122 (57%)	12/46 (26%)	3/53 (6%)	85/221 (38%)

(Adapted from Ref. 13).

that these gradients in survival created by the classification of clinical features were independent of those created by Duke's method of classifying rectal tumours applied to the same group of patients [16].

Breast cancer

Patients with carcinoma of the breast have been classified according to the growth rate of the tumour using 2 items of information from the patient's history [17]. These are the length of time for which symptoms are present, and whether or not changes in symptoms have occurred. Changes in symptoms are referred to as 'transition events' and include an increase in the size of a breast mass, an increase in the consistency of a breast mass, the development of other masses in the breast, the development of masses in supraclavicular fossae or axillae, and the development of changes in the skin such as ulceration, contraction or change in the shape of the breast. Retraction of the nipple, the development of skin nodules, or the development of pain or edema in the arm or chest wall are also classified as transition events.

The first report [17] partitioned the duration of symptoms into 3 intervals; less than 3 months, between 3 and 18 months, and greater than 18 months. In more recently studied patients, few were found to have symptoms of more than 18 months duration, and the classification was revised to a single partition at 4 months. Results obtained with this latter classification will be decribed here.

Patients in whom symptoms had been present for at least 4 months, but in whom no transition event had occurred, were designated as of 'slow' growth on the basis that this was the only mechanism that would allow a tumour to be present for a substantial period of time without undergoing change. Conversely, the group designated 'rapid', was formed by patients in whom symptoms had been present for less than 4 months but in whom a transition event had occurred during this time. Patients in the remaining 2 categories (those with symptoms of at least 4 months duration who had experienced a transition event, and those with symptoms for less than 4 months but in whom no transition event had occurred) are those in whom no definitive statement can be made about growth rate and these groups were combined to form a third category called 'intermediate'. A fourth category was formed of patients who had systemic symptoms of anorexia, fatigue or weight loss, or metastatic symptoms.

Fig. 1 shows the influence of these categories of growth rate on survival in patients classified according to the histological status of the axillary lymph nodes. In patients with negative nodes, the categories of growth rate created a monotonic gradient in survival, although survival in the slow and intermediate categories was similar. Survival in the rapid category was, however, considerably worse and was statistically significantly different from that of the intermediate class ($X^2 = 4.0$; $p < .05$). In patients with histologically-involved axillary nodes, the categories of

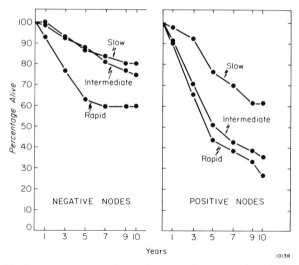

Figure 1. Survival in breast cancer according to lymph node status and clinical estimate of growth rate. (Adapted from Ref. 18).

growth rate again created a survival gradient that was statistically significant $(X^2 = 9.2; \ p < 0.02)$.

Further analyses also showed that the categories of growth rate created differences in survival within patient of the same anatomical stage, within patients of different menopausal status, and in tumours of different histologies. Growth rate retained its prognostic importance when considered in relation to the type of treatment that the patient had received [17, 18, 19].

These principles of classification were applied to 756 patients with breast cancer who were enrolled in a randomized control trial of adjuvant hormonal therapy The information from the patient's history that was required to estimate the growth rate of the tumour, was obtained from all patients at entry into the trial, thus allowing a prospective assessment of the prognostic importance of clinical estimates of growth rate, and comparison with other prognostic factors.

Fig. 2 shows the survival of this patient population, classified according to growth rate in the manner described above. The categories of growth rate were associated with survival differences that were consistent with the belief that they did indeed identify groups of patients with tumours of different biological potential. The overall trend in prognosis between the slow, intermediate, and rapid categories was statistically significant $(X^2 = 15.1, \ p < 0.001)$, as was the difference in survival between each of the individual categories.

The prognostic impact of the clinical estimation of growth rate in this patient population was compared with that of other prognostic factors, including lymph node status, clinical anatomical stage, and the histological grade of the tumour. When the prognostic effects of these factors were considered together with growth rate, each variable generally remained associated with substantial independence and statistically significant prognostic distinctions. Results are shown in Table 3

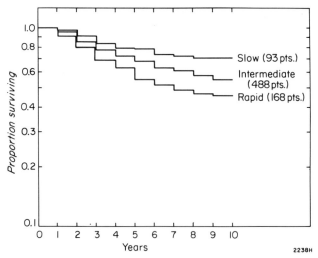

Figure 2. Survival in breast cancer according to clinical estimate of growth rate.

for patients classified according to both growth rate and axillary lymph node status.

Growth rate created gradients in survival for patients with and without lymph node involvement. In patients with negative lymph nodes there was a three-fold increase in death rate from the slowly growing to the rapidly growing group. The relative death rate for patients with either 1 to 3, or 4 or more involved nodes approximately doubled from the slow to the rapid category. There were also gradients in survival within the categories of growth rate that were created by the classification of lymph node status. The categories of growth rate remained associated with significant difference in survival ($X^2 = 10.10$; $p = 0.001$) after

Table 3. Relative death rates* according to growth rate and lymph node histology in breast cancer (The number of patients in each group is shown in parentheses.)

Growth rate	Lymph node histology		
Growth rate	Negative	1–3 nodes involved	≥4 nodes involved
Slow	0.20	0.58	0.99
	(17)	(45)	(22)
Intermediate	0.61	0.84	1.97
	(100)	(202)	(116)
Rapid	0.62	1.23	1.87
	(22)	(80)	(45)

* Relative death rates as the ratio (O/E) of observed deaths (O) within each category, to the number of deaths expected (E), calculated from the log rank test. The average death rate for the entire population is 1.00. Relative death rates less than 1.00 thus indicate survival that is better than average, and rates greater than 1.00 survival that is worse than average.

adjustments for differences in lymph node involvement, indicating that the prognostic effects of growth rate cannot be explained by differences in histological lymph node involvement between the groups [20].

Hodgkin's disease

The presence of systemic symptoms such as weight loss, night sweats and fever, is an unfavourable prognostic sign in patients with Hodgkin's disease and this information has been used in accordance with the principles described above to estimate growth rate and prognosis in patients with Hodgkin's disease. Patients were first classified according to the presence of absence of systemic symptoms.

Patients without systemic symptoms were classified into groups: (a) asymptomatic and found to have Hodgkin's disease during physical or radiographic examination performed for pre-employment, insurance of other routine purposes; (b) symptomatic (but without systemic symptoms) and symptoms were designated as *long* if they had been present for more than a year, and *short* if present for less than a year. Patients with systemic symptoms were classified according to the sequence in which the symptoms had developed. If the systemic symptoms had been the first manifestation of Hodgkin's disease, the classification was designated *initial*. If the systemic symptoms had occurred after the appearance of some other manifestation of the disease, such as lymphadenopathy, the term *subsequent* was used.

The 5 year survival rates for the 184 patients from whom this classification was derived were 100% for those who were asymptomatic, 90% for those with a long

Table 4. 5-Year survival rates according to Ann Arbor stage and symptom category in Hodgkin's disease

Symptom		Anatomic stage				
		Proportion (and %)				
		I	II	III	IV	Total
A	Asymptomatic or Long	7/7 (100)	10/11 (91)	7/7 (100)	0/1 (0)	24/26 (92)
	Short	26/36 (72)	15/26 (58)	14/29 (48)	1/4 (25)	56/95 (59)
B	Subsequent	0/1 (0)	4/7 (57)	7/18 (39)	2/8 (25)	13/34 (38)
	Initial	0/3 (0)	1/6 (17)	2/9 (22)	1/11 (9)	4/29 (14)
	Total	33/47 (70)	30/50 (60)	30/63 (48)	4/24 (17)	97/184 (53)

duration of primary symptoms but no systemic symptoms, 59% for those with a short duration of primary symptoms only, 38% for those in whom systemic symptoms occurred subsequent to some other manifestation of Hodgkin's disease, and 14% for those in whom systemic symptoms were the first manifestation of disease.

Comparison of these survival gradients with those created by the Ann Arbor method of anatomical staging is shown in Table 4. Among patients without systemic symptoms, in each of the anatomical Stages 1–3, wurvival in the asymptomatic or long group was substantially better than in the short group. The contrasting survival rates were respectively 100 and 72% in Stage 1, 91 and 58% in Stage 2 and 100 and 48% in Stage 3. In each of these instances the difference in the 5 year survival rate between the symptomatic categories within each stage were greater than the differences observed between adjacent anatomic stages. In Stage 4 no long-short gradient was seen but there were few patients in this group.

Among patients with systemic symptoms no survival difference was seen between the subsequent and initial groups in Stage 1, but the number in each category is small. In each of the other anatomic stages, however, patients with subsequent symptoms had better survival rates than patients with initial systemic symptoms. The contrasting rates were 57 versus 17% in Stage 2, 39 versus 22% in Stage 3, and 25 versus 9% in Stage 4. Classification according to histologic type of Hodgkin's disease and therapy also showed that the prognostic impact of these symptom categories was independent of these other prognostic influences [21].

The influence of these symptom categories on prognosis was confirmed in the study of 2 further patient populations. The information required to assign patients to symptom categories was extracted from medical records by observers who were 'blind' with respect to patient outcome [22].

The survival gradients showed that the 5 year survival rate in the asymptomatic and long category was 71%, 56% in the short category, 24% in the subsequent category and 0% in the initial category. The results obtained with the first patient population are substantially validated, both in terms of the quantitative result obtained, and the gradient in survival that is created by these symptom categories. The information required to stage these patients according to the Ann Arbor taxonomy was, however, not regularly available and the independence of the prognostic impact of these symptom categories from other prognostic factors could not be examined in this patient population.

Acute lymphoblastic leukemia

Morbidity in acute leukemia is chiefly attributable to infection and hemorrhage, and both of these variables are know to influence prognosis. The method of classifying morbidity in acute leukemia described here was developed to evaluate the resulting taxonomy as a possible means of prognostic staging for this disease [23]. It was developed in an inception cohort of patients with acute leukemia of both lymphoblastic and myeloblastic varieties but results will be given only for acute lymphoblastic leukemia.

Patients were classified according to the severity of infection and hemorrhage. The severity of infection was classified as follows: all infections that were deep involved parenchymal tissues or were associated with severe of extensive tissue distruction, were classified as *severe infections*. This category included septicemia, pneumonia, acute sinusitis associated with fever, abscess formation or extensive ulceration of the skin, oral pharynx, anorectal or vagical regions, or extensive areas of cellulitis. Patients without evidence of severe infection, but with localized or superficial infection, were classified as having *mild infection*. This category included those with oral or pharyngeal inflammation without ulceration, otitis media, roentgenographic evidence of sinusitis without fever, substantial bacteriuria without fever, localized superficial skin infections, or vaginal infections without ulceration or necrosis. Patients with none of the above manifestations were classified as having *no infection*.

Each patient was also classified separately according to the severity of any hemorrhage occurring before the initiation of antineoplastic therapy. Patients with intracranial bleeding, or those with severe blood loss from mucosal surfaces, were classified as having *severe hemorrhage*. This category included patients with cerebral or subarachroid hemorrhage, or hematemesis melena or epistaxis that was prolonged or severe enough to require blood rensfusions or surgical intervention. Patients with either mild mucosal bleeding, or with only cutaneous manifestations of hemorrhage were classified as having *mild hemorrhage*. This category included patients with occult gastrointestinal bleeding, with brief or mild epistaxis, or with only cutaneous manifestations of hemorrhage such as petechia, purpura of bruising. Patients with none of the above manifestations were classified as having *no hemorrgahe*.

Classification of the severity of infection and hemorrhage was then combined to create three stages: Stage 1 comprised patients in whom no infection or hemorrhage had been present, Stage 2 patients who had mild hemorrhage or mild infection or both, and Stage 3 patients with severe infection or severe hemorrhage or both.

The survival of patients with acute lymphoblastic leukemia, classified according to these stages, is shown in Fig. 3. The median survival of patients in Stage 1 was 64 months, 16 months for patients in Stage 2 and 10.5 months for patients in Stage 3. The prognostic impact of this classification of morbidity was evaluated further by partitioning the population according to morbidity and the other prognostic factors of age, total white blood count and platelet count. Table 5 shows the median duration of survival observed when patients were classified according to these prognostic factors. Each of the prognostic factors of age, white blood count and platelet count was associated with previously reported differences in survival,

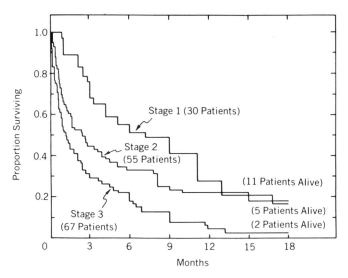

Figure 3. Survival in acute lymphoblastic leukemia according to severity of clinical morbidity.

but within the strata created by these variables, the classification of morbidity continued to show substantial gradients in median survival.

The excellent survival of patients with no morbidity appeared to be uninfluenced by other prognostic factors, and furthermore, no notable differences in survival were seen in any of the three groups of morbidity partirioned according to platelet count. The prognostic influence of the platelet count appeared to arise here from disproportionate distribution of morbidity so that the worst classes of morbidity contained a greater number of people with the lowest platelet counts. Analysis of the survival curves associated with the data shown in Table 5 revealed that the gradients created by the classification of morbidity within these strata were also, for the most part, statistically distinctive, and that the prognostic differences created by the classification of morbidity were larger and more statistically distinctive than those associated with the other prognostic factors.

On follow up, these differences in pretherapeutic morbidity in patients with acute lymphoblastic leukemia remained associated with differences in survival among patients who achieved complete remission. The prognostic distinctions associated with these differences in clinical morbidity are thus not entirely attributable to differences in immediate mortality, but appear to be due to differences in the biological potential of the tumour. Among patients achieving complete remission during their first course of antineoplastic treatment, the median survival of patients with no pre-treatment morbidity (Stage 1) exceeded 66 months, whereas the median surival of patients with mild morbidity (Stage 2) was 22 months, and that of patients with severe morbidity (Stage 3) was 14 months.

This taxonomy was applied to a second population of patients with childhood acute lymphoblastic leukemia. To avoid possible bias when these procedures in classification were applied to a second patient population, the data were extracted from medical records using the criteria for identifying the clinical phenomena described above, but without knowledge of the clinical taxonomy that was being tested. The data were subsequently coded and classified without knowledge of the patient's response to treatment or survival [24].

Similar results were obtained in the second patient population. Among those patients who achieved complete remission median survival was 55 months for those with no morbidity (Stage 1), 32 months for those with mild morbidity (Stage 2), and 18 months for those with severe morbidity (Stage 3). It was again possible to show that the prognostic influence of this clinical taxonomy was independent

Table 5. Acute lymphoblastic leukemia: Median survival (months) according to stage and other prognostic factors

Prognostic factor		Stage			
		1	2	3	Total
Age, yrs		>68.0	15.0	10.5†	13.5
	≤2	(5)*	(9)	(5)	(19)
		>65.0	25.0‡	19.4†	25.0§
	2≤10	(10)	(25)	(10)	(45)
		>67.0	11.3‡	2.0†	9.0§
	2<10	(2)	(24)	(8)	(34)
WBC count/cu mm	≥50,000	6.0	13.0	9.0	14.0
		(1)	(15)	(6)	(22)
		64.0	20.5‡	10.5†	20.0§
	<50,000	(16)	(43)	(17)	(76)
Platelet count/cu mmΠ	≥40,000	50.0	19.7‡	9.0†	22.5§
		(11)	(17)	(7)	(35)
		<60.0	15.5	11.0	14.0
	<40,000	(3)	(41)	(14)	(58)
Total		64.0	16.0‡	10.5†	19.0§
	(17)	(58)	(23)	(98)	

* Parenthetical numbers indicate number of patients in each group.
† Gradient is significant at P < .05.
‡ Gradient is significant at P < .05 between stages 1 and 2 in this category.
§ Gradient is significant at P < .05 for trend across the three stages in this category.
Π Platelet count unknown in five patients.

of that of the prognostic effects of other variables such as age, leukocyte count, granulocyte count, and platelet count.

Discussion

There are 3 issues which are often cited by those clinicians who express reservations about using the patient's clinical history for the purposes of classifying cancer. these reservations concern the reliability of information in the patient's history, the clinical significance of 'delay' in patients seeking medical advice for cancer, and the question of 'biological predeterminism' in cancer.

(1) All clinicians have from time to time encountered patients who were unable to give a consistent history of their illness. Concern about the unreliability of information derived from patients may make some reluctant to accept that such information could be used to assess the patient's prognosis. However, comparisons of the reliability of factors in the patient's history with the reliability of findings obtained by physical examination of patients by physicians, suggest that the information obtained from the patient's history is at least as reliable as that obtained on physical examination [25].

(2) In several instances cited in this review, patients with a long duration of primary symptoms prior to diagnosis and therapy have an outcome that is better than that of patients whose symptoms were of shorter duration. At first glance, this observation may seem to be at variance with the customary advice given to patients that they should promptly report any new symptoms. However, the better outcome associated with a long duration of primary symptoms does not, of course, imply that delay is advantageous. It means only that rapidly progressive tumours usually bring about rapid changes in a patient, while slowly growing tumours produce change more gradually. Patients are thus more likely to report early after the onset of symptoms from rapidly growing tumours. The observations linking the duration of symptoms and prognosis merely provide clinicians with a way of drawing inferences about the behaviour of tumours from the behaviour of patients, and do not constitute recommendations to patients.

(3) The use of information from the patient's history to determine prognoses indicates that in some circumstances, the biological potential potential of cancer can be determined before treatment and this raises the question of biological predeterminism in cancer [26]. However, by accepting the strong influence on outcome that is exerted by most prognostic factors in cancer and the relatively weaker effects of most treatments it does not imply that the clinical course of cancer cannot be influenced by therapy. In fact, an improved understanding of the clinical and biological properties that affect the outcome of cancer provides the clinician with knowledge that may help him to change the outcome of cancer in the individual.

Finally, it is obvious that much of the work presented here is the product of a relatively small number of investigators, many of whom have been associated with each other at one time or another. It appears that most clinicians concerned with the management of patients with cancer are not yet convinced that prognostically useful information can be obtained from such an approach. It is hoped that this review may prompt others to develop new methods for deriving such information in tumours so far unclassified, and to test and improve the methods described in the tumours reviewed above.

Conclusion

The results of the studies summarized in this chapter provide clear evidence that the clinical features elicited from the history of patients with cancer can provide prognostic information about the rate of growth of the tumour that is not discernible from staging systems based solely upon anatomical features. Information about the growth rate of the tumour is available from the routine clinical evaluation of patients and can be obtained without recourse to expensive diagnostic technology [27, 28] and at no additional cost or risk to the patient.

References

1. Feinstein AR: On classifying cancer while treating patients. *Arch Intern Med* 45 (10): 1879-1791, 1985
2. Zelen M: The importance of prognostic factors in planning therapeutic trials. In: *Cancer Therapy: Prognostic Factors and Criteria of Response*, Staquet MJ (ed.) New York: Raven Press, 1975, pp. 1–6
3. Simon R: Importance of prognostic factors in cancer clinical trials. *Cancer Treat Rep* 68 (1): 185–192, 1984
4. Feinstein AR: A clinical method for estimating the rate of growth of a cancer. *Yale J Biol Med* 41: 422–433, 1969
5. Feinstein AR: *Clinical Judgement*. Williams and Wilkins Co., 1967
6. Feinstein AR: Symptoms as an index of biological behaviour and prognosis in human cancer. *Nature* 209: 241–245, 1966
7. Feinstein AR, Prichett J, Schimph C: The epidemiology of cancer therapy: II. The clinical course: Data, decisions and temporal demarcations. *Arch Intern Med* 123: 323–343, 1969
8. Feinstein AR: The pretherapeutic classification of co-morbidity in chronic disease. *J Chronic Dis* 23: 455–468, 1985
9. Armitage P: *Statistical Methods in Clinical Medicine*. Blackwell Oxford, 1977
10. Sackett DL, Hayes B, Tigwell P: *Clinical Epidemiology. A Basic Science for Clinical Medicine*. Little Brown and Co., Boston and Toronto, 1985
11. Feinstein AR, Sosin DM, Wells CK: The Will Rodgers phenomenon. Stage migration and new diagnostic techniques as a source of misleading statistics for survival in cancer. *N Engl J Med* 312: 1604–1608, 1985
12. Feinstein AR: Symptomatic patterns biological behaviour and prognosis in cancer of the lung: Practical application of Boolean algebra and clinical taxonomy. *Ann Intern Med* 61 (1): 27–43, 1964

36

13. Feinstein AR: A new staging system for cancer and reappraisal of 'early' treatment and 'cure' by radical surgery. *N Eng J Med* 279 (14): 747–753, 1965
14. Chahinian P, Israel L: prognostic value of doubling time and related factors in lung cancer. In: *Lung Cancer*, New York: Academic Press, 1976
15. Zorzitto M, Germanson T, Cummings B, Boyd NF: A method of clinical prognostic staging for patients with rectal cancer. *Dis Colon Rectum* 25 (8): 759-765, 1982
16. Boyd NF, Cummings BJ, Harwood AR, Rider WD, Thomas GM: Observer variation in the assessment of patients with rectal cancer. *Dis Colon Rectum* 25 (7): 664–668, 1987
17. Charlson M, Feinstein AR: The auxometric dimension. A new method for using rate of growth in prognostic staging of breast cancer. *JAMA* 22 (2): 180–185, 1974
18. Charlson M. Feinstein AR: A new clinical index of growth rate in the staging of breast cancer. *Am J Med* 69: 527–535
19. Charlson M: Delau in treatment of carcinoma of the breast. *Surg Gynecol Obstet* 160: 393–399, 1985
20. Boyd NF, Meakin JW, Hayward J, Brown TC: Clinical estimation of the growth rate of breast cancer. *Cancer* 48 (4): 1037–1042, 1981
21. Boyd NF, Feinstein AR: Symptoms as an index of growth rates and prognosis in Hodgkin's disease. *Clin Invest Med* 1 (1): 25–31, 1978
22. Boyd NF, Pater JL, Ginsburg AD, Myers FW: Observer variation in the classification of information from medical records. *J Chronic Dis* 32: 327–332, 1978
23. Boyd NF, Clemens JD, Feinstein AR: Pre-therapeutic morbidity in the prognostic staging of acute leukaemia. *Arch Intern Med* 139: 324–328, 1979
24. Boyd NF, Coates E, Clemens JD, Ayoub J, Chevalier L: Pretreatment clinical morbidity as an index of the biologic potential of acute lymphoblastic leukaemia of childhood. *Leuk Res* 5 (2): 159–164, 1981
25. Yorkshire Breast Group: Observer variation in recording clinical data from women presenting with breast lesions. *Br Med J* 2: 1196–1199, 1977
26. McDonald IG: Biological predeterminism in human cancer. *Surg Gynecol Obstet* 92: 433–452, 1951
27. Feinstein AR: Clinical Biostatistics. Hard science soft data and the challenges of choosing clinical variables in research. *Clin Pharmacol Ther* 22: 485–498, 1983
28. Feinstein AR: An additional basic science for clinical medicine: IV. The development of clinimetrics. *Ann Intern Med* 99: 843–848, 1983

3. Clinical staging and its prognostic significance

A.H.G. PATERSON

In this chapter, clinical staging is taken to mean the anatomical extent of cancer as defined by means other than surgical exploration and post-operative pathological examination of tissues. In defining the extent of malignant disease in a patient, the clinical stage is the *expression* of biological processes such as the rate of cell division, the balance of cell proliferation and destruction, and the cancer's metastatic potential. Unlike the level of estrogen or progesterone receptor protein or the histological grade, clinical stage is not in itself a biological determinant of prognosis, although patients with limited extent of disease, when analysed as a group, generally survive longer than those patients with more extensive disease. The topic is discussed under the following headings;
– Systems and objectives of staging
– Components of staging
– Fallacies and limitations of staging
– Chronological or biological prognostic factor?

Systems and objectives of staging

Current staging classifications are based on a description of the extent of the disease, and use symbols for the rapid communication of clinical information. In the first part of this century, attempts were made to assess the operability or otherwise of the disease [1] but this soon gave way to staging systems accepted by several influential medical centres. For example, the International Federation of Gynecology and Obstretics (F.I.G.O.) Staging Systems have been in use, with modifications, since 1937, having been correlated in all important respects with the TNM system [2].

The classification of tumours according to the characteristics of the primary tumour (T), the draining regional lymph nodes (N), and distant metastases (M) – the TNM system of the U.I.C.C. – was introduced after the second world war and has gradually gained acceptance, at least in North America and Western

Europe. It is now used in the staging of solid tumors, particularly of the breast, head and neck, gastrointestinal tract and lung, although clinicians continue to think and talk in terms of stage rather than TNM system.

Nevertheless, there are several malignancies where the TNM descriptive system is impractical and melanoma is an example where prognosis is determined by the microanatomical level of spread [3] and depth of invasion [4]. Hodgkin's disease and non-Hodgkin's lymphoma also are not easily classified by the TNM system and the Ann Arbor modification of the Rye Staging System is more satisfactory [5], Colorectal carcinomas are usually staged by Duke's microhistological system [6] rather than a TNM system. It is rare to hear clinicians using the TNM system in brain tumors, preferring a description of the size, site, and histological grade of the tumour.

The staging of malignant disease has improved our ability to compare results from different centres. Batley [7] has written on the causes of inaccuracy in cancer statistics including variability of staging, where removal of a few patients from one stage to another will improve or worsen treatment results depending on which direction they are re-staged. If survival rates by stage are compared between centres, there may be gross differences in treatment results, yet if *all* the patients are evaluated and compared, the results become similar. Again, differences in results between centres may merely mean that there are a higher proportion of early cases in one centre, leading to apparently better results.

Clinical staging attempts to define the anatomical extent of a malignant disease process also for the purpose of choosing an appropriate treatment and predicting the likely course of the disease. In selecting suitable therapy, clinicians tend to think of staging as a guide to whether local or systemic therapy should be used. In malignancies which are only moderately sensitive to ionizing radiation or cytotoxic chemotherapy, the anatomical extent of disease does often determine the treatment modality, but if a cancer is very sensitive to drugs and has a propensity for early widespread dissemination, then these drugs should be used whatever the stage (eg. embryonal cell carcinoma of the testis).

In predicting the course of the disease in the individual, the reliability of clinical staging is less certain. The widespread assumption, that the greater the extent of the disease the poorer is the prognosis, is often invalid when prognosticating for the individual patient. Thus, a patient presenting with Stage IV breast cancer might outlive a patient presenting with Stage I disease. Stage is only one of an array of prognostic factors which must be assessed.

Very often, limited anatomical disease does reflect good prognosis but in many individual patients, stage does not necessarily correlate with outcome. In the Stage IV case of follicular lymphoma or the Stage IV breast cancer patient with indolent osteosclerotic metastases, stage might be an expression of the age of the tumour, in other words a 'chronological' prognostic factor. This concept is shown in the schematic diagram in Fig. 1.

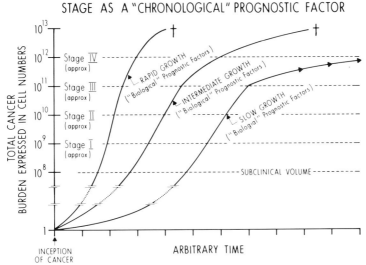

Figure 1. Hypothetical growth curves of three cancers: a rapidly growing cancer, one of intermediate growth, and a slowly growing cancer. The determinants of growth rate (e.g. histology, nuclear grade, rate of cell proliferation) might be termed prognostic factors of a biological nature. The total cancer burden of each malignancy (expressed as total number of cells in the tumour) might roughly equate with stage of disease. In this conceptual arrangement, stage reflects the age of the cancer within its own natural history. Some Stage IV cancers with slow growth can remain in this stage for long periods of time. High stage patients should not necessarily be regarded as having a poor prognosis since biological prognostic factors must be considered.

Components of staging

History

The clinical history is important and the presence or absence of sweats, fevers and a weight loss greater than ten percent over three-month period, may mean the difference between a patient with Hodgkin's disease receiving radiation therapy alone, or a six month's course of combination chemotherapy with or without radiation therapy. The presence of 'B' symptoms implies systemic Hodgkin's disease with a prognosis significantly poorer than in the absence of symptoms [8].

Manifestation of pain in a patient with apparently localized breast cancer may identify a patient with metastatic disease at presentation, and we have found a careful history to be as reliable a guide in diagnosing bone metastases as is routine bone scanning in patients with breast cancer [9]. Back pain is often found in young men with testicular tumours which involve the retroperitoneal lymph nodes. Bleeding in a primary malignant melanoma usually indicates a larger primary and a poorer prognosis [10]. The prognostic importance of clinical history is discussed in Chapter 2.

Physical examination

Traditionally, the clinician attempts to measure the size of the primary tumour, to detect the presence or absence of enlarged regional lymph nodes, and to identify associated clinical signs. But how accurate should one attempt to be? Which aspects of the clinical examination are particularly important and what is their influence on prognosis and treatment decisions in the face of so much diagnostic technology available today?

Clinical assessment of the dimensions of a primary mass are particularly important in the preoperative assessment of accessible solid tumours such as those in breast, head and neck and bone, and in the lymphomas. But there is often a surrounding tissue reaction which makes a measurement taken in the clinic spuriously large compared to the measured pathological dimensions. Primaries in less accessible areas, such as ovarian cancers, pose even greater problems for clinical measurement. Nevertheless, the maximum diameter of a primary tumour influences the choice of local treatment and is a prognostic factor for local recurrence, although it is not as major a prognostic factor for survival as, for example, the presence of involved regional lymph nodes [10, 11].

In the detection of cancer-involved regional lymph nodes, clinical examination is often grossly inaccurate. Palpably enlarged lymph nodes often turn out to be reactive hyperplasia, while lymph nodes which are clinically impalpable may be pathologically involved by cancer. Many studies have demonstrated the inaccuracy of clinical regional lymph node assessment [12]. This inaccuracy is in the region of 35% for both false positives and false negatives, rendering this clinical assessment of limited value in cases where lymph nodes are either impalpable, or enlarged but freely mobile.

The presence of fixed, hard lymph nodes is more accurately correlated with pathological involvement. This is borne out in the case of breast cancer, by a greater difference in survival between clinical Stage III and Stage II breast cancers, than between clinical Stage I and Stage II breast cancers [13].

Associated clinical features are often important for prognosis, and in some instances can be detected only in the clinic. The presence of erythema of the breast (indicating an inflammatory carcinoma of the breast) or skin nodules, can be detected only in the clinic, preferably in an examination room exposed to daylight. Peau d'orange and fixation of the tumour to the chest wall indicate inoperability and a poorer prognosis.

The detection of large abdominal masses (greater than 10 cm) in the diffuse lymphomas indicates a poorer prognosis despite a low clinical stage. Large mediastinal masses in Hodgkin's disease (greater than 6 cm) indicate a high likelihood of mediastinal recurrence unless added treatment is given.

Diagnostic investigations

New technology for localising tumour in inaccessible areas and more aggressive sampling of tissues, have led to a more precise evaluation of disease extent. More aggressive staging, with its tendency towards categorizing patients into more advanced stages, has led to an apparent improvement in survival results in all stages, even when no real change in survival has occurred. But more accurate staging does allow a more rational approach to therapy. This trend to more precise staging is likely to continue with improvements in diagnostic imaging devices, and with the use of tumour cell surface antigen-directed monoclonal antibodies, to detect the presence of malignant cells in tissues such as bone marrow or liver [14].

Lymphangiography allows detection of cancer-involved lymph nodes within the abdomen with an accuracy which (in the case of Hodgkin's disease) can occasionally challenge the ability of the surgeon and the pathologist to find involved lymph nodes [15]. Accuracy depends on the skill and experience of the radiologist in interpreting the lymphogram.

CT scanning is becoming increasingly important in identifying intrathoracic Hodgkin's disease, particularly pleural, pericardial and extranodal spread [16]. In many other anatomical sites, CT scanning is supplanting lymphography as the diagnostic technique of choice, although many radiologists still feel that CT scanning, like lymphography, is inadequate in detecting retroperitoneal upper abdominal lymph nodes. In intra-abdominal disease, CT scanning may be used instead of lymphography in patients with testicular tumors. Here, CT scanning together with tumour marker studies have a 90% accuracy in detecting retroperitoneal lymph node cancer deposits [17].

Radionuclide scanning is currently of variable importance in clinical staging. Bone scintigraphy is clearly the most accurate technique for detecting bone metastases [9] and we use it on all patients with node-positive breast cancer, as well as on those node-negative patients who have symptoms. On the other hand, routine radiocolloid liver scanning has limited value either as a preoperative staging procedure or as a method of following the course of the disease. Exceptions to this might be patients with gastrointestinal malignancies, small cell carcinoma of the lung and some paediatric tumors such as rhabdomyosarcoma and Wilm's tumour [18].

The use of tumour-seeking radiopharmaceuticals has been reported for detecting metastatic disease for staging purposes. On the whole, the results are disappointing [19], although [67]gallium citrate may occasionally be of value in detecting seminoma or Hodgkin's disease involving the mediastinum [20]. Ultrasound examination is of particular value in the detection of liver metastases, and in the demonstration of lymphadenopathy in the porta hepatis and splenic hilum [21]. It is also helpful in the staging and follow-up of pelvic tumors such as ovarian carcinomas and choriocarcinomas. Nuclear magnetic resonance imaging has promise of improving our ability to stage patients with tumours involving the difficult upper one-third of the abdomen.

Tumour markers

Tumour markers when present in the blood may reflect tumour bulk and activity, but only in a few tumours is this of practical value. Patients with embryonal cell carcinoma of the testis or gestational trophoblastic disease can be followed by measurement of the beta sub-unit of human chorionic gonadotrophin. Patients with choriocarcinoma are categorised into 'high risk', 'medium risk', or 'low risk' disease [22], and 'staging' is based as much on the assumed tumour bulk reflected in the level of β-HCG, as on precise anatomical location of tumour deposits.

The categorising of patients by combining biological prognostic factors and stage (which is predominantly a chronological prognostic factor) is often used by the practising clinician to distinguish 'curable' from 'sub-curable' cases [23]. In choriocarcinoma however, stage is submerged into the clinician's assessment of 'curability' and it is this 'curability' which determines the dosage and combination of drugs used.

Fallacies and limitations in staging

The more assiduous a clinician is in staging, the better will his results appear to be when analysed by stage [7]. For example, those who tend to find larger tumours than are in fact there, show better survival rates for each stage than the more liberal 'stagers'. As late as 1976, Chandler Smith argued that the practice of clinical staging was questionable as a means of assessing cancer treatment results [24]. This conclusion does not downplay the value of careful clinical staging, but emphasises possible reasons for differences in results between centres.

Another fallacy lies in the staging systems themselves, where subtle differences in interpretation of the accepted system can influence end-results. For example, there is often considerable discrepancy between centres in the staging of malignant diseases, e.g. categorizing a patient either to Stage IIE Hodgkin's disease or Stage IV, when nearby (but not contiguous) bone or lung lesions are under question. The choice of the higher stage will improve the overall survival rate for all the stages [25].

There is no basis for the assumption that all cancer patients progress through the various stages at roughly the same rate until death from distant metastases occurs, and that only timely intervention by the clinician prevents this process. There is considerable evidence however, of biological factors ('biological predeterminism') which influence the stage of disease at which patients present themselves to the clinician [26]. Thus, 'early' stage cancers may be small not necessarily because they are early, but because they are slowly growing. Conversely, large, 'late' stage cancers may be large not necessarily because the patients have presented late, but because they are rapidly growing cancers.

In the individual patient, the doctor who prognosticates from clinical staging evidence alone is risking serious inaccuracy unless he has observed the natural history of the disease in that patient. Common solid tumours where extensive disease is not incompatible with long survival are renal cell carcinomas, leiomyosarcomas and carcinomas of the breast and prostate. Careful consideration of the previous course of the disease in a Stage IV patient will avoid rash prognostic statements.

Merely because staging may include histopathological assessment does not necessarily make it more accurate. The pathological laboratory is often challenged, for example, in the relative accuracy of the lymphangiogram and pathological staging in Hodgkin's disease. In the final analysis, assessment of the accuracy of clinical and pathological staging often depends on retrospective analysis and this approach has faults of its own.

The limited accuracy of clinical staging is particularly well recognized in breast cancer. In patients with clinical Stage I cancer, approximately one-quarter of the patients have axillary lymph node metastases detected by the pathologist while in patients assigned to a clinical Stage II category, over one-third of the patients have no detectable axillary metastases on histology [27]. In fact, the clinical status of the axillary lymph nodes at presentation is not related to ten-year survival, provided they are found to be histologically negative [28].

In our own series of 869 analysable patients, we have found that pre-operative clinical staging of breast cancer gives a reasonable spread of survival rates at 10 years (Table I). There is a similar spread of survival rates when clinical and pathological information is combined. At 10 years, our relative survival rates for patients with Stage I disease in 92.2%, for Stage II disease 75.4%, for Stage III disease 44.8%, and for Stage IV disease 8.2% [29].

This relatively high 10 year survival rate illustrates a further problem of patient

Table 1. 10-Year survival rates for women in Northern Alberta with breast cancer diagnosed from 1971 through 1974 by stage at time of diagnosis

TNM Stage	No. of Women*	Actuarial Survival	Relative Survival Rate (%)
I	180	77	89
II	399	61	74
III	221	36	45
IV	69	6	8

* All patients

selection and variation in staging practices. The staging was performed by two experienced clinicians and the above survival rates are significantly higher than those reported elsewhere. And yet, when we examine our own patients by pathological node status, our survival rates come closer to most other centres, although they are still significantly higher than, for example, the NSABP ten year survivals [30]. This suggests either that there is observer variation even when pathological examination is used as the staging standard, or that breast cancer behaves differently in Alberta, or that we are looking at a selected group of patients. We believe that our survival rates reflect the behaviour of breast cancer in a community.

In Hodgkin's disease, there is a similar difficulty in assessing axillary nodes as in breast cancer. A clinically normal spleen will harbour Hodgkin's disease in some 25% of patients, whereas an enlarged spleen will be histologically normal in up to one-half of patients [31]. The advent of staging laparotomy and splenectomy in Hodgkin's disease has had the effect of advancing some 20-30% of patients to a higher stage than that based on clinical staging, and some 10-20% of patients to a lower stage than clinically suspected [31].

That increasing accuracy of clinical staging has improved survival rates is not easy to demonstrate, but there is no doubt that more accurate staging leads to more appropriate therapy in the higher stage patient and also avoids unnecessary morbidity when the tumour is localized.

Chronological or biological prognostic factor?

What information does clinical staging provide about the biological behaviour of the tumour and its relationship to the host? Is it a 'chronological' prognostic factor, or it is an expression of the intrinsic biological aggressiveness of the tumour within the host (a 'biological' prognostic factor) or is it a complex and variable combination of both?

One way of examining this question in breast cancer is to examine the survival of patients with recurrent disease according to the clinical stage at which they presented [32]. In Fig. 2 we see that the survival time from diagnosis of first recurrence is similar whether the patient presented initially with clinical Stage I disease or Stage III disease. Again, patients with recurrent disease who had histologically negative axillary lymph nodes at presentation survive a similar time to those who had positive axillary lymph nodes. But if we look at the disease-free survival of these patients (Table 2) we see a gradation in these times: Stage I patients have the longest disease-free survival and Stage III patients have the shortest. These results suggest that clinical stage (and axillary node status) are predominantly chronological prognostic factors expressing the age of the tumour.

Nevertheless, if we look only at patients presenting with local recurrence, there

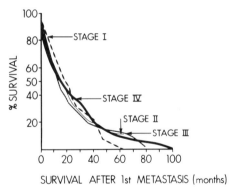

Figure 2. Survival after diagnosis of first distant metastases by clinical stage at presentation in 719 (of 896 patients) who had adequate documentation of clinical stage. Stage I, 75 patients; Stage II, 240 patients; Stage III, 218 patients, Stage IV, 186 patients. No significant difference was observed in survival (p = <0.50).

is a significant difference in survival for those patients who originally presented with clinical Stage I disease compared to those patients who originally presented with Stage III disease (Fig. 3). This would suggest an element of 'biological predeterminism' [26] so that the stage at which a patient presents with breast cancer is reflected in differing survivals after local recurrence.

Clinical stage in breast cancer, when examined in a large population of patients, therefore appears to be an expression both of the age of the tumour and of its biological growth characteristics. However, it is likely that in individual patients, one or other dimension of stage as a prognostic factor – chronological or biological – will dominate. We therefore need biological tests to determine which

Table 2. Relationship of prognostic factors to duration of disease-free survival in breast cancer.

	Total No. of patients who presented with primary breast cancer	No. developing metastasis (%) but not presenting with metastasis*	Median disease-free survival (months)	Statistical Significance	
Stage I	630	75 (12%)	24	NS	I vs II
Stage II	982	240 (24%)	23	P<0.001	I vs III
Stage III	463	218 (47%)	15	P<0.01	II vs III
0 Nodes	1144	46 (13%)	24	P<0.05	0 vs 1–3
I–3 Nodes	566	167 (30%)	20	P<0.001	0 vs >4
>4 Nodes	291	147 (51%)	17	NS	1–3 vs >4

* Patients presenting with distant metastases at time of diagnosis were excluded from this analysis, i.e. excluded were 186 stage IV patients, 5 patients with zero nodes, 17 with 1–3 nodes and 7 with >4 nodes.

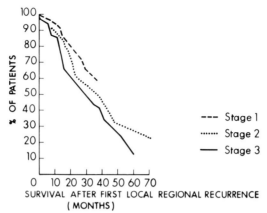

Figure 3. Survival after first loco-regional recurrence as site of first recurrence by clinical stage at presentation in 229 patients. Stage I, 51 patients; Stage II, 98 patients; Stage III, 80 patients. The trend of the survival curves was statistically significant. Test for trend (p = 0.008); test for heterogeneity (p = 0.027).

patients are harbouring slowly growing tumours and which are truly 'early.' This is particularly relevant for early diagnosis programmes, since many slowly growing small tumours may never become clinically metastatic, whereas 'early' tumours may be curable by removal.

Conclusion

Clinical staging is an important prognostic factor but of a different nature from biological factors such as histology or hormone receptor level. It can be regarded as an expression of the age of the tumour relative to its natural history, and therefore as a 'chronological' prognostic factor. Staging cannot be used in isolation in making prognostication. It cannot be assumed that tumours of low stage have been diagnosed early and that tumours of high stage are always late; the former may be slowly growing tumours and the latter rapidly growing, and in these cases, stage is predominantly a reflection of biological prognostic factors. More precise anatomical staging is helpful but must go hand in hand with research into biological prognostic factors.

Acknowledgement

My thanks to members of the Breast Unit, Cross Cancer Institute, and in particular to Drs. A.W. Lees and P.E. Burns for their advice and for the use of some of their unpublished work; to Mr. K. Leisner for preparing the illustrations and to Mrs. Shyrose Nurmohamed for preparing the manuscript.

References

1. McCann FJ: The Technique of the More Extensive Abdominal Operations for Cancer of the Womb. *Lancet*, 819–827, 1912
2. *Manual for Staging of Cancer*: American Joint Committee for Cancer Staging and End Result Reporting. American Joint Committee, Chicago, Illinois, 1977
3. Clark WHJr, Goldman LI, Mastrangelo MJ (eds.): *Human Malignant Melanoma*, Grune, New York 15–31, 1979
4. Breslow A: Tumour Thickness, Level of Invasion and Lymph Node Dissection in Stage I Cutaneous Melanoma. *Annals of Surgery* 182–572, 1975
5. Rosenberg SA: Report of the Committee on Staging of Hodgkin's Disease. *Cancer Research* 26: 1310, 1966
6. Dukes CE: 'The Classification of Cancer of the Rectum.' *J Pathology Bacteriology* 35:323, 1932
7. Batley F: The Dilemma of Cancer Statistics. *Archives Surgery* 88: 163–166, 1964
8. Carbone PP, Kaplan HS, Mushoff K, Smithers DW and Tubiana M: Report of the Committee on Hodgkin's Disease Staging Classification. *Cancer Research* 31: 1860, 1971
9. Lentle BC, Burns PE, Dierich H and Jackson FI: Bone Scintiscanning in the Initial Assessment of Carcinoma of the Breast. *Surgery, Gynaecology & Obstetrics* 141: 43–47, 1975
10. Fisher ER, Sass R, Fisher B: Pathologic Findings from the National Surgical Adjuvant Project for Breast Cancers (Protocol No. 4): Discriminants for Tenth Year Treatment Failure. *Cancer* 53: 712–723, 1984
11. Fisher B, Slack NH and Bross, IDJ: Cancer of the Breast: Size of Neoplasm and Prognosis. *Cancer* 24: 1071–1080, 1969
12. Langlands AO, Kerr G: On the Staging of Breast Cancer. *Clinical Radiology* 27: 17–19, 1986
13. MacKay EN, Sellars AH: A Clinical Trial of TNM Staging of Breast Cancer, Ontario 1960–62. *European Journal of Cancer* I: 515–524, 1966
14. Royston I, Sobol RE: Editorial: Monoclonal Antibody Immunocytology: Potential Application for Staging and Monitoring Malignant Disease Activity. *Journal of Clinical Oncology* 3:4:453–454, 1985
15. Glees JP, Gazet JC, MacDonald JS, Peckman MJ: The Accuracy of Lymphography in Hodgkin's Disease. *Clinical Radiology* 25: 5–11, 1974
16. Portlock CS, 'Hodgkin's Disease' p. 729–740. In: *Medical Clinics of North America* 68:3. W.B. Saunders Company, 1984
17. Venner P, Castor W: Personal Communication. 1986
18. Harbert JC: 'Efficacy of Liver Scanning in Malignant Disease.' *Seminars in Nuclear Medicine* 14: 287–295, 1984
19. Paterson AHG, McCready VR: Tumour Imaging Radiopharmaceuticals. *British Journal of Radiology* 48: 520–531, 1975
20. Paterson AHG, Peckham MJ, McCready VR: Value of Gallium Scanning in Seminoma of the Testis. *British Medical Journal* I: 1118–1121, 1975
21. Glees J, Taylor K, Gazet JC, Peckham MJ, McCready VR: Accuracy of Grey-Scale Ultrasonography of the Liver and Spleen in Hodgkin's Disease and the Other Lymphomas Compared with Isotope Scans. *Clinical Radiology* 28: 233–238, 1977
22. Begent RHJ, Bagshawe KD: Management of High-Risk Choriocarcinoma. *Seminars in Oncology* 9: 198–203, 1982
23. Fisher RI, Hubbard SM, Devita VT, Berard CW, Wesley R, Cossman J, Young RC: Factors Predicting Long-Term Survival in Diffuse Mixed, Histiocytic or Undifferentiated Lymphomas. *Blood:* 58: 45–51, 1981
24. Smith Chandler: The Questionable Practice of Clinical Staging. *Perspectives in Biology and Medicine* 273–277, 1976

25. Connors JM, Klimo P: Is It an E Lesion or Stage IV. An Unsettled Issue in Hodgkin's Disease Staging. *Journal of Clinical Oncology* 2: 1421–1423, 1984
26. MacDonald I: Natural History of Mammary Carcinoma. *American Journal of Surgery* III: 435–442, 1966
27. Atkins HA, Haywood JL, Klugman DJ, Wayte AB: Treatment of Early Breast Cancer: A Report After 10 Years of A Clinical Trial. *British Medical Journal* 2: 423–429, 1972
28. Hamilton T, Langlands AO and Prescott RJ: The Treatment of Operable Cancer of the Breast: A Clinical Trial in the South-East Region of Scotland. *British Journal of Surgery* 61: 758–761, 1974
29. Lees AW: Personal Communication, 1985
30. Fisher B: Ten Year Follow-up of Breast Cancer Patients in a Cooperative Clinical Trial Evaluating Surgical Adjuvant Chemotherapy. *Surgery Gynaecology & Obstetrics* 140: 528–534, 1975
31. Rosenberg SA: A Critique of the Value of Laparotomy and Splenectomy in the Evaluation of Patients with Hodgkin's Disease. *Cancer Research* 31: 1737–1740, 1971
32. Holland JF: Breaking the Cure Barrier. *Journal of Clinical Oncology* 1: 75–90, 1983

4. Prognostic significance of disease-free interval

J. ROSENMAN and M. VARIA

The disease-free interval (DFI) is the period of time between the primary treatment of a malignancy and the first sign of tumor recurrence. The recording of this interval is necessarily approximate, because detection of a recurrence depends on how symptomatic it is or on how diligently it is looked for. There is a widespread clinical impression that an extended disease-free interval is indicative of a slow rate of tumor growth, but few confirmatory studies have been done.

The significance of the DFI in modern oncologic treatment needs to be re-examined, even though recent interest in pointers to cancer prognosis has shifted from clinical to laboratory parameters. Many new treatment options for patients with recurrent cancer are accompanied by significant morbidity, and we need better predictors both for treatment response and long-term post-recurrence survival. If the length of the DFI is a measure of the *rate* of disease progression, then the DFI might be a predictor for the length of the post-recurrence survival (PRS) [1]. Such knowledge might help (a) In deciding how aggressive one should be in the treatment of a patient with tumor recurrence (b) In predicting response, as rapidly growing tumors may be more sensitive to chemotherapy or radiation therapy than are slowly growing tumors.

The inquiry will concentrate on cancers of the breast and uterine cervix because more information on the DFI is available for these tumors. Most publications concerning the DFI of other malignancies are limited to case reports of unusually late tumor recurrences and offer little insight into when and why they occur [2–7].

Breast cancer

That patients with breast cancer can suffer very late relapses was first reported in 1907 [8] and there followed many reports of recurrence after disease-free intervals of forty years or more [9–12]. Subsequently, Shimkin *et al.* [13] reported on 372 patients with recurrent breast cancer and concluded that there was a significant correlation between the DFI and post-recurrence survival. This correlation was especially strong for local-regional recurrences.

Goldenberg et al. [14] reported that for 610 woman with inoperable primary, locally recurrent, or metastatic breast cancer, the two-year survival rate rose from 20% for a DFI less than 12 months, to 50% for a DFI greater than 60 months. However, Papaioannou et al. [15] failed to find a significant difference in the median post-recurrence survival, between breast cancer patients with a DFI greater than five years and those with a DFI from one to two years (23 vs 17 months: $p = .09$).

As part of an American Joint Committee on Cancer Staging study, Culter et al. [16] reported on the survival of 888 patients with metastatic breast cancer. Patients with a DFI of greater than 5 years, 2–5 years, 1–2 years and less than 1 year were compared. Excluded were 111 patients given a 'dire' prognosis (recurrence in the liver, peritoneum, brain or spinal cord) and 20 other patients who relapsed at less than two months. The median survival times were found to be 26 months, 15 months, 11 months and 7 months respectively. However, in a group of patients with *isolated* breast cancer recurrences randomized to receive chemoimmunotherapy or placebo Buzdar et al. [17] reported that survival of the control group at one year and two years was found to be independent of the DFI.

Pater et al. [18] found that survival after relapse increased with increasing DFI but only up to two years, remaining constant after that. However, Pearlman and Jochimsen [19] reported that an increased disease-free interval was not predictive for increased post-recurrence survival until the DFI was greater than 48 months. These authors also noted that the time from first recurrence to second recurrence (R_1-R_2 interval) also increased with increasing DFI after 48 months.

Rosenman and Perrone [20] reported that the post-recurrence survival *for distant metastases only* was decreased only for a DFI less than 12 months, but update after four more years of follow-up now shows that the length of the DFI and post-recurrence survival are correlated ($p = .0045$) for *all* values of the DFI. More recently, Alanko et al. [21] reported that post-recurrence survival was very greatly increased if the DFI was greater than 18 months as opposed to less than 18 months ($p < .0001$). The effect was still present, but reduced, if the patients had been given adjuvant hormone therapy.

With regard to *locally* recurrent carcinoma of the breast, Chu et al. [22] noted an increasing median survival as a function of the DFI but the standard deviations were marked. Bedwinek et al. [23] also noted that survival after local-regional recurrence depended on the disease-free interval, with a five year survival of 56% for those with a DFI greater than 24 months and only 17% for a DFI less than 24 months.

Table 1. DFI as a predictor of post-recurrence survival (Breast cancer)

Years	Number	Median PRS for a DFI of:				Site of Failure	Sig	Ref
		<1 yr	1–2 yrs	2–5 yrs	>5 yrs			
1918–1947	98	13 mo		31 mo	58 mo	local	p<.05	13
»	83	14 mo		18 mo	20 mo	osseous	p<.05	
»	193	6 mo		10 mo	9 mo	soft tissue	p>.05	
1922–1961	610	n/a	n/a	n/a	24 mo	advanced	n/a	14
1954–1964	123	n/a	17 mo	n/a	23 mo	local & dist	p=.09	15
1950–1961	614	7 mo	12 mo	15 mo	25 mo	distant only	p=.001	16
1961–1970	456	11 mo	16 mo	22 mo	20 mo	local & dist	sig to 5 yrs	18
1961–1970	464	10 mo[b]	14 mo[b]	15 mo[b]	29 mo[b]	distant only	n/a	19
1971–1980	245	16 mo	22 mo	26 mo	35 mo	distant only	p=.005	20
1950–1970	215	27 mo[b]	30 mo[b]	38 mo[b]	50 mo[b]	local only	n/a	22

DFI: Disease-free interval
PRS: Post-recurrence survival
n/a: Data not available.

[a] Years in which the patient had the recurrence.
[b] Values read from graph.

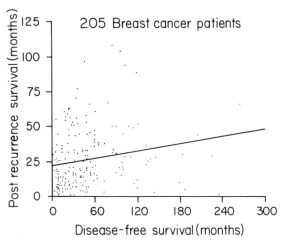

Figure 1. Relationship between disease-free interval and post-recurrence survival in 205 breast cancer patients.

A summary of all these findings (Table 1) suggests that the DFI *does* predict for post-recurrence survival, but certain observations are necessary:

(1) Although a correlation between DFI and post-recurrence survival is seen in most series, the variations are quite marked. Fig. 1 is a scattergram of the updated Massuchusetts General Hospital study of 205 patients [20]. The superimposed line is the least squares best fit. If $\overline{\text{PRS}}$ is the average post-recurrence survival then

$$\overline{\text{PRS}} = 21.9 + 0.09 * \text{DFI},\qquad(1)$$

where DFI and PRS are measured in months. Thus, the PRS rises from 21.9 months for immediate relapsers to 43.5 months for a DFI of 20 years.

(2) The DFI seems better correlated with the survival after local-regional recurrences than it does with survival after development of distan metastases. This was the explicit finding of Shimkin [13]. Bedwinek [23] reported a 56% five year survival for local-regional recurrences with a DFI greater than 24 months, but 17% for a DFI less than 24 months (p = .0001) while our data for distant metastases only [20] show corresponding five year survivals of 19.4% and 10.4% (p = .066). More data recurrence and distant metastases are needed to clarify this possible distinction between locoregional recurrence and distant metastases.

(3) The correlation between the DFI and PRS is reduced for recurrences in life-threatening locations such as the brain or liver. Our data support this observation in that the DFI was correlated with the PRS in 108 patients who recurred in bone (p = .014), but not in the 97 patients who initially recurred in non-osseous sites (p = .144).

(4) The duration of post-recurrence survival has steadily improved throughout

the years for all patient categories. This finding is in agreement with other reports [24-26] and is probably due to the earlier detection of recurrences and the use of post-recurrence chemotherapy. Thus, the significance of the DFI appears not to have changed over the many years spanned by these studies.

(5) The effect of different treatment regimens on the prognostic significance of the DFI must be taken into account. While there is good evidence that the systemic progression of breast cancer is not altered by the form of local treatment [27, 28], both hormonal manipulation and cytotoxic chemotherapy probably increase the disease-free interval and survival after recurrence [25]. It is therefore important to ask if the relationship between the DFI and PRS is altered by these treatments, and how far DFI is of predictive value for response to hormone or chemotherapy.

Veronesi et al. [29] showed that a DFI of less than two years was associated with a 20% response rate to oophorectomy, compared to 40% in patients with a DFI greater than two years. This finding was in accord with an earlier study by Fracchia [30] who showed that for 500 patients the response rate to adrenalectomy was 44% in patients with a DFI greater than two years, as opposed to 28% in those with a DFI less than two years. Henderson and Canellos [31] combining the results of 14 previous studies reported that response rates to any endocrine ablation range from 30% for patients with a DFI less than two years, to 56% for those with a DFI greater than five years. The correlation between DFI and response to additive hormonal therapy is however less clear and Lerner et al. [32] could not show a relationship between the DFI and response to tamoxifen therapy.

The value of the DFI in predicting post-recurrence survival appears unchanged by the administration of hormones; many of the patients summarized in Table 1 were in fact treated with high-dose estrogen after recurrence. Alanko et al. [21] specifically showed that survival after the first recurrence was more strongly correlated with the DFI than with estrogen or progesteron receptor status. However, in patients treated with hormones, positive double receptor status was a better prognostic indicator of post-recurrence survival.

The prognostic value of the DFI in predicting response to cytotoxic chemotherapy is unclear. Henderson and Canellos [31] in their review of 19 studies on 855 patients conclude that there is a tendency for those with a longer DFI to have a higher response rate to chemotherapy, although the highest response rate was seen in patients initially presenting with metastatic disease. However, Valagussa et al. [33] in a report on 318 patients (included in the Henderson series) reported that the lowest rate of response was seen in patients with a DFI greater than two years. Swenerton et al. [34], reporting on 619 patients (not included in the Henderson study), found no correlation between response rate and the DFI (63% for a zero DFI, 64% for a DFI less than two years and 66% for a DFI greater than two years). A modest increase in post-recurrence *survival* with increasing DFI was however seen.

To sum up the data presented suggest that the length of the disease-free interval reflects the rate of growth of breast cancer and as such may be predictive for post-recurrence survival. Such a conclusion is in accord with observations of Pearlman [19] that the DFI is predictive of the time from first recurrence to second recurrence and that this interval, too, is predictive of the PRS. However, breast cancer is a highly variable disease, and two patients with the same DFI could have widely different post-recurrence survivals. The significance of the DFI in the face of adjuvant cytotoxic or homonal therapy is uncertain but is probably maintained.

The DFI seems predictive of response to hormonal ablation but it is unclear whether this extends to additive hormonal therapy. The value of the DFI in predicting response to cytotoxic chemotherapy needs to be clarified.

Can the disease-free interval be predicted?

Because patients with large numbers of positive axillary lymph nodes (and to a lesser extent, large primary breast tumors) have a higher ultimate failure rate than those with less advanced disease, one would expect the length of the disease-free interval to decrease with advancing stage. This was first shown explicitly by Shimkin [13] for clinical staging and, in more detail by Rosenman and Perrone [20] for pathologic staging. In the latter study, a multivariate analysis showed that both the tumor size and number of positive axillary nodes can independently predict for the length of the disease-free interval (p = .004 and p = .037) respectively. The observation that the disease-free interval depends more on tumor size and less on the number of positive nodes may be related to the observation that the percentage of proliferating cells (expressed as the thymidine labeling index of the primary tumor) correlates better with tumor size than with lymph node status [35].

Other variables thought to correlate with the DFI are the thymidine labeling index (LI) itself and the presence of estrogen and/or progesterone receptors. The LI was found in one study to be especially low in patients with an extended DFI [36]. Alanko [21] cites ten reports that claim a correlation between the length of the DFI and the presence of estrogen or progesterone receptor and eight reports that claim the opposite.

Cancer of the uterine cervix

Like breast cancer, very late recurrences in cancer of the uterine cervix have been reported and the longest appears to be 34 years [37]. It is not certain if these are true recurrences, new primaries in the cervix, or new vaginal primaries because, unlike breast cancer, the disease-free interval in cervix cancer is usually very short, as is also post-recurrence survival.

Table 2. DFI and PRS in recurrences of cancer of the uterine cervix

Years[a]	Number	Stage	Median DFI	Longest DFI	Median PRS	Alive[b] >5 yrs	Ref
1969–1979	67	IB	13 mo	7½ yrs	13 mo	10%	38
1947–1964	65	I	18 mo	>10 yrs	n/a	11%	39
»	119	II	12 mo	>10 yrs	n/a		
1955–1964	134	all	18 mo	17 yrs	12 mo[c]	10%	40
1965–1977	40	IB, IIA	11 mo	> 5 yrs	10 mo	13%	41
1951–1962	193	all	n/a[e]	13 yrs	n/a[f]	4%	42
1964–1976	160	all	<12 mo	n/a	n/a	6%[g]	43
1960–1970	68	all	>12 mo	17 yrs	<12 mo	13%[h]	44
1948–1963	178	all	n/a	n/a	n/a	5%	45
1969–1980	35	IB	10½ mo	8½ yrs	5 mo	3%	UNC data
»	80	II	10 mo	8½ yrs	8 mo	3%	
»	127	III	7½ mo	8½ yrs	7 mo	1%	

DFI: Disease-free interval
PRS: Post-recurrence survival.

[a] Years in which the patient had the recurrence
[b] Percent of all recurrent cervix cancer patients
[c] Treated
[d] Untreated
[e] 81% by 2 years
[f] 90% dead by two years
[g] Alive > 3 years
[h] 17.6% for those with local recurrence only.

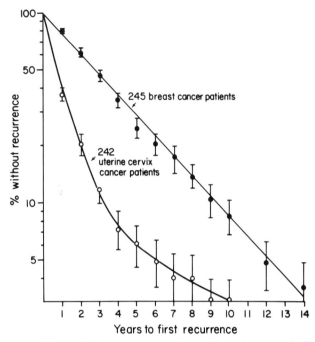

Figure 2. Comparison of disease-free interval in 242 patients with cervix cancer with that for 245 breast cancer patients.

In Fig. 2 the DFI for 242 patients with cervix cancer is compared to that for the 245 breast cancer patients previously discussed. The cervix cancer date comes from our experience at the University of North Carolina with more than 600 cervix cancer patients treated from 1969-1980 with radiation therapy. The data in Table 2 on median disease-free survival and survival after recurrence come from eight recent series [38–45].

The prognostic significance of the DFI in cervix cancer has not been extensively studied. Truelsen [46] reported on the recurrence patterns of 704 patients and concluded that there was no relationship between the DFI and PRS for cervix cancer. More recently Shingleton *et al.* [38] reported that for patients with stage IB carcinoma of the cervix the median post-recurrence survival was 9 months for those with a DFI less than 1 year compared to 14 months for those with a DFI greater than 1 year. Barber *et al.* [39], agree, and suggests that a DFI of less than 18 months implies a grave prognosis but present no data.

Halpin *et al.* [40], however, found no difference in the DFI between those patients having a post-recurrence survival of five or more years and those who had relapsed earlier. Krebs *et al.* [41] found a median post-recurrence survival of 12 months for those with a DFI greater than 6 months, versus 6 months for those with a DFI less than 6 months. In addition there were five patients alive more than five years after recurrence and all of them had a DFI greater than 6 months.

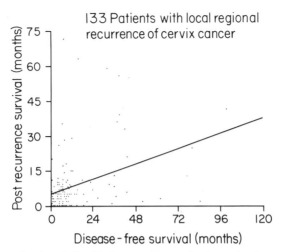

Figure 3. Scattergram showing relationship between diesease-free interval and post-recurrence survival in 133 patients with local regional recurrence of cervix cancer.

In the rather rare instances where the first and only recurrence of cervix cancer is in the lung, the median disease-free interval is about 30 months [47, 48]. Fuller *et al.* [47] reported that for these patients a prolonged DFI was associated with an improved duration of survival.

Because these data are not consistent, we analyzed our experience at the University of North Carolina in 242 patients with recurrent cancer of the uterine cervix who had been treated between 1969 and 1980 with radiation therapy. We found a strong correlation between the DFI and post-recurrence survival for patients whose first site of failure was in the pelvis (p < .001), but not for patients whose first site of failure was extrapelvic. Fig. 3 is a scattergram of the DFI versus post-recurrence survival for the 133 cervix cancer patients with pelvic recurrences. Linear regression analysis gives

$$\overline{PRS} = .277 * DFI + 4.72 \tag{4}$$

where both $\overline{PRS}$ and DFI are measured in months.

Selected patients who have suffered a recurrence of their cervix cancer can be retreated either with a pelvic exenteration [38] or with radiation therapy [49] and ultimately, up to 10% of all recurrences can be cured (see Table 2). Knowing that a long disease-free interval will select out for slowly growing disease is useful when trying to decide whether a given patient should be subjected to a hazardous retreatment.

As with breast cancer, cervix cancer patients with more advanced stage tumors recur earlier. In our series, stage I patients had a median DFI of 10½ months and 75% of the patients failed by 28 months. The corresponding figures for stage II patients are 10 months and 22 months, respectively, and for stage III patients, $7\frac{1}{2}$ months and $15\frac{1}{2}$ months.

Although all the patients in our series were treated primarily with radiation, Shingleton [38] showed that the ultimate recurrence rate and the recurrence rate/month of 37 stage IB patients treated with radiation was similar to that of 30 radical hysterectomy patients treated with of without radiation.

Renal adenocarcinoma

Renal adenocarcinoma is unusual for several reasons. Long disease-free intervals are not uncommon [50], there are case reports of patients living as long as 50 years with the disease [51], and spontaneous regression of metastases has been well documented [52]. While cytotoxic chemotherapy is generally ineffective, patients with solitary metastases can sometimes be cured with surgery [53]. For all these reasons it is of interest to examine the significance of the DFI in this disease.

Grabstald [54] noted that 5/13 (38%) of patients with a DFI greater than 18 months survived more than 24 months post-recurrence, versus only 7/50 (14%) surviving with a DFI less than 24 months. Similarly, Talley *et al.* [55] reviewed 72 patients and found that the median post-recurrence survival of those with a DFI greater than 18 months was 15 months, but only 8 months for those with a DFI less than 18 months. Rafla [56] reported on the diease-free interval and post-recurrence survival of 63 patients and our re-analysis of his date shows that the DFI and PRS are correlated at $p < .05$. On the other hand, Nichols *et al.* [57] reported on 28 patients who had extraordinarily long disease-free intervals of 10–24 years but our re-analysis shows no correlation between the DFI and PRS for these patients ($p = .28$).

O'Dea *et al.* [58] reported that 44 patients who presented with, or developed, *solitary* metastases and subsequently had them resected. For the 26 patients with a non-zero disease-free interval, the correlation between the DFI and PRS was suggestive but not significant ($p = .15$ by our re-analysis). If the additional 18 patients who presented with solitary metastases were included (DFI $= 0$), then the significance became $p = .003$ in our re-analysis. Only 1/19 (5.3%) of the patients with a zero DFI were cured, as opposed to 3/26 (11.5%) of those with a non-zero DFI. However, many of these patients lived five years or more before dying of their disease as opposed to a median PRS of less than five months for patients with multiple recurrences [55].

The median length of the DFI for renal adenocarcinoma is similar to that of cervix cancer. For those patients who do not *present* with metastatic disease, the disease-free interval is about a year [56], and the more advanced stage cancers fail most rapidly [57]. The average DFI for patients who developed only solitary metastases, is about 31 months [53].

Hodgkin's disease

Hodgkin's disease is unlike the previously discussed malignancies in that substantial numbers of patients can be cured even after a recurrence. Therefore the question is not so much how well the DFI predicts for post-recurrence survival, but rather how well it predicts for subsequent cure.

Kaplan [58] has shown that the chance of ultimate cure after relapse depends somewhat on the DFI. The subsequent three year survival of patients who had a DFI of one year or less was approximately 45%. The three year post-recurrence survival for patients who relapsed in the second year was about 60%. In a partial update of Kaplan's paper, Spittle *et al.* [59] reported on 114 stage I and II patients treated with radiation therapy who had suffered a recurrence. Of the 59 patients whose primary recurrence developed within a year, 61% were dead with disease at the time of publication. Of the 35 patients with a DFI of one to two years, 51% were dead with disease and among the 20 patients with a DFI greater than two years only 40% were dead of disease.

Spittle *et al.* [59] also compared the interval to first relapse (DFI) with the interval to second relapse (R_1-R_2 interval) for 57 patients. Our re-analysis of their published data shows that the DFI and R_1-R_2 interval are correlated at the $p = .117$ level, suggestive but not statistically significant. More patients would be needed to firmly establish the relationship.

Finally, Spittle *et al.* [59] clearly showed that the disease-free interval decreases both with increasing stage of presenting disease and increasing histological agressiveness. Thus, stage I patients had a mean DFI of 19.3 months, stage II-A a mean DFI of 16.9 months and stage II-B a mean DFI of 12 months. Patients with lymphocyte-predominate histology had a mean DFI of 30.3 months, those with nodular sclerosing histology 15.7 months, mixed cellularity 13.9 months, and lymphocyte-depleted 9.3 months.

Osteogenic sarcoma

Osteogenic sarcoma can respond dramatically to cytotoxic chemotherapy and it is therefore of interest to enquire whether the disease-free survival is predictive of either post-recurrence survival or response to drugs. Sutow *et al.* [60] examined this question by reviewing 106 patients with metastatic osteogenic sarcoma at the M.D. Anderson Hospital. They showed that the median post-recurrence survival of patients with a DFI of less than one year was seven months, as compared to 26 months for those with a DFI greater than a year. Furthermore, this effect was greater after 1971 when the patients were treated with more aggressive chemotherapy.

Prostatic cancer

Patients with metastatic carcinoma of the prostate have a widely variable survival with 10% surviving ten years or more [61]. A number of attempts have been made to identify patient characteristics predictive of such long-term survial [62–65] but we were unable to find any report on the significance of the disease-free interval in prostate cancer. Perhaps the reason is that the majority of stage D prostate cancer patients have metastatic disease on initial presentation and thus have a non-determinable DFI.

Other malignancies

Patients with cancers of the head and neck are so prone to develop new primaries that it is difficult to assess the significance of the disease-free interval. In patients with ovarian cancer a disease-free interval is again difficult to define because the typical state III patient ondergoes intitial staging laparotomy and debulking, many months of chemotherapy and frequently a 'second-look' laparotomy. Rubin and Green [66] have reviewed the natural history of patients with various solitary metastases and conclude that a longer DFI is a good prognostic sign for patients with solitary lung and liver metastases, but is probably irrelevant for patients with brain metastases.

Conclusion

The length of the DFI should be taken into account when a patient is being considered for aggressive treatment of recurrent disease. In the case of cervix cancer, aggressive local retreatment is a reasonable option if the disease is indolent and likely to be confined within the pelvis. On the other hand, a long disease-free interval may be a contraindication for aggressive chemotherapy in breast cancer, since such treatment is rarely curative and one might wish to withhold aggressive chemotherapy until metastases begin to grow rapidly. Aggressive resection of *solitary* metastases in renal and onther cancers has a higher cure rate if the disease-free interval is long [47, 48, 53, 66] and a short DFI is a strong relative contraindication for surgery.

The past decade has seen the introduction of more accurate methods of imaging recurrences, including bone scans, computerized tomography, nuclear magnetic resonance and labeled monoclonal antibody scans. In addition we are now developing more specific biochemical tests to detect recurrence, including carcino-embryonic antigen (CEA) and radioimmunoassay for prostatic acid phosphatase. As a result, the determination of the disease-free interval should be far more accurate than in the past. Many of the studies quoted in this chapter need to be repeated, and in the light of the findings, the prognostic significance of the DFI may change.

Acknowledgement

We wish to thank Dr. Gustavo Montana for his generous help in providing the data on patients with cervix cancer. We wish to thank Ms Carol Venuti at the Massachusetts General Hospital Tumor Registry for her help in providing an update on our breast cancer patients.

References

1. Malaise EP, Chavaudra N, Charbit A, Tubiana M: Relationship between the growth rate of human metastases, survival and pathological type, *Europ J Cancer* 10: 451–459, 1974
2. Warhol M, Nickoloff B, Weinberg D: Seminoma metastasis to the terminal ileum after a 17-year disease-free interval. *Cancer* 52: 1957–958, 1983
3. Briel HA, Beattie CW, Ronan SG, Chaudhuri PK, Das Gupta TK: Late recurrence of cutaneous melanoma. *Arch Surg* 118: 800–803, 1983
4. Burkett FE, Johnson RL: Carcinoma of the esophagus twelve years after curative resection for carcinoma of the esophagus. *Cancer* 51: 2327–2331, 1983
5. Sutherland CM, Krementz ET, Harkin JC, Culotta V Jr: Recurrence of neuroblastoma following prolonged remission. *Arch Surg* 116: 474–475, 1981
6. King GA, Sagerman RH: Late recurrence in medulloblastoma. *Am J Roentgenol Radium Ther Nucl. Med* 123: 7–12, 1975
7. Morton JJ, Morton JH: Cancer as a chronic disease. *Ann Surg* 137: 683–703, 1953
8. Ransohoff J: Very late recurrences after operation for carcinoma of the breast. *Ann Surg* 46: 72–80, 1907
9. Woosley G: Late recurrence after radical operation for carcinoma of the breast. *Ann Surg* 80: 932–938, 1924
10. Steward FJ: Cancer of the breast: recurrence 31 years after operation. *Brit M J* 1: 156–157, 1925
11. Chilko AJ, Quastler H: Delayed metastases in cancer of the breast. *Am J Surg* 55: 75–82, 1942
12. Doyle JC, Hummer GJ: Peritoneal carcinomatosis forty-one years after radical mastectomy. *JAMA* 149: 1543–1545, 1952
13. Shimkin MB, Lucia EL, Low-Beer VA, Bell HG: Recurrent cancer of the breast. Analysis of frequency, distribution, and mortality at the University of California hospital, 1918 to 1947, inclusive. *Cancer* 7: 29–46, 1954
14. Goldenberg IS, Bailar JC, Lowry RH: Survival of women with hormonally treated breast cancer. *Surg Gynec Obst* 119: 785–789, 1964
15. Papaioannou AN, Tanz FJ, Volk H: Fate of patients with recurrent carcinoma of the breast. *Cancer* 20: 371–376, 1967

16. Cutler SJ, Asire AJ, Taylor SG: Classification of patients with disseminated cancer of the breast. *Cancer* 24: 861–869, 1969

17. Buzdar AU, Blumenschein GR, Smith TL, Tashima CK, Hortobagyi GN, Yap HY, Gutterman JU, Hersh EM, Gehan EA: Adjuvant chemoimmunotherapy following regional therapy for isolated recurrences of breast cancer (stage IV NED). *J Surg Oncol* 12: 27–40, 1979

18. Pater JL, Mores D, Loeb M: Survival after recurrence of breast cancer. *CMA Journal* 124: 1591–1595, 1981

19. Pearlman NW, Jochimsen PR: Recurrent breast cancer: factors influencing survival, including treatment. *J Surg Oncol* 11: 21–29, 1979

20. Rosenman J, Perrone T: The metastasis-free interval following curative treatment for breast cancer. *Int J Rad Oncol Biol Phys* 10: 63–67, 1984

21. Alanko A, Heinonen E, Scheinin T, Tolppanen EM, Vihko R: Significance of estrogen and progesterone receptors, disease-free interval, and site of first metastasis on survival of breast cancer patients. *Cancer* 56: 1696–1700, 1985

22. Chu FCH, Lin FJ, Kim JH, Huh SH, Garmatis CJ: Locally recurrent carcinoma of the breast. *Cancer* 37: 2677–2681, 1976

22. Bedwinek JM, Lee J, Fineberg B, Ocwieza: Prognostic indicators in patients with isolated local-regional recurrence of breast cancer. *Cancer* 47: 2232–2235, 1981

24. Todd M, Shoag M, Cadman E: Survival of women with metastatic breast cancer at Yale from 1920 to 1980. *J Clin Oncol* 1: 406–408, 1983

25. Kaufman RJ: Advanced breast cancer-additive hormonal therapy. *Cancer* 47: 2398–2403, 1981

26. Ahmann Frederick: Chemotherapy and hormonal therapy of advanced breast cancer. In: *Breast Carcinoma; Current Diagnosis and Treatment*, Feig SA and MCLelland R (eds.) New York: Masson Publishing, 1983, pp 533–540

27. Fisher B, Bauer M, Margolese R, Poisson R, Pilch Y, Redmond C, Fisher E, Wolmark N, Deutsch M, Montague E, Saffer E, Wickerham L, Lerner H, Glass H, Shibita H, Deckers P, Ketcham A, Oishi R, Russell I: Five year results of a randomized clinical trial comparing total mastectomy and segmental mastectomy with or without radiation in the treatment of breast cancer. *New Eng J Med* 312: 664–673, 1985

28. Fisher B, Redmond C, Fisher E, Bauer M, Wolmark N, Wickerham L, Deutsch M, Montague E, Margoles R, Foster R: Ten-year results of a randomized clinical trial compring radical mastectomy and total mastectomy with or without radiation. *New Eng. J Med* 312: 674–681, 1985

29. Taylor SG: Endocrine ablation in disseminated mammary carcinoma. *Surg Gynecol Obstet* 115: 443–448, 1962

30. Fracchia aa, Randall HT, Farrow JH: The results of adrenalectomy in advanced breast cancer in 500 consecutive patients. *Surg Gynecol Obstet* 125: 747–765, 1967

31. Henderson IC, Canellos GP: Cancer of the breast: The past decade (second of two parts). *N Eng J Med* 302: 78–90, 1980

32. Lerner HJ, Band PR, Israel L, Leung BS: Phase II study of tamoxifen: report of 74 patients with stage IV breast cancer. *Cancer Treat Rep* 60: 1431–1435, 1976

33. Valagussa P, Brambilla C, Bonadonna G: Advanced breast cancer: Are the traditional stratification parameters still of value when patients are treated with combination chemotherapy? *Europ J Cancer* 15: 565–571, 1979

34. Swenerton KD, Legha SS, Smith T, Hortobagyi GN, Gehan EA, Yap HY, Gutterman JU, Blumenschein GR: Prognostic factors in metastatic breast cancer treated with combination chemotherapy. *Cancer Res* 39: 1552–1562, 1979

35. Silvestrini R: The cell kinetics of breast cancer. In: *Breast carcinoma; Diagnosis and Management*. Bonadonna G (ed). New York: John Wiley & Sons, 1984, pp 5–13

36. Tubinana M, Pejovic MJ, Renaud A, Contesso G, Charaudra N, Givanni J, Malasise EP: Kinetic parameters and the course of the disease in breast cancer. *Cancer* 47: 937–943, 1981

37. Covington EE: Recurrence of carcinoma in the cervix after 15 years. *Am J Obstet Gynecol* 87: 471–477, 1963

38. Singleton HM, Gore H, Soong SJ, Orr JW Jr, Hatch KD, Austin JM JR, Partridge EE: Tumor recurrence and survival in stage IB cancer of the cervix. *AM J Clin Oncol* 6: 265–272, 1983

39. Barber HRK, O'Neil WH: Recurrenct cervical cancer after treatment by a primary surgical program. *Obstet Gynecol* 37: 165–172, 1971

40. Halpin TF, Frick HC, Munnell EW: Critical points of failure in the therapy of cancer of the cervix: A reappraisal. *Am J Obstet Gynecol* 114: 755–764

41. Krebs HB, Helmkamp BF, Sevin BU, Poliakoff SR, Nadji M, Averette HE: Recurrent cancer of the cervix following radical hysterectomy and pelvic node dissection. *Obstet Gynecol* 59: 422–427, 1982

42. Calame RJ: Recurrent carcinoma of the cervix. *Am J Obstet Gynecol* 105: 380–385, 1969

43. Van Nagell JR, Rayburn W, Donaldson ES, Hanson M, Gay EC, Yoneda J, Marayuma Y, Powell DF: Therapeutic implications of patterns of recurrence in cancer of the uterine cervix. *Cancer* 44: 2354–2361, 1979

44. Prasasvinichai S, Glassburn JR, Brady LW: Treatment of recurrent carcinoma of the cervix. *Int J Rad Biol Phys* 4: 957–961, 1978

45. Colpitis RV, Rogers RE: Recurrent carcinoma of the cervix at the University of Texas, M.D. Anderson Hospital and Tumor Institute at Houston. In: *Cancer of the Uterus and Ovary*. Chicago: Year Book Medical 1969, pp 269–282

46. Truelsen F: *Cancer of the Uterine Cervix*. Clinical features with particular reference to the results of radiotherapy. A report of 2918 cases. London: H. K. Lewis, 1949, pp 278–289

47. Fuller AF, Scannel JG, Wilkins: Pulmonary resection for metastases from gynecologic cancers: Massachusetts General Hospital Experience, 1943–1982. *Gynecol Oncol* 22: 174–180, 1985

48. Tellis CJ, Beechler CR: Pulmonary metastasis of carcinoma of the cervix. *Cancer* 49: 1705–1709, 1982

49. Prempree T, Amornmarn R, Villasanta U, Kwon T, Scott R: Retreatment of very late recurrent invasive squamous cell carcinoma of the cervix with irradiation. *Cancer* 54: 1950-1955, 1984

50. Donaldson JC, Slease RB, DuFour DR, Saltzman AR: Metastatic renal cell carcinoma 24 years after nephrectomy. *JAMA* 236: 950–951, 1976

51. Water CW, Gillespie DR: Metastatic hypernephroma of fifty years duration. *Minn Med* 43: 123–125, 1960

52. Middleton RG: Surgery for metastatic renal cell carcinoma. *J Urol* 97: 973–977, 1967

53. O'Dea MJ, Zincke H, Utz DC, Bernatz P: The treatment of renal cell carcinoma with solitary metastases. *J Urol* 120: 540–542, 1978

54. Grabstald H: Renal-cell cancer III. Types of treatment. *New York J Med* 64: 2771–2782, 1964

55. Talley RW, Moorhead EL, Tucker WG, Emiliana L, Brennan MJ: Treatment of metastatic hypernephroma. *JAMA* 207: 322–328, 1969

56. Rafla S: Renal cell carcinoma. Natural history and results of treatment. *Cancer* 25: 26–40, 1970

57. McNichols DW, Segura JW, DeWeerd: Renal cell carcinoma: Long-term survival and late recurrence. *J Urol* 126: 17–23, 1981

58. Kaplan HS: Prognostic significance of the relapse-free interval after radiotherapy in Hodgkin's Disease. *Cancer* 22: 1131–1136, 1968

59. Spittle MF, Harmer CL, Cassady, Kaplan HS: Analysis of primary relapses after radiotherapy in Hodgkin's Disease. *Natl Cancer Inst Monogr* 36: 497–508, 1973

60. Sutow WW, Herson J, Perez: Survival after metastasis in osteoarcoma. *Natl Cancer Inst Monogr*. 56: 227–231, 1981

61. Jordan WP Jr, Blackard CE, Byar DP: Reconsideration of orchiectomy in the treatment of advanced prostatic carcinoma. *South Med J* 70: 1411–1413, 1977

62. Reiner WG, Scott WW, Eggleston JC, Walsh P: Long-term survival after hormonal therapy for stage D prostatic cancer. *J of Urol* 122: 183–184, 1979

63. van der Werf-Messing BH, Menon RS, van Putten WL: Prostatic cancer treated by external irradiation at the Rotterdam Radiotherapy Institute. *Stahlentherapie* 160: 293–300, 1984

64. Byar DP, Corle DK: Analysis of prognostic factors for prostate cancer in the VACURG studies. in: *Controlled Clinical Trials in urologic Oncology*, Denis L, Murphy GP, Prout GR, Schroder F (eds.) New York: Raven Press, 1982, pp 147–169

65. Emrich LJ, Priore RL, Murphy GP, Brady MF: Prognostic factors in patients with advanced stage prostate cancer. *Cancer Res* 45: 5173–5179, 1985

66. Rubin P, Green J: *Solitary Metastases*. Springfield Illinois: Charles C. Thomas Publisher., 1968, pp 14–16, 63–65, and 98

5. Prognostic significance of response to therapy

M. HARDING and S.B. KAYE

Standardised criteria for classification of tumour response to treatment in advanced breast cancer have been recommended by the UICC [1] and gained almost universal acceptance. The duration of a complete response is measured from the first observation of complete tumour regression to the first documented recurrence. In contrast, partial response and stable disease durations are timed from initiation of treatment to recognition of progressive disease. The UICC criteria do not specify the minimal duration of response but a four week period is generally accepted.

This classification does not include the 'minor response' category of a 25–50% reduction in tumour area, nor 'symptomatic response' which refers to patient benefit without measurable tumour regression. While these categories are regularly employed in clinical reports, they are more accurately included in the stable disease category.

The prognostic significance of response to therapy in various types of cancer will be considered under the following headings;
– Limitations of response assessment
– Response to chemotherapy in advanced disease
– Response to hormone therapy in advanced disease
– Impact of adjuvant therapy on survival
– Importance of drug resistance.

Limitations of response assessment

Inherent inaccuracy of tumour measurement

Cutaneous lesions are accepted as the most easily measurable by clinical examination yet, in a simulated exercise assessing the size of lucite balls under foam rubber, serial measurements by the same observer revealed false categorisation of response in a single lesion (diameter 1.0–2.6 cm) in 12.6% of instances [2].

There was also marked variability in measurement of metastatic nodal disease and hepatomegaly, but evaluation of radiologically well-defined pulmonary lesions was more consistent. As the observers were trained oncologists, and fully aware of the purpose of the study, these results have disconcerting implications for the validity of clinical response assessment.

In most studies, response evaluation is performed prior to each treatment, usually at 3 or 4 weekly intervals. Documentation of a partial response of 4 weeks duration may therefore be based on a single measurement at 4 weeks being different from the pre-treatment and 8-week tumour dimensions. In some rapidly growing but responsive malignancies, treatment late in the disease may result in such a transient remission, but the majority of adult solid tumours do not regress and subsequently progress within an 8-week period. In view of the possible observer variation in tumour measurement, such data are open to question.

Lack of correlation between biological and clinical response

Measured tumour volume includes not only the population of malignant cells, a variable proportion of which will be biological end-stage cells capable of only limited division, but also fibroblasts, macrophages and lymphocytes. Additionally, areas of necrosis, oedema and non-malignant tissue from which the tumour originates will be included. Cytotoxic or cytostatic treatment can influence only the population of dividing cells which, in many tumours, constitutes a small fraction of the measured tumour volume. While a clinical response is believed to reflect significant cell loss from the neoplastic growth fraction, its degree is unquantifiable except in the minority of hormone- or oncofoetal antigen-secreting tumours.

An apparent partial response could result from spontaneous infarction and subsequent clearence of necrotic debris by the reticuloendothelial system. Reduction of local oedema in response to steroids may also be documented erroneously as a chemotherapeutic remission. Conversely, significant response to treatment could be masked if a solid tumour mass becomes cystic without sufficient change in dimensions for response to be recognised.

Complete response is accepted as indicating a high degree of sensitivity to therapy. However, a mass < 1 cm in diameter, comprising 10^9 cells, is not reliably detected by physical examination or standard radiology, and technological advances in ultrasonography and computerised tomography have only reduced the limit of resolution to 2 mm (2.5×10^8 cells). It has been calculated, by comparison of tumour-secreted human chorionic gonadotrophin levels and estimation of cell numbers in surgically-removed gestational trophoblastic tumours, that the minimal detectable cell number is 10^5, and therefore, as measured clinically, radiologically or biochemically, a complete response is far from a total eradication of biologically-active tumour.

A complete biological remission can be accepted retrospectively only in those patients where clinically complete response is durable. The disease-free interval which is considered equivalent to cure varies according to the tumour type. Rapidly growing malignancies (high grade lymphoma and small cell lung cancer) usually relapse within 2 years, so that a majority of patients free from recurrence at this time will be long term survivors. In contrast, the natural history of breast cancer in some patients is so long, that the point at which disease-free survival equates with cure may well be indefinable.

Prognostic significance of response to chemotherapy in advanced disease

The clinical impact of chemotherapy on a particular tumour type is initially assessed in advanced, measurable disease. On this basis, tumours can be classified as highly, moderately or minimally drug sensitive, and the effect of treatment on patient survival might be expected to correlate with intrinsic tumour responsiveness. However, within each disease type, recognised parameters of prognostic significance can be defined, which may be independent predictors of either response or survival.

Highly responsive tumours

The most chemosensitive adult solid tumours are the teratomas, gestational trophoblastic tumours and lymphomas. Currently available intensive combination chemotherapy regimes give response rates in excess of 80% for advanced teratoma [3], choriocarcinoma [4], Hodgkin's disease [5] and high grade non-Hodgkin's lymphoma [6]. The majority of remissions are complete and of these most are durable, with a proportion of patients (varying from 50% with non-Hodgkin's lymphomas to 70% with teratomas) remaining long term disease-free survivors. Most studies [3–6] emphasise that achievement of a complete response is the most important prognostic factor for prolonged survival.

However, subsequent relapse occurs in a proportion of patients and there is no evidence that prolonged maintenance chemotherapy prevents this [3, 5]. The relapse rate correlates with pretreatment tumour burden in Hodgkin's disease [5], and the stage of disease at presentation also influences the complete remission rate in these tumours [4–6]. Because of the adverse prognostic effect of high tumour burden, it is current practice to initiate treatment at diagnosis, irrespective of symptomatology.

In the group of highly chemosensitive tumours, the numbers of patients with partially or non-responsive disease may be small. Although median survival among partial responders exceeds that of patients whose tumours do not respond to initial therapy [3, 5, 6], this difference does not invariably reach statistical significance.

In a few instances a clinical 'partial' response may mask pathologically complete remission and on resection, a residual tumour mass is found to contain only necrotic material. A policy of post-chemotherapy surgery is employed mainly in teratoma, and it may convert a pathologically partial response into a complete remission in a minority of patients, with the consequent potential for long term survival [7].

The low grade non-Hodgkin's lymphomas are clearly biologically different from their high grade counterparts. Spontaneous remission is infrequently seen. A high complete response rate may result from single-agent therapy, but relapse is common and there is no convincing evidence that survival advantage accrues from either attainment of a complete remission or from early treatment of asymptomatic disease [8].

Moderately responsive tumours

This broad category includes tumours with response rates to chemotherapy in advanced disease of between 40% and 75%. The highest response rates (60–75%) are seen in small cell lung and in ovarian carcinomas, although only about half the remissions are complete. A minority of these patients may become long term disease-free survivors. The most important prognostic indicators are the extent of tumour prior to chemotherapy: absence of visceral metastasis in small cell lung carcinoma [9] and bulk residual ovarian carcinoma [10]. In addition to these, attainment of a pathologically confirmed complete response is of prognostic significance [9, 10].

For the majority of patients with moderately responsive tumours, chemotherapy is palliative. Nevertheless, there is often a significant survival advantage for responders over non-responders [9–11]. It is not possible to prove that this prolonged survival is a direct consequence of tumour response, as it is not considered ethical to perform randomised trials with a non-treatment arm in these malignancies. However, in the prechemotherapy era, the survival of patients with metastatic small cell lung cancer was so poor that treatment responders are unlikely to be a selected group with a biologically-determined good prognosis.

On the other hand, survival of patients with metastatic breast cancer varied widely before the advent of systematic therapy, and doubt remains as to whether chemotherapy confers any survival advantage in this disease [12, 13]. Current data suggest that there may be a strong correlation between favourable prognostic factors (long disease-free interval from mastectomy to metastasis, post-menopausal status and bone or soft tissue disease only) and oestrogen ± progesterone receptor status [14]. Although this does not influence response to chemotherapy [15], it is possible that the relatively long survival of some patients is a biological characteristic and that the effect of treatment response may be minimal. However, most trials of chemotherapy as initial systemic therapy for breast cancer are not stratified for these variables, so the relative contributions of tumour biology and tumour responsiveness to survival remain uncertain.

A feature of breast cancer is that the prognosis associated with prolonged disease stabilisation appears similar to that of a partial response [16]. It is uncertain whether this reflects the inadequacy of response criteria, or identification of a very slowly progressive tumour subgroup. However, the survival of patients with either stable disease or a partial response is shorter than that of those who achieve a complete remission, indicating that tumour responsiveness is of prognostic significance in an unselected patient population.

Although moderately responsive tumours usually respond well to initial optimal chemotherapy, treatment of recurrent disease is generally disappointing in terms of response rate and duration, and the effect of a second response on overall survival is limited. (Conversely, if primary treatment is suboptimal, the influence of a response to salvage therapy may be substantial). As survival data are generally reported in relation to initial treatment, it may appear that primary response does not influence survival in some trials. In ovarian cancer, for example, fewer responses result from single alkylating agent therapy than from platinum-containing combinations, yet patient survival in one randomised trial was similar [17]. However, a 30% response rate to the platinum-based regime as second line therapy in chlorambucil-treated patients may account for the apparent disparity between response to initial therapy and survival.

Some tumours exhibit moderate chemosensitivity in the response of locally recurrent or metastatic disease, yet in the past, the impact of chemotherapy on length of survival has been modest. Newer drug combinations are improving response rates in gastric [18] and bladder [19] carcinomas, and these may lead to a survival advantage in the future. Again, the full potential of chemotherapy may be realised if effective regimes are employed as initial treatment for locally advanced tumours. This approach already appears promising in Stage III and IV cervical carcinoma, though it is premature to conclude that the high response rate (55% after four weeks of platinum-based combination chemotherapy, 90% post-irradiation) will necessarily prolong survival (R.P. Symonds: personal communication). In head and neck cancers, early chemosensitivity is an independent prognostic variable for survival following radiotherapy and further cytotoxic treatment [20].

Similar combined modality therapy is becoming accepted practice in osteosarcoma. Initial chemotherapy was introduced in the hope that response at the primary site might facilitate limb-conserving surgery, and that early systematic therapy would be more effective in micrometastatic disease thereby improving survival. The early response rate, as assessed by $\geqslant 90\%$ necrosis in the resected primary lesion, is high: furthermore, most of the patients who subsequently relapsed were among the non-responders [21].

Poorly responsive tumours

Poorly responsive tumours are here defined as those in which current chemotherapy gives measurable responses in <40% of unselected patients. Tumours falling within this category include renal, pancreatic, colorectal and non-small cell lung carcinomas, together with melanoma and soft tissue sarcomas. With such low response rates, and few if any complete remissions, it is not surprising that the impact of chemotherapy on patient survival is limited. Among the few controlled, randomised trials undertaken in these tumour types, there is no observed survival benefit for treatment in non-small cell lung cancer [22] but possibly prolonged survival in pancreatic cancer [23].

Most non-controlled studies show that responding patients outlive those with progressing colorectal [24] and non-small cell lung [25] tumours. However, it has yet to be shown conclusively that the observed response is responsible for the survival advantage. Other factors of prognostic significance (especially performance status, weight loss and extent or site of disease) may influence the response rate and may be equal, or more important, determinants of survival [24–27]. Multivariate analysis of large studies is required.

Prognostic significance of response to hormone therapy in advanced disease

Manipulation of the hormonal environment by ablative surgery or additive hormone therapy leads to tumour regression in approximately 30% of breast cancer patients [28] and no single treatment is shown to be consistently superior to another. Hormone responsiveness is associated with prolonged survival and moreover, is predictive of further response to second-line hormonal therapy [29].

The biological basis of the hormone response has been clarified by demonstration of oestrogen and progesterone receptors in breast carcinomas [14]. Remissions are seen in 70% of oestrogen receptor positive patients but only in <10% of those with oestrogen receptor negative tumours. (The influence of progesterone receptor positivity on response is less clearly defined). Therefore, hormone responsiveness and detectable cytoplasmic oestrogen receptor are not independent prognostic variables, and most studies correlate the latter with prolonged survival. However, there is evidence that, in the receptor positive subgroup, a response to hormone therapy enhances the survival benefit conferred by the presence of oestrogen receptors [30].

Objective responses to orchidectomy or oestrogen therapy are documented in 40% of patients with metastatic prostatic cancer. Subjective improvement is significantly more frequent, reflecting in part the difficulty of proving response in skeletal disease. Although therapy may delay the appearance of metastases when used for locally advanced tumours and may cause regression in established metastases, there is no proven survival advantage from early hormone therapy [31], as opposed to delayed treatment when metastatic disease becomes symptomatic. However, preliminary data on the combined use of LHRH agonists and antiandrogen therapy indicate that higher response rates are achievable than with orchidectomy or oestrogen alone and this may translate into early survival benefit [32]. This therapeutic combination also results in a significant proportion of complete responses (25%) and further data from such treatment may confirm the currently circumstantial association between response (particularly CR) and prolonged survival.

Impact of adjuvant therapy on survival

Adjuvant treatment is based on the thesis that micrometastases, present at the time of primary tumour resection, have a higher growth fraction than larger, clinically detectable metastases and should therefore be more susceptible to cytotoxic therapy. In current trials of adjuvant treatment, response is not assessable directly for the individual patient, and can only be inferred retrospectively. Partial response in micrometastases would manifest by delayed appearance of overt metastatic disease, resulting in prolonged disease-free survival. Complete remission of micrometastases would equate with cure, but the observation period necessary to define this may be very long, particularly in breast cancer.

In order to demonstrate survival benefit from adjuvant therapy (and by inference, partial or complete tumour response) randomised, controlled trials are mandatory. Furthermore, the most meaningful data will be produced from trials which are stratified for the major prognostic variables found in advanced disease.

Chemotherapy

It might be assumed that the best results from adjuvant chemotherapy would be achieved in the most chemosensitive tumours, but this is not necessarily the case. Adjuvant treatment of irradiated localised Hodgkin's disease certainly prolongs disease-free survival, but there is no overall survival benefit owing to the effectiveness of salvage chemotherapy [33].

Among moderately sensitive tumours, breast cancer has attracted most research since the preliminary reports of prolonged relapse-free intervals in patients receiving adjuvant therapy for node-positive tumours [34, 35]. This benefit becomes less marked as the observation period lengthens and retains statistical significance only for certain subgroups [36, 37]. These studies show that survival advantage is associated with a prolonged relapse-free interval, but other controlled trials fail to demonstrate that prolongation of the disease-free interval translates into overall survival benefit [38, 39].

Evidence is accumulating that survival advantage from adjuvant chemotherapy may be confined to breast cancer patients with poorly differentiated [40, 41] and oestrogen receptor-negative [39, 41] tumours. Most currently reported trials do not specify the proportions of patients with these variables in the control population and treatment group, and it is possible that despite randomisation these characteristics may be unequally represented in the two arms. This may account for the apparent discrepancy between trials in terms of survival advantage, which disappears when data from many trials is compared. An analysis of all reported randomised, controlled trials indicates significant prolongation of survival for premenopausal patients receiving adjuvant chemotherapy [42].

The maximum survival difference between treated and control groups occurs in premenopausal patients with 1–3 positive nodes and is approximately 20% at 5 years [36, 37]. If, by inference, this reflects the response rate of micrometastatic breast tumors, it is substantially inferior to the 40-70% response rate to chemotherapy in measurable metastatic disease [11, 15, 16]. It is possible, since the proportion of complete remissions is relatively high, that the 20% of patients with a prolonged disease-free survival may be cured but in view of the long natural history of breast cancer, such a conclusion is premature.

With regard to other moderately chemosensitive tumours, randomized postoperative adjuvant chemotherapy trials have proved disappointing in bladder cancer [43], and results have been conflicting in gastric and head and neck carcinomas [44, 45]. For stage I ovarian cancer, adjuvant chemotherapy still requires proper evaluation, and this will require randomized trials stratified for variables such as histological tumour grade and capsule penetration.

Treatment results in operable osteogenic sarcoma have improved in recent years, and although doubt has been expressed over the contribution of adjuvant chemotherapy to these results [46], recently published randomized trials do indicate a significant improvement in relapse-free survival, even though patient numbers are relatively small [47, 48]. Controversy persists over the contribution that neoadjuvant (preoperative) chemotherapy makes to improved survival, but the approach has the great merit of making limb-sparing surgery a possibility for many patients.

Among tumours which are poorly responsive to chemotherapy, the results of adjuvant chemotherapy have been disappointing, although positive survival advantages have been claimed when adjuvant treatment has included both chemotherapy and radiotherapy. This applies to recent studies in carcinoma of the rectum [49], and also to adenocarcinoma or anaplastic large cell carcinoma of the lung [50].

Hormone Therapy

Early results of adjuvant ovarian ablation in premenopausal patients with breast cancer were relatively disappointing, although benefit from a combination of ovarian irradiation and prednisolone in certain subgroups has been reported [51]. The relative non-toxicity of tamoxifen has encouraged further studies of adjuvant hormone therapy in this disease and several prospectively randomised, controlled trials show a significantly increased relapse-free survival in post-menopausal, node-positive patients [52, 53]. In some trials, tamoxifen appears to influence loco-regional recurrence only and not systemic metastasis, while in others a significant improvement in both relapse-free and overall survival is seen [54].

There is controversy over the significance of oestrogen receptor assay in predicting the outcome of adjuvant tamoxifen therapy, although the balance of evidence suggests that it is an important variable [55, 56]. In view of the long treatment period and relatively early reporting of all these trials, it is not possible to predict whether tamoxifen only delays recurrence (micrometastatic partial response) or may be curative (complete response). An important factor to consider in analysis of randomized trials involving tamoxifen is the first therapy given for relapse in control-arm patients. Since this will frequently be tamoxifen, many trials will in fact be comparing immediate with delayed tamoxifen treatment for primary breast cancer, and survival data should be carefully examined with this in mind.

With regard to prostatic cancer, sequential trials from the Veterans Administration Co-operative Urological Research Group showed that adjuvant stilboestrol in the dose originally used (5 mg daily) actually caused an excess cardiovascular mortality in the treated patient group, despite a trend in favour of reduced cancer deaths. A lower hormone dose (1 mg daily) avoided the excess cardiovascular deaths, but did not significantly prolong overall survival [31].

In summary, therefore, the theoretical advantages of adjuvant therapy have yet to be realised in most adult cancers. Chemotherapy is not without toxicity and is clearly unnecessary in the most responsive tumour types. For the remainder, the relatively low complete response rates in measurable disease may be reflected in significantly prolonged survival for only a minority of treated patients. Under these circumstances, the toxicity: benefit ratio becomes important. In this respect, hormone therapy has significant advantages but is relevant only in a few tumour types.

Importance of drug resistance

We have noted that some survival advantage can usually be shown for patients whose tumours respond to therapy, but that major benefit (i.e. survival measured in years for patients with advanced disease) is uncommon outside the highly responsive tumour category. This reflects the short duration of partial remissions, particularly those resulting from chemotherapy. Complete responses tend to be more durable and for any given tumour type, an increase in the complete remission rate should be paralleled by a greater survival advantage.

Following an objective response, drug resistance is apparent when continuation of effective therapy fails to convert a partial to a complete remission or to prevent disease progression. What is more, the apparent growth rate of relapsing tumours frequently exceeds that of the disease prior to initial therapy and this accelerated growth phase may negate any potential survival benefit resulting from the primary response. Therefore, drug resistance is a major factor responsible for failure to prolong survival to a significant extent in most cases. The mechanisms of drug resistance are discussed in another chapter.

Conclusion

1. Accurate clinical assessment of response has inherent limitations. The minimal duration of a meaningful response might usefully be increased beyond the currently accepted 4 week period.

2. In many tumours there is an association between response and survival. Where chemotherapy is potentially curative, the prognostic significance of a complete remission is unequivocal. In the palliative situation, there is reasonable evidence that the modest survival benefit conferred by a response results from the treatment-induced remission in moderately sensitive tumours. Such a causal relationship is less clearly established for the poorly responsive tumour types.

3. A similar association should exist between inferred micrometastatic response and prolonged survival in the adjuvant situation. However, despite the number of randomised controlled trials in this field, the subgroups most likely to benefit have yet to be clearly defined.

Acknowledgements

We are grateful to Mrs M McLeod for typing the manuscript and the Cancer Research Campaign for support.

References

1. Hayward JL, Carbone PP, Heuson J-C, Kumaoka S, Segaloff A, Rubens RD: Assessment of response to therapy in advanced breast cancer. *Cancer* 39: 1289–1294, 1977
2. Warr D, McKinney S, Tannock I: Influence of measurement error on assessment of response to anticancer chemotherapy: Proposal for new criteria of tumour response. *J Clin Oncol* 2: 1040–1046, 1984

3. Einhorn LH, Williams SD, Troner M, Birch R, Greco FA: The role of maintenance therapy in disseminated testicular cancer. *N Engl J Med* 305: 727–731, 1981

4. Begent RHJ, Bagshawe KD: The management of high-risk chorio-carcinoma. *Semin Oncol* 9: 198–203, 1982

5. De Vita V, Simon RM, Hubbard SM, Young RC, Berard CW, Moxley JH, Frei E, Carbone PP, Canellos GP: Curability of advanced Hodgkin's disease with chemotherapy. Long term follow-up of MOPP-treated patients at the National Cancer Institute. *Ann Intern Med* 92: 587–595, 1980

6. Fisher RI, De Vita VT, Hubbard SM, Longo DL, Wesley R, Chabner BA, Young RC: Diffuse aggressive lymphomas: Increased survival after alternating flexible sequences of ProMACE and MOPP chemotherapy. *Ann Intern Med* 98: 304–309, 1983

7. Tait D, Peckham MJ, Hendry WF, Goldstraw P: Post-chemotherapy surgery in advanced non-seminomatous germ-cell testicular tumours: The significance of histology with particular reference to differentiated (mature) teratoma. *Br J Cancer* 50: 601–609, 1984

8. Rosenberg SA: The low-grade non-Hodgkin's lymphomas: challenges and opportunities. *J Clin Oncol* 3: 299–310, 1985

9. Comis RL: Small cell carcinoma of the lung. *Cancer Treat Rev* 9: 237–258, 1982

10. Vogl SE, Pagano M, Kaplan BH, Greenwald E, Arseneau J, Bennett B: Cis-platin based combination chemotherapy for advanced ovarian cancer: High overall response rate with curative potential only in woman with small tumour burdens. *Cancer* 51: 2024–2030, 1983

11. Swenerton KD, Legha SS, Smith T, Hortobagyi GN, Gehan EA, Yap H-Y, Gutterman J.U, Blumenschein GR: Prognostic factors in metastatic breast cancer treated with combination chemotherapy. *Cancer Res* 39: 1552–1562, 1979

12. Powles TJ, Smith IE, Ford HT, Coombes RC, Jones JM, Gazet J-C: Failure of chemotherapy to prolong survival in a group of patients with metastatic breast cancer. *Lancet* i: 580–582, 1980

13. Ross MB, Buzdar AU, Smith TL, Eckles N, Hortobagyi GN, Blumenschein GR, Freireich EJ, Gehan EA: Improved survival of patients with metastatic breast cancer receiving combination chemotherapy. *Cancer* 55: 341–346, 1985

14. McGuire WL: Hormone receptors: their role in predicting prognosis and response to endocrine therapy. *Semin Oncol* 5: 428–437, 1978

15. Rubens RD, King RJB, Sexton S, Minton MJ, Hayward JL: Oestrogen receptor status and response to cytotoxic chemotherapy in advanced breast cancer: *Cancer Chemother Pharmacol* 4: 43–45, 1980

16. Howell A, Wagstaff JM, Harland RNL, Jones M, Wilkinson MJ: The significance of the 'No Change' category of response in patients treated with endocrine therapy and chemotherapy for advanced carcinoma of the breast. *Proc 3rd European Conference on Clinical Oncology* Abstract 635, 1985

17. Williams CJ, Mead GM, MacBeth FR, Thompson J, Whitehouse JMA, MacDonald H, Harvey VJ, Slevin ML, Lister TA, Shepherd JH, Golding P: Cisplatin combination chemotherapy versus chlorambucil in advanced ovarian carcinoma: Mature results of a randomised trial. *J Clin Oncol* 3: 1455–1462, 1985

18. Klein HO, Wickramanayake PD, Dieterle F, Mohr R, Oerkermann H, Gross R: High-dose MTX/5-FU and adriamycin for gastric cancer. *Semin Oncol* 10: (suppl. 2) 29–31, 1983.

19. Harker WG, Meyers FJ, Freiha FS, Palmer JM, Shortliffe LD, Hannigan JF, McWhirter KM: Torti FM: Cisplatin, Methotrexate and Vinblastine (CMV): an effective chemotherapy regimen for metastatic transitional cell carcinoma of the urinary tract. A Northern California Oncology Group Study. *J Clin Oncol* 3: 1463–1470, 1985

20. Hill BT, Price LA, Busby E, MacRae K, Shaw HJ: Positive impact of initial 24-hour combination chemotherapy without cis-platinum on 6 year survival figures in advanced squamous cell carcinomas of the head and neck. In: *Adjuvant Therapy of Cancer* IV, Jones SE, Salmon SE (eds). Orlando: Grune & Stratton, pp 97–106, 1984

21. Rosen G, Nirenberg A: Chemotherapy for primary osteogenic sarcoma. Ten year evolution and current status of pre-operative chemotherapy. In: *Adjuvant Therapy of Cancer* IV, Jones SE, Salmon SE (eds). Orlando: Grune & Stratton, pp 593–600, 1984

22. Woods RL, Levi JA, Page J, Raghavan D, Byrne M, Fox R, Tattersall M, Stuart-Harris R: Non-small cell cancer: A randomised comparison of chemotherapy with no chemotherapy. *Proc Am Soc Clin Oncol* 4: Abstract C–691, 1985

23. Mallinson CN, Rake MO, Cocking JB, Fox CA, Cwynarski MT, Diffey BL, Jackson GA, Hanley J, Wass VJ: Chemotherapy in pancreatic cancer: Results of a controlled, prospective, randomised, multicentre trial. *Br Med J* 281: 1589–1591, 1980

24. Herrmann R, Spehn J, Beyer JH, Von Franqüe U, Schmieder A, Holzmann K, Abel U: Sequential methotrexate and 5-fluorouracil: Improved response rate in metastatic colorectal cancer. *J Clin Oncol* 2: 591–594, 1984

25. Elliott JA, Ahmedzai S, Hole D, Dorward AJ, Stevenson RD, Kaye SB, Banham SW, Stack BHR, Calman KC: Vindesine and cisplatin combination chemotherapy compared with vindesine as a single agent in the management of non-small cell lung cancer: a randomised study. *Eur J Cancer Clin Oncol* 20: 1025–1032, 1984

26. Lavin P, Mittelman A, Douglass H, Engstrom P, Klaassen D: Survival and response to chemotherapy for advanced colorectal adenocarcinoma. *Cancer* 46: 1536–1543, 1980

27. Stanley KE: Prognostic factors for survival in patients with inoperable lung cancer. *J.N.C.I.* 65: 25–32, 1980

28. Kennedy BJ, Fortuny IE: Therapeutic castration in the treatment of advanced breast cancer. *Cancer* 17: 1197–1202, 1964

29. Harris AL, Powles TJ, Smith IE: Aminoglutethimide in the treatment of advanced postmenopausal breast cancer. *Cancer Res* (suppl.) 42: 3405s-3408s, 1982

30. Howell A, Harland RNL, Bramwell VHC, Swindell R, Barnes DM, Redford J, Wilkinson MJS, Crowther D, Sellwood R: Steroid hormone receptors and survival after first relapse in breast cancer. *Lancet* i: 588–591, 1984

31. Byar DP, Corle DK: Analysis of prognostic factors in prostatic cancer in the VACURG studies. In: *Controlled Clinical Trials in Urologic Oncology*, Denis L, Murphy GP, Prout GR, Schröder F (eds) New York: Raven Press, 147–169, 1984

32. Labrie F, DuPont A, Belanger A, Lefebvre FA, Cusan L, Raynaud JP, Husson JM, Fazekas AT: New hormonal therapy in prostate cancer: combine use of a pure antiandrogen and an LHRH agonist. *Horm Res* 18: 18–27, 1983

33. Anderson H, Deakin DP, Wagstaff J, Jones JM, Todd IDH, Wilkinson PM, James RD, Steward WP, Blackledge G, Scarffe JH, Crowther D: A randomised study of adjuvant chemotherapy after mantle radiotherapy in supradiaphragmatic Hodgkin's disease PSIA-IIB: A report from the Manchester Lymphoma Group. *Br J Cancer* 49: 695–702, 1984

34. Fisher B, Carbone P, Economou SG, Frelick R, Glass A, Lerner H, Redmond C, Zelen M, Band P, Katrych DL, Wolmark N, Fisher ER: L-Phenylalanine mustard (L-PAM) in the management of primary breast cancer: A report of early findings. *N Engl J Med* 292: 117–122, 1975

35. Bonadonna G, Brusamolino E, Valagussa P, Rossi A, Brugnatelli L, Brambilla C, De Lena M, Tancini G, Bajetta E, Musumeci R, Veronesi U: Combination chemotherapy as an adjuvant treatment in operable breast cancer. *N Engl J Med* 294: 405–410, 1976

36. Fisher B, Redmond C, Fisher ER: A summary of findings from NSABP trials of adjuvant therapy. In: *Adjuvant Therapy of Cancer* IV, Jones SE, Salmon SE (eds) Orlando: Grune & Stratton, pp 185–194, 1984

37. Bonadonna G, Rossi A, Tancini G, Brambilla C, Valagussa P: Adjuvant chemotherapy trials in resectable breast cancer with positive axillary nodes. The experience of the Milan Cancer Institute. In: *Adjuvant Therapy of Cancer* IV, Jones SE, Salmon SE (eds). Orlando: Grune & Stratton, pp 195–207, 1984

38. Howell A, George WD, Crowther D, Rubens RD, Bulbrook RD, Bush H, Howat JMT, Sellwood

RA, Hayward JL, Fentiman IS, Chaudary M: Controlled trial of adjuvant chemotherapy with cyclophosphamide, methotrexate and fluorouracil for breast cancer. *Lancet* ii: 307–311, 1984

39. Taylor SG, Olsen JE, Cummings FJ, Knuiman M for the ECOG: Observation compared to adjuvant chemo-hormone-therapy in postmenopausal breast cancer. *Proc Am Soc Clin Oncol* 4: Abstract C-235, 1985

40. Fisher B, Fisher E, Redmond C: Long term survival with adjuvant chemotherapy related to tumor differentiation: the NSABP experience. *Proc Am Soc Clin Oncol* 4: Abstract C-252, 1985

41. Jakesz R, Kolb R, Reiner G, Rainer H, Schemper M, Moser K: Effect of adjuvant chemotherapy in Stage I and II breast cancer is dependent on tumor differentiation and estrogen receptor status. *Proc Am Soc Clin Oncol* 4: Abstract C-265, 1985

42. U.K. Breast Cancer Trials Co-ordinating Sub-Committee and U.I.C.C. Project on Controlled Therapeutic Trials: Review of mortality results in randomised trials in early breast cancer. *Lancet* ii: 1205, 1984

43. Smith PH, Child JA, Mulder JU, Van Oosterom AT, Martinez-Pineiro J, Richards B, Stoter G, Dalesio O, De Pauw P, Sylvester R: Co-operative studies of systemic chemotherapy – a review of the work of the EORTC Urological Group. *Cancer Chemother Pharmacol* 11 (suppl): 25–29, 1983

44. Ogawa M, Taguchi T: Upper gastro-intestinal tumours. In *Cancer Chemotherapy* 7, Pinedo H, Chabner B (eds) Amsterdam: Elsevier, pp 322–331, 1985

45. Taylor SG: Head and neck cancer. In: *Cancer Chemotherapy* 7, Pinedo H, Chabner B (eds) Elsevier, Amsterdam, pp 287–301, 1985

46. Carter SK: Adjuvant chemotherapy in osteogenic sarcoma: the triumph that isn't? *J Clin Oncol* 2: 147–148, 1984

47. Link MP: Adjuvant therapy in the treatment of osteosarcoma. In: *Important Advances in Oncology*, De Vita VT, Hellman S, Rosenberg SA, (eds) Philadelphia: Lippincott, 193–207, 1986

48. Eilber FR, Eckhardt J: Adjuvant therapy for osteosarcoma: a randomised prospective trial. *Proc Am Soc Clin Oncol* 4: Abstract C-561, 1985

49. Gastrointestinal Tumour Study Group: Prolongation of the disease-free interval in surgically treated rectal carcinoma. *N Engl J Med* 312: 1465–1472, 1985

50. Holmes EC, Hill LD, Gail M and the Lung Cancer Study Group: A randomised comparison of the effects of adjuvant therapy on resected stages II and III non-small cell carcinoma of the lung. *Ann. Surg* 202: 335–341, 1985

51. Meakin JW, Allt WEC, Beale FA, Brown TC, Bush RS, Clark RM, Fitzpatrick PJ, Hawkins NV, Jenkin RDT, Pringle JF, Reid JG, Rider WD, Hayward JL, Bulbrook RD: Ovarian irradiation and prednisolone therapy following surgery and radiotherapy for carcinoma of the breast. *Can Med Assoc J* 120: 1221–1229, 1979

52. Pritchard KI, Meakin JW, Boyd NF, Ambus U, De Boer G, Dembo AJ, Paterson AHG, Sutherland DJA, Wilkinson RH, Bassett AA, Evans WK, Beale FA, Clark RM, Keane TJ: A randomised trial of adjuvant tamoxifen in postmenopausal women with axillary node positive breast cancer. In: *Adjuvant Therapy of Cancer* IV, Jones SE, Salmon SE (eds). Orlando: Grune & Stratton, pp 339–347, 1984

53. Gelber RD for the Ludwig Breast Cancer Study Group: Adjuvant therapy for postmenopausal women with operable breast cancer. II Randomised trials comparing endocrine therapy with surgery alone. In: *Adjuvant Therapy of Cancer* IV, Jones SE, Salmon SE (eds). Orlando: Grune & Stratton, pp 393–404, 1984

54. Baum M, Brinkley DM, Dossett JA, McPherson K, Patterson JS, Rubens RD, Smiddy FG, Stoll BA, Wilson A, Richards D, Ellis SH: Controlled trial of Tamoxifen as single adjuvant agent in management of early breast cancer. *Lancet* i: 836–839, 1985

55. Fisher B, Redmond C, Brown A, Wickerham DL, Wolmark N, Allegra J, Escher G, Lippman M, Savlov E, Wittliff J: Influence of tumour estrogen and progesterone receptor levels on the response to tamoxifen and chemotherapy in primary breast cancer. *J Clin Oncol* 1: 227–341, 1983

56. Rose C, Andersen KW, Mouridsen HT, Thorpe SM, Pedersen BV, Blichert-Toft M, Rasmussen BB: Beneficial effect of adjuvant tamoxifen therapy in primary breast cancer patients with high oestrogen receptor values. *Lancet* i: 16–19, 1985

6. Clinical pointers to prognosis in terminal disease

A.M. HOY

The evolution of the Hospice Movement during the last twenty years has focussed attention on the difficulty of prognostication in patients dying of cancer, and on the definition of the terminal phase of malignancy. Although a 'terminal care period' is recognised by most doctors and nurses caring for cancer patients, remarkably few attempts have been made to categorise the clinical pointers used to assess prognosis within that terminal period. This chapter aims to review the various factors used to prognosticate in terminal cancer, and also to assess the accuracy of such predictions.

Accuracy of assessment

A definition of terminal disease is when 'the advent of death is felt to be certain and not too far off' or when 'medical effort has turned away from therapy and become concentrated on the relief of symptoms' [1]. More recently, McCusker [2] has included the effect of therapy and defined the terminal period as: 'the period during which there is evidence of progressive malignancy, and in which therapy cannot realistically be expected to prolong survival significantly'. However, the existence of two mutually exclusive phases (one of active treatment and one of terminal care) is an oversimplification and there is, in practice, considerable overlap [3]. This imprecise definition of terminal disease reflects uncertainty, not only in prognostication but also of the clinical factors which will determine response to active treatment.

Parkes [4] assessed the accuracy of survival prediction in patients admitted to St. Christopher's Hospice for terminal care. He found that admitting physicians, nurses and referring general practititiones were equally liable to inaccuracy in their predictions, and that over half of the estimates were wrong by a factor of two or more. Of these 'errors', 87% were in an overoptimistic direction. Reassessment one week after admission improved the accuracy of nurses' estimates but not those of doctors. Byar et al. [5] suggested that an average prediction with upper and lower limits might be more accurate because death is usually due to a single event. But how useful or comprehensible is a prediction such as 'an average of three weeks, but death may occur at any time between now and nine weeks'?

Scotto and Schneiderman [6] reported the results of physicians' predictions of survival in patients with lung cancer on entry to a controlled trial of chemotherapy. They found that estimated survival in weeks of 8 or less, 12 or less, 16 or less and 20 or more, corresponded quite well with actual median survival of 6, 12, 19 and 22 weeks respectively. As well as being more accurate than in Parkes' study, the physicians' errors in estimates were more evenly distributed between optimism and pessimism for all groups. (Although these patients had advanced cancer they were not terminally ill by some criteria, and therefore it could be argued that the course of their disease was more predictable).

The development of hospice programmes throughout North America has stimulated discussion of prognostic indicators in terminal cancer for eligibility for Medicare reimbursement. Physicians have been required to state that a patient's live expectancy is six months or less. Brody and Lynn [7] point out that the field is underinvestigated and that 'physicians in general perform poorly'. Mount and Scott [8] go further and suggest that such an arbitrary limit to the terminal care period is contrary to the spirit of hospice care and is not borne out by their experience that 20% of hospice home care patients live longer than 6 months. Notwithstanding financial expediency, it would clearly be of practical value in planning terminal care facilities and priorities to have techniques available for more accurate prognostication [9].

Clinical pointers in terminal disease include assessments of physical status, psychological status and performance as a whole. Under physical status it is relevant to consider the likely precipitants of death in cancer patients. If it is possible to anticipate the onset of these precipitants, then it might be possible to prognosticate more accurately.

Precipitants of death in cancer patients

The final commom pathway of the dying process in cancer patients is brain stem failure, resulting in cessation of respiratory drive and consequent asystole due to myocardial anoxia. There have been few studies of the antecedent causes of this failure of homeostasis. Inagaki et al. [10] showed that the major causes of death in a large series of patients with cancers other than haematological malignancies were infections (47%), organ failure (25%), infarction (11%), haemorrhage (7%) and a category labelled carcinomatosis (10%), characterised by severe emaciation and widespread metastatic disease in the absence of specific organ failure.

The fatal infections were predominantly septicaemia and pneumonia, and to a lesser extent, peritonitis. Different types of infection tend to be characteristic of particular sites of primary tumours. Thus, genitourinary and gastrointestinal tumours were associated with septicaemia whereas pulmonary, head and neck and melanomatous tumours were associated with pneumonia. The incidence of infection as the precipitant of death in patients with leukaemia and lymphoma is higher still. Ketchel and Rodriguez [11] reviewed the literature and reported that 74% of leukaemia patients and 51% of lymphoma patients died of acute infection. Similarly, septicaemia is the cause of death in at least 60% of patients with multiple myeloma [12]. The mechanism is presumably immune paresis due both to treatment and the disease process itself.

The clinical signs of life-threatening infections such as septicaemia, pneumonia and peritonitis are well known. Pyrexia is caused by pyrogens liberated from bacteria and also present in white blood cells. These act by stabilizing the central thermodetector neurones of the hypothalamus, which results in alteration of the 'setting' of the body temperature [13]. If the temperature is too high, reflex sweating occurs. However, pyrexia and sweating may also occur in the absence of obvious infection. Occult tumour is a cause of pyrexia of unknown origin, and some tumours have been associated with characteristic patterns of fever and sweating. Disorders of thermo-regulation are rarely caused by direct central effects but, in the context of advanced cancer, may be of complex aetiology [14]. Many terminal care physicians recognise pyrexia, sweating and clammy skin as a bad prognostic omen [15].

Fever results in increased fluid loss through sweating. This may cause considerable fluid depletion which may be difficult to overcome in seriously ill patients. There may be mechanical barriers to oral rehydration, the bowel may be obstructed by tumour, or the patient may be nauseated or vomiting for reasons such as uraemia, hypercalcaemia or drugs causing emesis. Simple fever may, therefore, be associated with hypovolaemia. The option to treat infection actively with antibioties and to rehydrate the patient intravenously is important, but may be inappropriate. The key consideration is whether such treatment would aid symptom control, despite the knowledge that treating the infection and hypovolamia could improve the short term outlook.

Organ failure as the precipitant of death is mainly caused by tumour invasion except in cases of cardiac insufficiency, where more than half of the patients are found to have evidence of arteriosclerosis at post morten examination [10]. Organ failure involves lungs, heart, liver, central nervous system and kidneys, in that order of frequency. Although individual organ failure is easily distinguished, it may be difficult to separate a malignant basis from other pathology, especially in the case of respiratory and neurological signs. Thus, chronic obstructive airway disease may co-exist with pulmonary tumour (primary or secondary) making the clinical picture very complex. Similarly, progressive focal neurological deficit may be due to tumour but can also be caused by vascular disease or a combination of the two. The best guide is usually the time-scale of progression of symptoms and signs, and a history of previous pulmonary or cerebral disease unrelated to the cancer.

An enlarging, irregular and often tender liver is less easily confused with non-malignant pathology. With advanced hepatic metastases, a mixed obstructive and hepato-cellular derangement of liver functions tests usually completes the picture. However, obstructive jaundice due to gall stones will occasionally be found in patients with metastatic cancer [16]. It is also not uncommon for a deeply jaundiced patient to live several weeks before dying from hepatic failure due to metastases.

When renal failure is the cause of death, this is frequently due to post-renal obstructive uropathy. This is common with gynaecological and bladder cancers, and when retro-peritoneal spread has occurred. The serum levels of urea and creatinine are useful prognostic indicators, provided the patient does not have pre-existing chronic renal failure from other causes.

Clinical and radiological evidence of extensive bone metastases is not in itself a useful prognostic indicator [17]. At least some patients will show a long survival in the presence of multiple bone metastases because the tumour is hormone sensitive and responds to manipulation of the hormonal environment (e.g. breast and prostatic cancers). Additional factors predicting outcome include the number of bone lesions, the predominance of bone lesions over deposits in other systems, the rate of tumour growth, evidence of sclerotic reaction within the bone and the presence of biochemical or haematological characteristics. Stoll [17] has proposed statification of patients with bone metastases into favourable risk categories based on the clinical history and findings (Table I). To a large extent this is an assessment of the biological aggressiveness of the tumour and therefore the tempo of the disease (see Chapter I).

Haemorrhage as a cause of death was comparatively rare (7%) in the series of Inagaki *et al.* [10]. The site of bleeding was most frequently in the gastro-intestinal tract or brain, but major blood vessel rupture occurred in some patients, especially those with a head and neck primary tumour. Spontaneous haemorrhage as opposed to vessel rupture may be regarded as organ failure affecting the marrow. Clinical pointers to the likelihood of bleeding will therefore include an assessment of marrow function and reserve.

Some tumour types such as leukaemia and lymphoma, are particularly associated with marrow failure not only because of the natural history, but also because of previous chemotherapy and radiotherapy. However the common solid tumours frequently metastasize to the bone marrow even when overt bony secondaries are not demonstrable radiologically [18]. Marrow failure may involve any of the cell lines leading to pancytopaenia, but leukoerythoblastic anaemia is the classical finding in the peripheral blood picture [19]. This is characterised by immature white cells, nucleated erythoblasts and giant platelets. Red cell morphology is often abnormal, showing anisocytosis and poikilocytosis, and if fragmented red cells are present on the film, this suggests microangiopathic haemolytic anaemia (MHA). MHA is an indicator of the terminal phase of marrow failure [20].

Infarction, usually of the lungs or myocardium, occurred in 11% of patients in the series of Inagaki *et al.* [10]. Of the lung-damaged patients, half were caused by emboli from venous thrombosis and half by direct tumour effects. Most of the myocardial damage with organ failure was related to arteriosclerosis. Although thromboembolic disease is frequently associated with advanced cancer the likelihood of fatal pulmonary embolism or myocardial infaction is essentially unpredictable.

Cancer cachexia is important prognostically in cancer patients. De Wys *et*

Table 1. Stratification of bone metastases into risk categories (Adapted from Ref. 17)

Unfavourable

Clinical history
Aggressive primary tumour site (e.g. lung or stomach cancer)
Poorly differentiated primary tumour histologically
Short recurrence-free interval after primary treatment (less than 1 year)
No bone sclerosis radiographically when metastases first noted
No evidence of bone sclerosis in lytic lesions after systemic therapy

Clinical findings
Multiple bone lesions in scan, or 'permeative' holes in radiographs
High overall tumour burden clinically (i.e. multiple systems involved by metastases)
High overall tumour burden biologically (i.e. high levels of hydroxyproline excretion, serum acid phosphatase, carcinoembryonic antigen, etc.)
Vital organs overtly involved by metastases (e.g. brain, liver, spinal cord, peritoneum)
Poor general condition or evidence of leukoerythroblastic anaemia, pathological fracture of long bones, cord compression, or hypercalcaemia

Favourable

Clinical history
Indolent primary tumour site (e.g. prostatic cancer)
Well-differentiated primary cancer histopathologically
Long recurrence-free interval after primary treatment (over 3 years)
Sclerosis radiographically when metastases first presented
Sclerosis of lytic lesions following systemic therapy

Clinical findings
Solitary bone lesion in scan, or large 'geographic' hole with sharply defined edge in radiographs
Low overall tumour burden clinically (i.e. bone is dominant metastasis)
Low overall tumour burden biologically (i.e. low levels of tumour 'markers')
No vital organs overtly involved by metastasis
Good general condition and no evidence of leukoerythroblastic anaemia or hypercalcaemia

al. [21] have shown that weight loss carries a poor prognosis prior to chemotherapy. The characteristic features of cancer cachexia are anorexia and early satiety, weight loss and marked muscle weakness, anaemia of nonspecific type, and an altered metabolism often associated with a raised basal metabolic rate [22]. The aetiology of cachexia is complex but will usually reflect a poor nutritional intake, increased nutrient consumption by the tumour and sometimes remote metabolic effects of the tumour on the host, mediated by presumed humoral agents [23, 24].

Brennan has calculated that a debilitated patient with a large tumour mass (2 kg) could lose as much as 67% of his daily calorie intake assuming 1200 cal/day [24]. In such an extreme case, rapid weight loss will reflect both a high tumour burden and a poor prognosis. Cachexia is difficult to overcome in the terminal phase of cancer [16] and some have argued that it may represent a 'last ditch' mechanism of the host defences against the tumour [25].

Performance status and psychological status

The degree of disablement and a cancer patient's dependency are closely related. Attempts have been made to quantify disablement as performance status and this criterion was first used by Karnofsky and Burchenal in the evaluation of benefit from chemotherapeutic agents [26]. Yates *et al.* [27] suggested that Karnofsky Performance Status (KPS) score (Table 2) correlated reasonably well with variables related to physical functions such as the ability to balance or manage stairs, but less with happiness or other measures of psychological well being. When Yates *et al.* related KPS score to survival time it was found that a low initial score correlated well with early death, but that a high initial score did not necessarily predict long survival. Only one patient out of 11 who had a score of less than 50 survived more than six months. If repeated KPS scores showed rapidly dropping values, this could predict death to a limited extent (i.e. within 2 months of death).

Evans and McCarthy [28] have shown more recently that the KPS score is more accurate in predicting survival in terminally-ill cancer patients than the informed guesses of members of a community-based terminal care support team (nurse, doctor and social worker). No significant differences in accuracy were found between team members or disciplines. An upper and lower limit estimate of survival were recorded as well as KPS score and it was noted that nearly half of the initial survivors were outside the limits, and that these limits were usually overoptimistic. Although some doubt has been cast on the scientific validity and reproducibility of KPS scores [29], the above studies from Vermont and London suggest that their use is more accurate than clinical impression alone.

McCusker [2] has applied a different functional status scale to a retrospective study of the terminal care period of cancer. This was based on the Eastern Cooperative Oncology Group performance scale. There was a statistically significant correlation between functional ability at the onset of the terminal care period and survival. Other indices such as presence of pain, age, sex and the site of the cancer could not be so correlated.

There is a popular belief that a patient's state of mind may be reflected in his physical state and may even influence prognosis. Various links between will-to-live and survival have been postulated, and are reviewed by Maguire [30]. There are also several studies in which expected mortality is compared with actual mortality of bereaved spouses [31–33]. Excess mortality of the spouses was noted, particularly in the first six months when it would seem to be due mainly to coronary heart disease [34]. A striking case history reported by Lieberman emphasises the life-threatening nature of morbid grief [35], but Ward [36] has been unable to confirm excess mortality in bereavement.

Many studies of cancer patients over the last 30 years have sought to correlate length of survival with psychological status. Most of these have been retrospective and have suggested an association between poor prognosis and inability to express feelings of anger and depression, hopelessness, lack of fighting spirit, low socio-economic class and low verbal intelligence [30, 37, 38]. This type of study presents formidable problems of methodology. The various tests of psychological status include the Minnesota Multiphasic Personality Inventory (MMPI), the Rorschach ink blot interpretation test and the Wechsler Intelligence Scale. Depending on test conditions, these scales tend to be subjective and prone to observer bias. Even when studies were prospective in nature and the testing was performed at diagnosis, there was no certainty that the psychological status remained the same throughout the illness until death. Because these studies have been initiated by psychologists rather than oncologists, tumour staging is often unsophisticated. There could be disease-related variables which influence prognosis far more strongly than psychological status [30].

Even if it is accepted that psychological status can be correlated with prognosis in cancer, there remain problems of causation. Stoll [38] points out that there are at least two possible explanations: psychological stress may, in some cases,

Table 2. Karnofsky performance status scale

100	Normal, no complaints, no evidence of disease
90	Able to carry on normal activity, minor signs or symptoms of disease
80	Normal activity with effort, some signs or symptoms of disease
70	Cares for self. Unable to carry on normal activity or to do active work
60	Requires occasional assistance, but is able to care for most of his needs
50	Requires considerable assistance and frequent medical care
40	Disabled, requires special care and assistance
30	Severely disabled, hospitalization is indicated although death is not imminent
20	Hospitalization necessary, very sick, active supportive treatment necessary
10	Moribund, fatal processes progressing rapidly
0	Dead

shorten the expectation of life; but equally, psychological distress (such as depression) may be a manifestation of more advanced disease (possibly occult). It is also possible that a third unknown factor could be responsible for both the psychological state and the prognosis. Although it is not difficult to postulate neuro-endocrine mechanisms by which these effects might be mediated, there is no firm evidence that state of mind alters, or has a consistent predictive value in, cancer prognosis.

Clinical indications of death

Since the advent or organ transplantation, the need for cadaveric organ donors has made it essential to reconsider both the definitions and clinical characteristics of death. While this re-examination is most important when discussing discrete single-event causes of brain death such as trauma, the concepts that have arisen also have applications to prognostication in advanced malignancy that will progress to a fatal conclusion.

Because independent life is a complex of interrelated organ functions, death is rarely an event but a process [39]. Traditionally, death has been diagnosed when cardio-respiratory arrest occurs, but modern intensive care allows artificial respiratory support, and in some cases full recovery is possible. The old criteria of cessation of breathing and heart-beat are clearly inadequate [39], and merely indicate a step towards definitive (and irreversible) brain stem death. There is now acceptance of the concept of whole brain death, and care must be taken to distinguish whole brain death [40] from both coma and the so-called vegetative state [41].

Coma is deep sleeplike unconsciousness from which the patient cannot be roused. True coma never lasts more than about three weeks when asystole may supervene. Alternatively the patient may open his eyes and regain consciousness, or he may pass into a vegetative state. Coma is short-lived but a vegetative state may last for months or even years. Whole brain death is present when the brain stem fails to support respiration. Without artificial ventilation, this soon results in cardiac arrest. A suitable definition of whole brain death therefore is 'the irreversible loss of the capacity for consciousness, combined with the irreversible loss of the capacity to breathe' [40].

Clinical pointers which indicate abnormalities in both the conscious level and the capacity to breathe are likely to be important as indications of imminent whole brain death. However, it must be established that the underlying malignancy is progressive, and that it is responsible for the deterioration. If this cannot be established then there is a danger of mistaking signs of a single-event, cerebral lesion such as a cerebro-vascular accident, for deterioration due to the malignancy.

It is rare for consciousness to be lost resulting in a persistent vegetative state in terminally-ill cancer patients. Other deterioration of function such as failure of the swallowing reflex or Cheyne-Stokes respiration usually accompanies any clouding of consciouness. However, there are various clinical prodromes to this state of brain stem malfunction. The problem of prognostication is the difficulty in evaluating the many clinical features days, weeks and months before the occurrence of brain stem death.

Conclusion

The assessment of clinical pointers to prognosis in terminal malignant disease requires an understanding that death from cancer is a process rather than an event. This process leads to whole brain death, and is precipitated by a relatively small number of clinical situations. However, the interpretation and weighting of the many variables of physical and psychological status is complex and ill-understood. Without more precise staging and stratification, the prognosis of any individual is likely to be either better or worse than the median of a group of patients at the same stage of the same disease [42].

References

1. Holford JM: *Terminal Care. Care of the Dying.* Proceedings of a national symposium held on 29/11/72. HMSO London, 1913
2. McCusker J: The terminal period of cancer: definition and descriptive epidemiology. *J Chron Dis* 37: 377–385, 1984
3. Saunders CM: Appropriate treatment, appropriate death. In: *The Management of Terminal Malignant Disease*, Saunders CM (ed). London: Edward Arnold, 1984, pp 1–10
4. Parkes CM: Accuracy of predictions of survival in later stages of cancer. *Br Med J* 2: 29–31, 1972
5. Byar DP, Mantel N, Hankey BF: Predicting survival in terminal cancer: *Br Med J* 1: 611, 1973
6. Scotto J, Schneiderman MA: Predicting survival in terminal cancer. *Br Med J* 4: 50, 1972
7. Brody H, Lynn J: The physicians responsibility under the new Medicare reimbursement for hospice care. *N Eng J Med* 310: 920–922, 1984
8. Mount BM, Scott JF: Whither hospice evaluation. *J Chron Dis* 36: 731–736, 1983
9. Gotay CC: Research issues in palliative care. *J Palliative Care* 1: 24–31, 1985
10. Inagaki J, Rodriguez V, Bodey GP: Causes of death in cancer patients. *Cancer* 33: 568–573, 1974
11. Ketchel J, Rodriguez V: Acute infections in cancer patients. *Sem Oncol* 5: 167–179, 1978
12. Bergsagel DE, Bailey AJ, Langley GR *et al.*: The chemotherapy of plasma-cell myeloma and the incidence of acute leukaemia. *N Eng J Med* 301: 743–748, 1979
13. Livingstone RB: Visceral control mechanisms. In: Best and Taylor's *Physiological Basis of Medical Practice*, West JB (ed). 11th Ed. Baltimore: Williams and Wilkins, 1985, pp 1211–1234
14. Beeson PB: Pyrexia of uncertain origin. In: *Oxford textbook of Medicine*, Wetherall DJ, Ledingham JGG, Warrell DA (eds). Oxford University Press, 1983, pp 5.469–5.472
15. Doyle D, *Coping with a Dying Relative*. Edinburgh: MacDonald, 1983, pp 88–90
16. Calman KC, Welsh J: Physical aspects. In: *The Management of Terminal Malignant Disease*, Saunders CM (ed). London: Edward Arnold, 1984, pp 31–42

88

17. Stoll BA: Natural history, prognosis and staging of bone metastases. In: Bone metastasis: monitoring and treatment, Stoll BA, Parbhoo S (eds). New York: Raven Press, 1983, pp. 1–20

18. Di Stefano A, Toshima CK, Yap HY, Hortobagyi GN: Bone marrow metastases without cortical bone involvement in breast cancer patients. *Cancer* 44: 196–198, 1979

19. Delsol G, Guiu-Godfrin B, Guiu M, Pris J, Corberand J, Fabre J: Leukoerythroblastosis and cancer frequency, prognosis and physiopathologic significance. *Cancer* 44: 1009–1013, 1979

20. Hilgard P: Monitoring marrow failure in bone metastasis. In: *Bone Metastasis: Monitoring and Treatment*, Stoll BA, Parhoo S (eds). New York: Raven Press, 1983, pp 263–270

21. De Wys WD, Begg C, Lavin PT *et al.*: Prognostic effect of weight loss prior to chemotherapy in cancer patients. *Am J Med* 69: 491–497, 1980

22. Calman KC: Cancer cachexia. *Br J Hosp Med* 27: 28–34, 1982

23. Coombes RC: Metabolic manifestations of cancer. *Br J Hosp Med* 27: 21–27, 1982

24. Brennan MF: Supportive care of the cancer patient. In: *Cancer Principles and Practice of Oncology*, DeVita VT, Hellman S, Rosenberg SA (eds). 2nd Ed Philadelphia: Lippincott, 1985, pp 1907–1920

25. Murray MJ, Murray AB: Cachexia: a 'last ditch' mechanism of host defence? *J Roy Coll Phys Lond* 14: 197–199, 1980

26. Karnofsky DA, Burchenal JH: The clinical evaluation of chemotherapeutic agents in cancer. In: *Evaluation of Chemotherapeutic Agents*, Macleod CM (ed). New York Columbia University Press, 1949, pp 191–205

27. Yates JW, Chalmer B, McKegney P: Evaluation of patients with advanced cancer using Karnofsky performance status. *Cancer* 45: 2220–2224, 1980

28. Evans C, McCarthy M: Prognostic uncertainty in terminal care: can the Karnofsky index help? *Lancet* 1: 1204–1206, 1985

29. Hutchinson TA, Boyd NF, Feinstein AR: Scientific problems in clinical scales as demonstrated in the Karnofsky index of performance status. *J Chron Dis* 32: 661–666, 1979

30. Maguire P: The will to live in the cancer patient. In: *Mind and Cancer Prognosis*, Stoll BA (ed). Chichester: John Wiley and Sons, 1979, pp 169–182

31. Young M, Benjamin B, Wallis C: The mortality of widowers. *Lancet* 2: 454–456, 1963

32. Cox PR, Ford JR: The mortality of widows shortly after widowhood. *Lancet* 1: 163–164, 1964

33. Rees WD, Lutkins SG: Mortality of bereavement. *Br Med J* 4: 13–16, 1967

34. Parkes CM, Benjamin B, Fitzgerald RG: Broken heart: a statistical survey of increased mortality among widowers. *Br Med J* 1: 740–743, 1969

35. Lieberman S: Life threatening symptoms due to morbid grief. *Br Med J* 286: 702, 1983

36. Ward AWM: Mortality of bereavement. *Br Med J* 1: 700–702, 1976

37. Miller T, Spratt JS: Critical review of reported psychological correlates of cancer prognosis and growth. In: *Mind and Cancer Prognosis*, Stoll BA (ed). Chichester: John Wiley and Sons, 1979, pp 31–37

38. Stoll BA: Will to live and survival time in cancer. In: *Prolonged Arrest of Cancer*, Stoll BA (ed). Chichester: John Wiley and Sons, 1982, pp 117–134

39. Conference of Medical Royal Colleges and their Faculties in the United Kingdom. Diagnosis of death. *Br Med J* 1: 332, 1979

40. Pallis C: Whole-brain death reconsidered – physiological facts and philosophy. *J Med Ethics* 9: 32–37, 1983

41. Pallis C: ABC of the brain stem death: Reappraising death. *Br Med J* 285: 1409–1412, 1982

42. Selawry OS: The individual and the median. In: *Mind and Cancer Prognosis*, Stoll BA (ed). Chichester: John Wiley and Sons, 1979, pp 39–43

II. Biological pointers to prognosis

7. Biological markers of aggressiveness and invasiveness

M. TUBIANA

Considerable progress has been made in the search for prognostic indicators in patients with cancer. First, multivariate analysis has provided statistical tools which can help to identify the relevant prognostic factors and to assess their independent impact on the course of the disease [1, 2]. Prognostic factors which were previously used were often inadequate or even misleading.

A second source of progress has been the improved understanding of the natural history of cancer. It is now recognised that new variants may appear during the course of the disease and cause a progression from 'bad to worse'. This diversification is caused by the genetic instability of tumor cells. Clinical data strongly suggest that the degree of genetic instability varies widely with tumor type, since the incidence of tumor progression differs greatly among the various types of human tumors [3]. Some tumors do not show clinical evidence of progression, and in approximately 80% of human cancers, the tumor doubling time remains constant throughout the *clinical* course of the disease [4].

Three major clinical parameters are correlated with the degree of malignancy – the growth rate, the size of the primary tumor at the time of distant spread [3, 5], and the response to treatment. After surgery, the likelihood of local recurrence is linked to local invasiveness while after radiotherapy another factor is the intrinsic radiosensitivity of the neoplastic cells [6]. (Factors in resistance to chemotherapy are reviewed fully in Chapter 12).

The first section of this chapter will consider the biological markers which are correlated with the tumor growth rate and the kinetics of cell proliferation. The second will discuss those related to cell DNA content and the karyotype. The third group of prognostic indicators comprises those which are linked to cell differentiation or dysdifferentiation while the fourth comprises other indicators related to cell biology. (Factors associated with the development of metastasis are discussed fully in Chapter II and will be only briefly mentioned here).

Growth rate and tumor cell proliferation

The growth rate of a tumor is correlated with the time intervals between (a) treatment of the primary tumor and detection of the first distant metastasis (b) detection of first metastasis and death [4]. Thus, a correlation between the clinical tumor doubling time and the time interval between initial treatment and appearance of distant metastases has been observed for tumors such as osteosarcoma, embryonal carcinoma of the testis, soft tissue sarcoma, breast cancer [4, 5–14].

Labeling Index

The labeling index (LI) measures the proportion of cells which are synthesizing DNA at a given time, and is therefore related to the proportion of proliferating cells. Two techniques have been used for the measurement of LI. One is based on the use of tritiated thymidine which is a specific precursor of DNA, the cells being labelled either by an intravenous injection of tritiated or by *in vitro* incubation of tumor specimens. The labelled cells are the identified by autoradiography on sections or cell smears of the tissue. Another technique is based on cytofluorometry and incorporation of bromodeooxyuridine (Brdu) [15].

Although LI and clinical doubling time (DT) are correlated [16], they are not directly related because the amount of cell loss is variable and reduces the net increase in cell number per unit time. Overall, LI is a good parameter of the proliferation rate, provides an insight into cell kinetics and from a biological point of view, has more significance that the DT, which is largely influenced by the amount of cell loss.

Patients with acute leukemia on whom thymidine labeling have been performed, show a negative correlation between the duration of remission and the labeling index [12]. In 130 patients with with breast cancer whose LI had been measured at time of initial treatment and who were followed for at least 10 years [7, 17, 18], a statistically significant correlation was found between the LI and two time intervals: 'initial treatment to appearance of first metastasis' and 'first metastasis to death' [17].

A further observation not predicted by the model was that the probability of metastasis is lower in the group with a low LI, indicating that dissemination was more likely to occur for tumors with a high proliferation rate. This was confirmed when the same data were updated with a follow-up longer than one decade [18] and suggests that the difference is not due simply to a rapid growth rate of occult metastases in the high LI subgroups [18]. The finding is consistent with experimental data [4], and a similar trend is observed in studies with a shorter follow-up on breast tumors [19, 20, 21, 22], head and neck tumors [4, 23], and non-Hodgkin lymphoma [24].

Although some slowly growing tumors metastasize frequently (e.g. prostatic, kidney and thyroid carcinomas), the above observations suggest that rapid growth of the primary tumor favors metastatic spread. Other data support this conclusion, and in patients with non small cell bronchial carcinoma, a short DT indicated a poor prognosis whether applied to small or large tumors [25, 26]. It has also been reported that individuals with bronchial carcinoma whose DT was less than 6 months were all dead within 52 months, but the few whose DT exceeded 6 months survived for longer than 52 months [27]. Again, following surgical resection of pulmonary metastases, the long term survival rate is strikingly higher in patients with a long DT, suggesting that these patients were less likely to have metastatic lesions at sites such as liver, brain or bone [28, 29].

Nevertheless, LI is correlated with several other prognostic variables, and we need to examine whether the correlation found between LI and probability of relapse or dissemination might not be due to a coincidental correlation between LI and other prognostic indicators. In our study on breast cancer, Cox model analysis showed that LI is, with histologic grading, one of the two independent variables which are most highly correlated with probability of relapse [17,18]. Meyer *et al.* [22] also analysed their breast cancer data with the Cox model [2] and found that LI was, with axillary lymph node status, one of the two most predictive variables. They reported that the probability of relapse was significantly related to the LI, independent of TNM stage, axillary lymph node status, estrogen receptor content or menopausal status. Similarly, Gentili *et al.* [19] reported a correlation between LI and relapse rate independent of axillary lymph node involvement.

Studies have also shown an unfavorable prognostic significance for a high pretreatment LI in other solid tumors [21, 30], multiple myeloma [31] or leukemia [32]. The poor prognosis of tumors with a high Li when treated by cytotoxic therapy may appear paradoxical, since most tumors with a large proportion of proliferating cells are chemosensitive [4, 16, 30, 33, 34]. However, a high LI is only one of the factors which affect chemosensitivity so that for example in the acute phase of chronic leukemia, the cells proliferate much more rapidly, yet the leukemia is much less chemosensitive than during the chronic phase [35].

A likely explanation for the prognostic significance of LI is that increased LI is an index of dysdifferentiation. It was shown that the highest LI measurements were observed in undifferentiated tumors [33] and that within tumors of a given histological type, those tumors with the highest cell density [36] had the highest LI, suggesting the existence of a link between lack of cell contact inhibition and LI. Moreover, some data suggest that the increase in LI after irradiation is higher in tumors with an initial low LI and a low cell density, that is, those tumors most resembling normal tissues [36, 37].

In human tumors, the most rapidly proliferating subclone becomes the predominant one and this increased rate of proliferation results from an impaired control mechanisms. Evidence is accumulating that several oncogenesplay an important role in this control [38]. Thus, the correlation between the impaired control of cell proliferation (as shown by increase in LI or shortenig of DT) and the malignant potential of the tumor, is not surprising.

Cell DNA content and karyotype

Methodology

Measurement of the cell DNA classifies normal cells into three groups: (a) Diploid cells – not engaged in a cell cycle or in the G_1 post mitotic, presynthetic phase of the cell cycle and with a 2 n DNA content; (b) tetraploid cells– diploid cells which are in the G_2 post synthetic premitotic phase of the cell cycle and with a 4 n DNA content; (c) Cells with an intermediate DNA content because they are in the S phase.

In a normal cell population, there is a good correlation between the proportion of cells with an intermediate DNA content and the labeling index because the nuclear DNA content is strictly controlled. In a neoplastic cell population, however, the nuclear DNA content is often increased, or less frequently, decreased. The measurement of the DNA content distribution provides two distinct observations – the presence of ploidy abnormalities and the approximate proportion of tumor cells in the various phases of the cell cycle. Two techniques have been used for the measurement of the nuclear DNA content distribution in human tumors:

Image cytometry (ICM) has been used over two decades [39] and is relatively easy to perform on smears of dispersed cells stained according to the Feulgen technique [40]. On tissue sections, the technique is hampered by inherent limitations because DNA measurements are dependent upon the section thickness and the level of sectioning of each nucleus. It is difficult to calculate the distribution of DNA content intact nuclei from the distribution of nuclear DNA content in sections several cells thick, and stereoscopic methods have been used for this purpose [41, 42]. However, many authors simply compare the DNA content in tumor cell sections with that in sections of normal diploid cells (fibroblasts or endothelial cells) adjoining the tumor. The median DNA value of the normal cells is defined as 2 C and the tumor cell DNA is expressed in C units.

Despite its relative inaccuracy and the low resolution of the distribution obtained, ICM has three advantages: it allows estimation of DNA content in the microscopically identified part of the tumor; it enables a comparison between the morphological characteristics of a cell and its DNA content so that it is possible to exclude the non-neoplastic cells present in the tumor; it is a useful method for retrospective studies of patients with a long follow-up. Particularly because of the two last points, techniques have been developed for the preparation of single nuclei [43] or cell suspensions [44] from paraffin-embedded tissue blocks.

The use of automated ICM permits one to analyse only cells which are machine-selected according to well defined morphologic criteria. This markedly increases the number of tumor cells studied, and avoids the statistical bias associated with the measurement of a small number of cells [40, 50].

Flow cytometry (FCM) has several advantages [46]: it is less time-consuming than ICM and allows the analysis of a large number of cells in a short time: the resolution of the DNA profile is high and relatively minor ploidy abnormalities can be detected: the proportions of $G_0 + G_1$ and of G_2 cells can be calculated with fair accuracy. Until recently, FCM was carried out only on a fresh suspension of cells, but now it can be performed on nuclei isolated from paraffin-embedded material, although in this technique the high and varying fractions of cell debris may constitute a source of artefact [40].

In conclusion, FCM and ICM are competitive techniques but have complementary specificities. Comparisons of the two methods show that either one can determine the grade of ploidy [47, 48, 49].

DNA content

A large number of studies using FMC or ICM, have analysed the DNA content distribution in several thousand human tumors [46, 49, 50, 51]. In studies where a large number of primary human tumors were assayed, about 60% of them showed an aneuploid DNA content, although this proportion varied widely with the histological type of tumor and its site. For the same type of tumor, the proportion also varied among the different investigators.

The proportion of aneuploid cells is higher in metastatic tumors, but the differences are relatively small. In 656 human solid tumors studied by Frankfurt *et al.* [50] with flow cytometry, the overall frequency of aneuploidy was 61% and 71% respectively for primary and metastatic tumors (p > 0.05). For malignant melanoma, Mauro *et al.* [51] reported the frequencies to be 41% and 75% respectively. Thus, over one third of human tumors have a diploid cell DNA content, yet are capable of invasive and metastatic behaviour [52].

Solid cancers show a striking non-random distribution of ploidy abnormalities. The significance of each abnormality is not yet clear but in general, aneuploid tumors have more aggressive properties than diploid tumors [46, 49–64]. A large body of convergent data shows that changes in ploidy are correlated with the incidence of local recurrences and with metastasizing ability and resistance to treatment. Thus, it is generally agreed that aneuploidy can be a powerful prognostic indicator and even at an early stage of tumor growth (for example, *in situ* cancers of the urinary bladder) DNA analysis is useful for identification of tumors with a tendency to progress [60]. However, for some types of tumors, no obvious relationship between DNA content and prognosis was reported [65], although the number of patients studied and/or the duration of the follow-up are often insufficient to warrant definitive conclusions.

The incidence of aneuploidy was found to be correlated with other tumor characteristics in various types of human cancers: thus correlation was seen with histopathological grading in cancers of the breast [66, 50], ovary [67], sarcoma [50], bladder [60], non-Hodgkin lymphomas [68] and colorectal carcinomas [54, 56]; with nuclear volume [69]; with clinical stage in cancers of the colon [54], ovary, bladder [50] and prostate [50]; with local invasion in melanomas or bladder cancer [60]; with degree of undifferentiation in bladder [50, 60] and prostate cancers [50]; and with the growth rate or the growth fraction [51, 57, 67]. Breast tumors with near-diploid DNA levels tended to be of low histological grade and estrogen receptor-rich, whereas those with higher ploidy were more anaplastic and poorer in estrogen receptor protein [47, 70].

These findings show that multivariate analysis of prognostic factors is needed to assess the independent prognostic value of DNA content, but unfortunately, few studies of this type have been reported. For example, in one study of adult acute leukemia, the poor prognosis of cases with aneuploid patterns was reported as due to a different distribution of other prognostic factors [71], thus illustrating the limitations of univariate factor analysis. In several types of tumor, no correlation was looked for between the cell DNA content and other prognostic variables.

Although a linear correlation between DNA content and chromosomal abnormalities (Karyotype Index) has been noted [46], the proportion of discordances is significant. This suggests that the assay of cell DNA content by morphometry or flow cytometry is not sensitive enough to detect all genomic abnormalities. Moreover, there is no correlation between the degree of aneuploidy and the prognosis [46, 50]. Since there is a significant correlation between aneuploidy and the percentage of cells in S phase in lung, ovarian and breast carcinomas, we need to examine whether the unfavourable prognostic variable is aneuploidy or else a high proportion of proliferative cells. Some data [72] suggest that poor prognosis is linked to the higher growth fraction rather than to aneuploidy, but this data is not yet conclusive.

In research on carcinogenesis and progression, the assay of cell DNA content has proved valuable. Aneuploidy is never observed in normal tissues but it is often observed in precancerous lesions such as atrophic gastritis, angio-immunoblastic lympho-adenopathy [51] and in precancerous nasal epithelium dysplasia [73]. In colo-rectal adenomas the progressive increase in ploidy abnormality with size and histological type strongly supports the sequence from adenoma to carcinoma, and suggests that aneuploid lesions have a relatively high potential for progression to invasive cancer [54]. A progressive increase in the degree of ploidy was reported also in other types of human tumors and was confirmed in experimental carcinogenesis studies [73].

The proportion of aneuploid cells and the degree of aneuploidy are higher in small invasive cancers than in precancerous lesions, and are further increased in the advanced stage [54]. However, in the great majority of patients with breast cancer [74], papillary thyroid carcinoma [75] or ovarian cancer [53], the DNA histogram exhibited a high degree of stability during the course of the disease, and a change from an euploid type in the primary tumor to an aneuploid type in the metastases was observed in only a small proportion of patients [50, 53, 74].

The incidence of multiclonality varies widely among the various types of human cancers, from approximately 7% in basal cell carcinoma of the skin, to 50% in small cell lung cancers [51]. Stemlines with different DNA contents found in a primary tumor may have different metastatic potential. The presence of several aneuploid subpopulations in a tumor suggests a marked genetic instability and this multiclonality appears to be a reliable indicator of poor prognosis; possibly because the occurrence of resistant cell variants is also associated with genetic instability [3].

In conclusion, cell DNA content already appears to be a powerful prognostic indicator but further investigations are needed. From a technical point of view, progress in the sensitivity and resolution of the methods should eliminate neoplastic tumors with a normal DNA content, and lead to a better understanding of the discrepancy between an apparently normal karyotype and an abnormal DNA content [46]. The introduction of parameters other than DNA content (such as nuclear chromatin texture or morphometric features) may also facilitate the interpretation of the information collected. In diploid tumors, the prognostic significance of individual cells with hypertetraploid DNA content or an increased proportion of tetraploid cells [40], should be further investigated. Prospective studies combining an assay of cell DNA content, the measurement of BrdU-labeled cells [15] and automated morphometric studies, should provide further information.

Karyotype and chromosome aberration

Detailed karyotyping is a more refined technique than is estimation of DNA content but it is time-consuming, requires fresh tissue samples and gives information only on cells capable of mitotic division *in vitro*. A large number of specific chromosomal aberrations are reported in various types of cancers but correlations between specific cytogenetic abnormalities and prognosis have been most studied in leukemias [46, 71, 76, 77]. Clonal chromosome abnormalities were variously reported in 50% and 100% of acute non-lymphocytic leukemia patients [76, 78] and in two thirds of patients with acute lymphocytic leukemia [79]. Both in children and adults, the various non-random cytogenetic abnormalities were found to be associated with specific histologic subtypes, with etiology, with treatment success and with ultimate outcome after therapy [76, 77,

80, 81]. In a large number of hospitals, karyotyping is now routinely performed during the work-up patients with acute non-lymphocytic leukemia.

Non-random chromosomal aberrations have also been observed in non Hodg-kin lymphoma [82]. For example, Burkitt's disease is defined by specific translo-cations which have helped to recognize the nature of the disease, despite differing clinical presentations and whether or not the Epstein-Barr virus was associated in its development. The various translocations which have been reported show that chromosome 8 is the consistent and therefore significant one [83]. In some non-Hodgkin lymphomas the presence of numerical and/or structural chromo-some abnormalities, varying from one cell to another in the same tumor, suggests a karyotypic instability which might itself have a prognostic significance [84]. In contrast with leukemia and lymphoma, the karyotype has been studied in only a relatively small number of solid tumors and no prognostic study has yet been performed.

Biological markers of cell differentiation

The histopathological grading of tumors gives useful prognostic information and in general, histologically undifferentiated tumors have a poor prognosis. Howev-er, the morphologic features of the cells do not identify all their biological properties (see Chaper 8). Since neoplastic change is generally associated with a block in the differentiation process (or dysdifferentiation), the study of biological markers of cell differentiation can provide prognostic information.

Steroid receptors in breast cancer

The ability of the mammary epithelium to synthesize estrogen receptor(ER) is a manifestation of biochemical differentiation and additional information can be gained by analysis of progesterone receptor (PR) content, as this receptor repre-sents an end-result of a functioning ER mechanism. In a normal mammary gland, the concentration of PR is regulated by serum estrogen [85] and this applies also in a large proportion of tumors. In general, PR concentration is related to age and menopausal status [86, 87], but administration of antiestrogens such as tamoxifen may provoke an increase in PR concentration [88].

ER and PR assays have been used also as an index of hormonal dependency and a guide for treatment selection [89, 90], but here we shall discuss the attempts to assess the prognostic significance of ER and PR. It is difficult for two reasons. (a) It requires a large number of breast cancer patients with a sufficiently long follow-up, since the time interval between treatment and relapse is different in patients with or without receptors. (This is not surprising since, as we have seen, the presence of receptors is correlated with the growth rate or the LI). (b) The presence of receptors is correlated with several other prognostic indicators so that the independent prognostic value of the receptor assays can be assessed only by multivariate analyses and only few studies of this type have been reported.

The presence of ER and PR is correlated with differentiated histologic and cytologic features [93, 94, 95], in particular with ultrastructural differentiation of tumor cells [96, 97], as well as with the size of the cell or nucleus [98], or with aneuploidy [99]. Although the Scarff-Bloom histopathological gradingis correlated with the presence of ER [94, 95, 96], only the architectural pattern component is related to the presence of PR [96].

The absence of receptors is correlated with unfavorable clinical indicators such as the presence of an inflammatory reaction [100], but is not related to axillary lymph node involvement [94]. A large number of univariate statistical analyses have shown that breast cancer patients with ER + and/or PR + tumors have a better prognosis than those with a low receptor content and that PR is a better prognostic indicator than ER [100–107]. A few multivariate analyses suggest that ER has an independent impact but that PR has a more powerful prognostic independent significance [94, 95].

In the multivariate analysis carried out at Villejuif on 438 patients with a follow-up of more than 5 years, the most powerful prognostic indicator was the absence of axillary lymph node involvement, the second was PR and the third was histological grading while ER had no independent prognostic impact [108]. However, we need more information on the *long-term* prognostic significance of the presence of receptors, and on the paradoxical problem of ER − PR + tumors. The level beyond which the amount of receptor should be considered significant is also in doubt.

One limitation of a biochemical assay when performed on a single sample of a tumor is the variability of ER levels in different regions of the same tumor. Tumor heterogeneity is clearly seen in multiple microsamples of a tumor [109] or by histochemical techniques. The latter have their own problems, one being that there are several types of estrogen binding sites [110]. The various fluorescent ligands which have been used in histochemical assays recognize separate binding sites, and although there is some degree of commonality and positive interaction between these multiple estrogen binding sites [111, 112], for a optimal hormone response all sites may be necessary [111].

The presence within a human tumor of different cell clones varying in their receptor content and probably also in their rate of proliferation, explains the variations in receptor content which have been demonstrated by sequential receptor measurements [113]. Overall, there is a lower percentage of receptor positive assays in metastatic tissue than in primary tumors [114, 115]. This would suggest either that when tumors become more aggressive and metastasize, there may be a trend for cells to lose receptors, or else that the most malignant sublines (that is those which are receptor negative) may have a higher tendency to disseminate.

It remains to be seen to what extent this loss of receptor as a result of a tumor progression affects the long-term prognostic value of positive receptors. Further investigation will also show whether the histochemical methods, which both determine the presence of ER receptor and provide an index of tumor cell heterogeneity, have a greater prognostic significance than do biochemical methods.

Receptors in other tumors

Steroid receptors have been found in cancers of the prostate, uterus, kidney, colon and pancreas [49] but there is not yet a clear demonstration of their prognostic significance. Assays of TSH receptor have been performed in differentiated thyroid cancers [116]. The highest amount was found in well differentiated cancers and the lowest in moderately differentiated cancers, which have a much poorer prognosis. However, papillary thyroid cancers have a prognosis equal to that of well differentiated cancers, although their content of TSH receptor is much lower. Thus the amount of receptor, although associated with the degree of differentiation, does not appear to have a reliable prognostic value.

Surface markers

The study of immunological cell markers has enabled us to establish the origin of the tumor cells and to analyse the maturation arrests which characterize several types of solid tumors, leukemias and lymphomas [117]. Thus, the use of surface markers has demonstrated the heterogeneity of hematological diseases that previously appeared homogeneous on morphological grounds. For example, it has been possible to distinguish chronic lymphocytic leukemias of T or B nature, or to identify several subtypes of large cell non-Hodgkin lymphomas [118]. The prognostic value of immunotyping, while still doubtful in adults, is recognized in childhood lymphomas. In children, a management strategy based on the study of surface antigens with a panel of monoclonal antibodies has proved to be of value [119, 120]. The cell lineage and the status of differentiation appear to have a greater significance than the clinical presentation [120].

Immunotyping has also clarified the natural history of some neoplastic diseases. For example in chronic granulocytic leukemia, the study of blood lymphocytes has shown that B-lymphocytes are involved in the leukemic clone. Moreover the blast crisis often involves leukemic cells of the pre-B phenotype [117]. This suggests that a neoplastic precursor can differentiate into both myeloid and B-lymphoid lines [117] and helps us to understand so-called tumor dedifferentiation. Acute leukemia blast cells displaying both lymphoid and myeloid characteristics have been described; such coexistence which is never observed in normal cells, may be due to aberrant gene expression and an abnormal differentiation program, and may be of prognostic significance [121]. Acute myeloid leukemia-(AML) blast cells with erythropoietic marker and markers associated with either megakaryocytes or B-lymphoid lineages have also been reported.

This simultaneous expression of markers specific for two different pathways demonstrates what is called 'lineage infidelity' [35]. It could be predicted that such deviation from normal differentiation program should exist in the most malignant clones, and in fact, in AML the response to therapy was much poorer in patients with blasts that exhibited lineage infidelity than in those where this was not identified (p = 0.02). However, in acute lymphocytic leukemia the impact of lineage infidelity is much smaller [35].

In normal tissues, cell multiplication and differentiation are coupled in the progeny of a stem cell [35, 122]. The factors which induce cell division also induce cell maturation and thereby a loss of the ability of the cell to proliferate, particularly because the arrest of cell multiplication occurs as a part of the program of terminal differentiation of mature cells. In neoplastic cell lines, an uncoupling of growth and differentiation is observed, and in some systems, the data suggest that this uncoupling is caused by inbalance of specific genes due to chromosome changes [122].

In several tumors, cancer progression appears to involve a loss of differentiated features. This might be due either to an inability of the non-stem cell descendants to progress along the differentiation pathways as much as in a differentiated tumor, or by a decrease in the proportion of non-stem cells produced during the division of stem cells [123] (increased propensity for self-renewal rather than provision of cells for differentiation). Whatever the case, this maturation block causes an apparent dedifferentiation of the tumor which may result in the emergence of the tumor stem cell morphological characteristics, and in a change towards a higher histologic grade. A direct consequence of this dysdifferentiation is an increase in the proportion of stem cells in the tumor and thereby a marked enhancement of the resistance of the tumor to ionizing radiations or to cytotoxic drugs.

Prognostic indicators associated with tumor cell biology

New prognostic indicators linked with the nature of the disease have been described in several types of tumors. For exemple, in acute myeloblastic leukemia-(AML) a measure of the *in vitro* renewal capacity of blast progenitors was shown to be a more significant prognostic variable than either patient age or percentage of blast cells in the marrow [35].

Dysregulation of gene expression

Abnormal activation of dormant parts of the cellular genome may lead to the synthesis in the tumor cell of products which are normally not synthesized by these cells. For example, ectopic hormone production in tumor cells is the consequence of an abnormality in the regulation of the gene which controls the synthesis of this hormone [124]. Altough we are not clear as to the prognostic significance of such production, in certain tumors it appears to be a consequence of dedifferentiation and embryonic cell expression. For example, pancreatic tumors may secrete gastrin like an embryonal (but not an adult) pancreatic cell. However, the best example of abnormal activation of dormant parts of the cellular genome is the production of oncofoetal oncogens such as alphafetoprotein (AFP) or carcino-embryonic antigen (CEA) (see Chapter 10).

Oncogenes and molecular biology

Increased knowledge of the molecular changes associated with the development of cancer has given rise to more basic parameters of prognosis, although they lack specificity. For exemple, the c-myc oncogene which is normally expressed when normal cells are triggered into proliferation, appears to be associated, when expressed in a tumor, with a poor prognosis. Seeger *et al.* [125] have reported that an amplification of the N-myc oncogene (which is a c-myc related sequence) is observed in 50% of patients with stage III or IV neuroblastomas, but in only a small proportion of stage II cases and renew in stage I. Analysis of relapse-free survival revealed that among patients of a given stage, amplification of N-myc was associated with the worst prognosis. N-myc is correlated with the ability to grow *in vitro* as an established line, a feature which is always associated with a poor prognosis [3].

An outstanding study in this field is that of Riou *et al.* at Villejuif [126, 127] who showed that in cervical cancer the amplification of the c-myc oncogene and its expression are greater in advanced than in early stages. There are two possible explanations. The first is that while a tumor grows from stage I to stage III, it frequently progresses towards a more malignant type. The other possibility is that the less malignant tumors remain longer in the early clinical stages, whereas the more malignant tumors progress rapidly to the more advanced stages. The latter hypothesis is consistent with what has been observed. Out of 75 stage I + II cases, only 32% had an increased expression of myc; but at 18 months follow-up, the relapse-free survival rate was 36% in those with elevated c-myc RNA levels and 91% in those with normal levels (p < 0.001) (Rion *et al.*, in press).

Another example is a reported case of papillary thyroid carcinoma, a part of which had become anaplastic [128]. In the undifferentiated zone an increased expression of the c-myc gene was found, whereas this gene was not expressed in the other regions of the tumor. These data strongly suggest that when DNA probes are available for *in situ* histologic studies, they will provide vital information both for diagnosis and prognosis in cancer patients.

Interchromosomal translocations and intrachromosomal inversions and deletions play an important role in malignant transformation. Fragments of DNA derived from regions of the genome containing the rearranging loci can be prepared by molecular cloning and used as hybridization probes. Such specific markers have been used for characterization of B and T cell lymphomas. They have already led to findings of widespread dissemination of occult tumor to lymph nodes in mycosis fungoides, and a high incidence of circulating tumor cells in patients with low grade lymphomas [129].

Conclusion

These last studies illustrate the current trend in the search for prognostic indicators. The aggressiveness of a tumor is related to the acquisition by tumor cells of new abilities, for example the capacity for hematogenous spread and seeding in other tissues. Knowledge of the changes at the genomic or the membrane level which are the cause or consequence of these new properties, will allow the introduction of more specific and more reliable markers. Close cooperation between clinical and fundamental research will be needed.

References

1. Armitage P, Gehan EA: Statistical methods for the identification and use of prognostic factors. *Int J Cancer* 13: 16–36, 1974
2. Cox DR: Regression model and life tables. *J Royal Stat Soc* 34: 187–202, 1972
3. Tubiana M: The growth and progression of human tumors. Implications for the management strategy. *Radiotherapy & Oncology* 6: 167–184, 1986
4. Tubiana M: Cell kinetics and radiation oncology. *Int J Radiat Oncol Biol Phys* 8: 1471–1489, 1982
5. Koscielny S, Tubinana M, Lê MG, Valleron AJ, Mouriesse H, Contesso G, Sarrazin D: Breast cancer: relationship between the size of the primary tumour and the probability of metastatic dissemination. *Br J Cancer* 49: 709–715, 1984
6. Fertil B, Malaise EP: Intrinsic radiosensitivity of human cell lines is correlated with radioresponsiveness of human tumors. *Int J Radiation Oncol* 11: 1699–1707, 1985
7. Tubiana M, Chauvel P, Renaud A, Malaise EP: Vitesse de croissance et histoire naturelle du cancer du sein. *Bull Cancer* 62: 341–358, 1975
8. Collins VP, Loeffler RK, Tivey H: Observations on growth rates of human tumours. *Am J Roentgenol* 76: 988–1000, 1956
9. Spratt JS, Spratt TL: Doubling time of pulmonary metastases and host survival. *Ann Surg* 159: 161–171, 1964
10. Breur K: Growth rate and radiosensitivity of human tumours. 1-Growth rate of human tumours. *Eur J Cancer* 2: 157–171, 1966

11. Malaise EP, Chavaudra N, Charbit A, Tubiana M: Relationship between the growth rate of human metastases, survival and pathological type. *Eur J Cancer* 10: 451–459, 1974

12. Pearlman AW: Breast cancer. Influence of growth rate on prognosis and treatment evaluation. A study on mastectomy scar recurrences. *Cancer* 38: 1826–1833, 1976

13. Cohen P: Het osteosarcoom van de Lange Pijnbeenderen (189 cases of osteosarcoma of the limb). Thesis. Amsterdam, 1974

14. Jeffrey GM, Price CHG, SissonsHA: The metastatic patterns of osteosarcoma. *Br J Cancer* 32: 87–107, 1975

15. Dean PN, Dolbeare F, Gratzner H, Rice GC, Gray, JW: Cell-cycle analysis using a monoclonal antibody to BrdU. *Cell Tissue Kinet* 17: 427–436, 1984

16. Malaise EP, Chavaudra N, Tubiana M: The relationship between growth rate, labelling index and histological type of human solid tumours. *Eur J Cancer* 9: 305–312, 1973

17. Tubiana M, Péjovic MH, Renaud A, Contesso G, Chavaudra N, Gioanni J, Malaise EP: Kinetic parameters and the course of the disease in breast cancer. *Cancer* 47: 937–943, 1981

18. Tubiana M, Péjovic MH, Chavaudra N, Contesso G, Malaise EP: The long-term prognostic significance of the thymidine labelling index in breast cancer. *Int J Cancer* 33: 441–445, 1984

19. Gentili C, Sanfilippo O, Silvestrini R: Cell proliferation and its relationship to clinical features and relapse in breast cancers. *Cancer* 48: 974–979, 1981

20. Gioanni J, Farges MF, Asin C, Lalanne CM: L'index de marquage dans les cancers du sein et des voies aérodigestives supérieures. *Bull Cancer* 66: 479–484, 1979

21. Meyer JS: Cell kinetics measurement of human tumors. *Human Pathology* 13: 874–877, 1982

22. Meyer JS, Friedman E, McCrate MM, Bauer WC: Prediction of early course of breast carcinoma by thymidine labelling. *Cancer* 51: 1879–1886, 1983

23. Chauvel P, Demard F, Gioanni J, Vallicioni J: Valeur pronostique de l'index de marquage dans les cancers des voies aéro-digestives supérieures (à propos de 60 observations). Forum de Cancérologie. Association Française pour l'Etude du Cancer, 1er juin 1981

24. Costa A, Bonadonna G, Villa E, Valagussa P, Silvestrini R: Labeling index as a prognostic marker in non-Hodgkin's lymphomas. *J Natl Cancer Inst* 66: 1–5, 1981

25. Meyer JA: Growth rate versus prognosis in resected primary bronchogenic carcinoma. *Cancer* 31: 1468–1472, 1973

26. Steele JD, Buell P: Asymptomatic solitary pulmonary nodules. *J Thorac Surg* 65: 140–151, 1973

27. Weiss W: Tumor doubling time and survival of men with bronchogenic carcinoma. *Chest* 65: 3–8, 1974

28. Joseph WL, Morton DL, Adkins PC: Prognostic significance of tumor doubling time in evaluating operability in pulmonary metastatic disease. *J Thorac Cardiovasc Surg* 6: 23, 1971

29. Morton DL, Joseph WL, Ketcham AS, Geelhoed GW, Adkins PC: Surgical resection and adjunctive immunotherapy for selected patients with multiple pulmonary metastases. *Ann Surg* 178: 360–366, 1973

30. Shackney SE, MCCormack GW, Cuchural GJ: Growth rate patterns of solid tumors and their relation to responsiveness to therapy. *Ann Intern Med* 89: 107–121, 1978

31. Durie BG, Salmon SE, Moon TE: Pretreatment tumor mass, cell kinetics, and prognosis in multiple myeloma. *Blood* 55: 364–372, 1890

32. Scarffe JH, Hann IM, Evans DIK, Morris Jones P, Palmer MK, Lilleyman JS, Crowther D: Relationship between the pretreatment proliferative activity of marrow blast cells and prognosis of acute lymphoblastic leukemia of childhood. *Br J Cancer* 41: 764–771, 1980

33. Tubiana M, Malaise E: Comparison of cell proliferation kinetics in human and experimental tumors: response to irradiation. *Cancer Treat Rep* 60: 1887–1895, 1976

34. Sasaki T, Sakka M: Implications of thymidine labeling index in the growth kinetics of human solid tumors. *Gann* 72: 181–188, 1981.

35. McCulloch EA: Stem cells in normal and leukemic hematopoiesis. *Blood* 62: 1–13, 1983

36. Courdi A, Tubiana M, Chavaudra N, Malaise EP, Lefur R: Changes in labeling indices of human tumors after irradiation. *Int J Radiat Oncol Biol Phys* 6: 1639–1644, 1980
37. Silvestrini R, Molinari R, Costa A, Volterrani F, Gardini G: Short term variation in labeling index as a predictor of radiotherapy response in human oral cavity carcinoma. *Int J Radiat Oncol* 10: 965–970, 1984
38. Calabretta B, Kaczmarck L, Ming PL, AU F, Ming SC: Expression of c-myc and other cell-cycle dependent genes in human colon neoplasia. *Cancer Res* 46: 6000–60004, 1985
39. Caspersson T, Lomakka G, Caspersson O: Quantitative cytochemical methods for the study of tumour cell populations. *Biochem Pharmacol* 4: 113–127, 1960
40. Cornelisse CJ: DNA cytometry of solid cancers. In: *Quantitative Image Analysis in Cancer Cytology and Histology*, Mary JY, Rigaut JP (eds). Amsterdam: Elsevier, 1986, pp 225–233
41. Mc Cready RW, Papadimitriou JM: An analysis of DNA cytophotometry on tissue sections in a rat liver model. *Analytical and Quantitative Cytology J* 5: 117–123, 1983
42. Bins M, Takens F: A method to estimate the DNA content of whole nuclei from measurements made in thin tissue sections. *Cytometry* 6: 234–237, 1985
43. Hedley DW, Friedlander ML, Taylor IW, Rugg CA, Musgrove EA: Method for analysis of cellular DNA content of paraffin-embedded pathological material using flow cytometry. *J Histochem Cytochem* 31: 1333–1335, 1983
44. Van Driel-Kulker AMJ, Mesker WE, Van Valzen I, Tanke HJ, Feichtinger J, Ploem JS: Preparation of monolayer smears from paraffin-embedded tissue for image cytometry. *Cytometry* 6: 268–272, 1985
45. Ploem JS: Preparation and staining of specimens for automated image analysis. In: *Quantitative Image Analysis in Cancer Cytology and Histology*, Mary JY, Rigaut JP (eds). Amsterdam: Elsevier, 1986, pp 3–17
46. Barlogie B, Raber MN, Schumann J, Johnson TS, Drewinko B, Swartzenbruder DE, Gohde W, Andreeff M, Freireich EJ: Flow cytometry in clinical cancer research. *Cancer Res* 43: 3982–3997, 1983
47. Auer G, Tribukait B: Comparative single cell and flow DNA analysis in aspiration biopsies from breast carcinomas. *Acta Pathol Microbiol Scand* 88: 355–358, 1980
48. Kreicbergs A, Cewrien G, Tribukait B, Zetterberg A: Comparative single cell and flow DNA analysis of bona sarcoma. *Anal Quant Cytol J* 3: 121–127, 1981
49. Wilking N, Gunven P, Theve NO: Biological characterisation of the tumour. In: *Screening and Monitoring of Cancer*, Stoll BA (ed). Chichester: John Wiley, 1985, pp 317–334
50. Frankfurt OS, Slocum HK, Rustum YM, Arbuck SG, Pavelic ZP, Petrelli N, Huben RP, Pontes EJ, Greco WR: Flow cytometric analysis of DNA aneuploidy in primary and metastatic human solid tumors. *Cytometry* 5: 71–80, 1984
51. Mauro F, Teodori L, Schumann J, Göhde W: Flow cytometry as a tool for the prognostic assessment of human neoplasia. *Int J Radiat Oncol Biol Phys* 12: 625–636, 1986
52. Greenebaum E, Koss LG, Elequin F, Silver CE: The diagnostic value of flow cytometric DNA measurements in follicular tumors of the thyroid gland. *Cancer* 56: 2011–2018, 1985
53. Friedlander ML, Hedley DW, Taylor IW, Russell P, Coates AS, Tattersall MH: Influence of cellular DNA content on survival in advanced ovarian cancer. *Cancer Res* 44: 397–400, 1984
54. Van den Ingh HF, Griffioen G, Cornelisse CJ: Flow cytometric detection of aneuploidy in colorectal adenomas. *Cancer Res* 45: 3392–3397, 1985
55. Blöndal T, Bengtsson A: Nuclear DNA measurements in squamous cell carcinoma of the lung: a guide for prognostic evaluation. *Anticancer Res* 1: 79–86, 1981
56. Wolley RC, Schreiber K, Koss LG, Karas M, Sherman A: DNA distribution in human colon carcinomas and its relationship to clinical behavior. *J Natl Cancer Inst* 69: 15–22, 1982
57. Abe S, Makiruma S, Itabashi K, Nagai T, Tsuneta Y, Kawakami Y: Prognostic significance of nuclear DNA content in small cell carcinoma of the lung. *Cancer* 56: 2025–2030, 1985

58. Tribukait B, Gustafson H, Esposti PL: The significance of ploidy and proliferation in the clinical and biological evaluation of blader tumors: a study of 100 untreated cases. *Brit J Urol* 54: 130–135, 1982

59. Atkin NB, Kay R: Prognostic significance of modal DNA value and other factors in malignant tumours, based on 1 465 cases. *Br J Cancer* 40: 210–221, 1979

60. Gustafson H, Tribukait B, Esposti PL: DNA pattern, histological grade and multiplicity related to recurrence rate in superficial bladder tumours. *Scand J Urol Nephrol* 16: 135–139, 1982

61. Tallroth E, Backdahl M, Auer G, Forsslund G, Granberg PO, Lundell G, Lowhagen T: Prognostic impact of nuclear DNA content in medullary carcinoma; a retrospective pilot study. *Radiotherapy and Oncology* 4: 225–230, 1985

62. Auer G, Eriksson E, Azavedo E, Caspersson T, Wallgren A: Prognostic significance of nuclear DNA content in mammary adenocarcinoma in humans. *Cancer Res* 44: 394–396, 1984

63. Kreicbergs A, Boquist L, Borssen B, Larsson SE: Prognostic factors in chondrosarcoma: a comparative study of cellular DNA content and clinico-pathologic features. *Cancer* 50: 577–583, 1982

64. Zetterberg A, Esposti PL: Prognostic significance of nuclear DNA levels in prostatic carcinoma. *Scand J Urol Nephrol* (Suppl) 55: 53–58, 1980

65. Tribukait B: Clinical DNA flow cytometry. *Med Oncol Tumor Pharmacother* 1: 211–218, 1984

66. Cornelisse CJ, Tanke HJ, De Koning H, Brutel de la Rivière G: DNA ploidy analysis and cytologic examination of sorted cell populations from human breast tumors. *Anal. Quant Cytol* 5: 173–183, 1983

67. Erba E, Vaghi M, Pepe S, Amato G, Bistolfi M, Ubezio P, Mangioni C, Landoni F, Morasca L: DNA index of ovarian carcinomas from 56 patients: in vivo in vitro studies. *Br J Cancer* 52: 565–573, 1985

68. Adler CP, Riede UN, Wurdak W, Zugmaier G: Cytophotometric measurements in Hodgkin lymphomas and non Hodgkin lymphomas. *Path Res Pract* 178: 579–589, 1984

69. Rigaut JP, Margules S, Boysen M, Chalumeau MT, Reith A: Karyometry of pseudostratified, metaplastic, and dysplastic nasal epithelium by morphometry and stereology. *Path Res Pract* 174: 342–356, 1982

70. Olszewski W, Darzynkiewicsz Z, Rosen PP, Schwartz MK, Melamed MK: Flow cytometry of breast carcinoma. Relation of DNA ploidy level to histology and estrogen receptor. *Cancer* 48: 980–984, 1981

71. Keating MJ, Smith TL, Gehan EA, Mc Credie KB, Bodey GP, Freirech J: A prognostic factor analysis for use in development of predictive models for response in adult acute leukemia. *Cancer* 50: 457–465, 1982

72. Tribukait B: Diagnostic and prognostic significance of modal DNA values and proportion of S-phase cells in human carcinoma of the bladder. In: *Quantitative Image Analysis in Cancer Cytology and Histology*, Mary JY, Rigaut JP (eds). Amsterdam: Elsevier, 1986, pp 315–317

73. Rigaut JP, Boysen M, Reith A: Karyometry of pseudostratified, metaplastic and dysplastic nasal epithelium by morphometry and stereology. 2. Automated image analysis (IBAS) of the basal layer of nickel workers. *Path Res Pract* 180: 151–160, 1985

74. Auer GU, Fallenius AG, Erhards KY, Sundelin BSB: Progression of mammary adenocarcinomas as reflected by nuclear DNA content. *Cytometry* 5: 420–425, 1984

75. Backdahl M, Cohn K, Auer G, Forsslund G, Granberg P, Lundell G, Löwhagen T, Willems J, Zetterberg A: Comparison of nuclear DNA content in primary and metastatic papillary thyroid carcinoma. *Cancer Res* 45: 2890–2894, 1985

76. Woods WG, Nesbit ME, Buckley J, Lampkin BC, McCreadie S, Kim TH, Piomelli S, Kersey JH, Feig S, Bernstein I, Hammond D: Correlation of chromosome abnormalities with patient characteristics, histologic subtype, and induction success in children with acute nonlymphocytic leukemia. *J Clin Oncol* 3: 3–11, 1985

77. Chilcote RR, Brown E, Rowley JD: Lymphoblastic leukemia with lymphomatous features associated with abnormalities of the short arm of chromosome 9. *New England J Med* 313: 286–291, 1985

78. De la Chapelle A, Berger R: Report of the committee on chromosome rearrangement in neoplasia and on fragile sites. Human gene mapping 7. *Cytogenet Cell Genet* 37: 274–311, 1984

79. Third international workshop on chromosome in leukemia. *Cancer Genet Cytogenet* 4: 95–142, 1981

80. Yunis JJ, Brunning RD, Howe RB, Lobell M: High-resolution chromosomes as an independent prognostic indicator in adult acute nonlymphocytic leukemia. *N Engl J Med* 311: 812–818, 1984

81. Williams DL, Tsiatis A, Brodeur GM, Look AT, Melvin SL, Bowman WP, Kalwinsky DK, Riviera G, Dahl GV: Prognostic importance of chromosome number in 136 untreated children with acute lymphoblastic leukemia. *Blood* 60: 864–871, 1982

82. Bloomfield CD, Arthur DC, Frizzera G, Levine EG, Peterson BA, Gajl-Peczalska KJ: Nonrandom chromosome abnormalities in lymphoma. *Cancer Res* 43: 2975–2984, 1983

83. Berger R, Bernheim A: Cytogenetics of Burkitt's lymphoma-leukaemia: In: *Burkitt's Lymphoma*, Lenoir G, O'Connor G, Olweny CLM (eds). IARC Scientific publication n° 60, Lyon 1985, pp 65–80

84. Kaneko Y, Rowley JD, Variakojis D, Haren JM, Ueshima Y, Daly K, Kluskens LF: Prognostic implications of karyotype and morphology in patients with non-Hodgkin lymphoma. *Int J Cancer* 32: 683–692, 1983

85. Houdebine LM, Teyssot B, Devinoy E, Ollivier-Bousquet M, Djiane J, Kelly PA, Delouis C, Kann G, Fevre J: Role of the progesterone in the development and the activity of the mammary gland. In: *Progesterone and Progestins*, Bardin CW, Milgrom E, Mauvais-Jarvis P (eds). New York: Raven Press, 1983, pp 297–319

86. Clark G, McGuire WL: Estrogen receptor content of human breast cancer tumors is related to age independently of menopausal status, but progesterone receptor is related to both age and menopausal status. *Proc Am Soc Clin Oncol* 2: C-392, 1983 (abstract)

87. Clark GM, McGuire WL: Progesterone receptors and human breast cancer. Breast *Cancer Res Treat* 3: 157–163, 1983

88. Namer M. Lalanne C, Baulieu EE: Increase of progesterone receptor by tamoxifen as a hormonal challenge test in breast cancer. *Cancer Res* 40: 1750–1752, 1980

89. Osborne CK: Combined chemohormonal therapy in breast cancer. A hypothesis. *Breast Cancer Research and Treatment* 1: 121–6, 1981

90. Jensen EV: Hormone dependency of breast cancer. *Cancer* 47: 2319–2326, 1981

91. Hartveit F, Dobbe G, Thoresen S, Dahl O, Tangen M, Thorsen T: The changing pattern of recurrence in oestrogen receptor positive and negative breast cancer with nodal spread, related to efferent vascular invasion. *Oncology* 40: 81–84, 1983

92. Von Maillot K, Horke W, Prestele H: Prognostic significance of the steroid receptor content in primary breast cancer. *Arch Gynecol* 231: 185–190, 1982

93. Antoniades K, Spector H: Correlation of estrogen receptor levels with histology and cytomorphology in human mammary cancer. *Am J Clin Pathol* 71: 497–503, 1979

94. Contesso G, Delarue JC, Mouriesse H, May-Levin F, Garnier H: Anatomopathologie du cancer du sein et récepteurs hormonaux. *Path Biol* (Paris) 31: 747–754, 1983

95. Lesser ML, Rosen PP, Senier RT, Duthie K, Menendez-Botet C, Schwartz MK: Estrogen and progesterone receptors in breast carcinoma: correlations with epidemiology and pathology. *Cancer* 48: 299–309, 1981

96. Le Doussal V, Pichon MF, Pallud C, Hacene K, Gest J, Milgrom E: Relationship between ultrastructure and receptor content of human primary breast cancer. *Histopathology* 8: 89–103, 1984

97. Stegner HE, Bahnsen J, Trams G: Correlation of estrogen and progesterone receptor status with ultrastructural differentiation in breast tumors. *J. Ster Biochem* 19: 297–303, 1983

98. Guazzi A, Bozzetti C, Riva I, Zaffe D, Cocconi G: Relationship between estrogen receptor concentration and cytomorphometry in breast cancer. *Cancer* 56: 1972-1976, 1985

99. Kute TE, Muss HB, Anderson D, Crumb K, Miller B, Burns D, Dube LA: Relationship of steroid receptor, cell kinetics, and clinical status in patients with breast cancer. *Cancer Res* 41: 3524–3529, 1981

100. Delarue JC, May-Levin F, Mouriesse H, Contesso G, Sancho-Garnier H: Oestrogen and progesterone receptors in clinically inflammatory tumours of the human breast. *Brit J Cancer* 44: 911–916, 1981

101. Goldolphin W, Elwood JM, Spinelli JJ: Estrogen receptor quantitation and staging as complementary prognostic indicators in breast cancer: a study of 583 patients. *Int J Cancer* 28: 677–683, 1981

102. Hartveit F, Dobbe G, Thoresen S, Dahl O, Tangen M, Thorsen T: The changin pattern of recurrence in oestrogen receptor positive and negative breast cancer with nodal spread, related to efferent vacular invasion. *Oncology* 40: 81–84, 1983

103. Von Maillot K, Horke W, Prestele H: Prognostic significance of the steroid receptor in primary breast cancer. *Arch Gynecol* 231: 185–190, 1982

104. McGuire WL, Clark GM: The prognostic role of progesterone receptors in human breast cancer. *Seminars in Oncology* 10 (suppl 4) 2–6, 1983

105. Saez S, Pichon MF, Cheix F, Mayer M, Pallud C, Brunet M, Milgrom E: Progesterone receptors and prognosis in early breast cancer: the experience of two centers. In: *Progesterone and Progestins*, Bardin CW, Milgrom E, Mauvais-Jarvis P (eds). New York: Raven Press, 1983, pp 355-366.

106. Stewart JF, Rubens RD, Millis RR, King RJB, Hayward JL: Steroid receptors and prognosis in operable (stage I and II) breast cancer. *Eur J Cancer Clin Oncol* 19: 1381–1387, 1983

107. Crowe JP, Hubay CA, Pearson OH, Marshall JS, Rosenblatt J, Mansour EG, Hermann RE, Jones JC, Flynn WJ, McGuire WL and participating investigators: Estrogen receptor status as a pronostic indicator for stage I breast cancer patients. *Breast Cancer Res Treat* 2 171–176, 1982

108. May-Levin F, Delarue JC, Contesso G, Sancho-Garnier H: Prognostic factors in breast cancer. *Breast Cancer Res Treat* 8, 100–106, 1986

109. Van Netten JP, Algard FT, Coy P, Carlyle SJ, Brigden ML, Thornton KR, Peter S, Fraser T, To MP: Heterogeneous estrogen receptor levels detected via multiple microsamples from individual breast cancers. *Cancer* 56: 2019–2024, 1985

110. Clark JH, Watson CS, Markarevich BM, Syne JS, Panko WB: Heterogeneity of estrogen binding sites in mammary tumors. *Breast Cancer Res Treat* 3: 61–65, 1983

111. Pertschuk LP, Eisenberg KB, Carter AC, Feldman JG: Heterogeneity of estrogen binding sites in breast cancer: morphologic demonstration and relationship to endocrine response. *Breast Cancer Res Treat* 5: 137–147, 1985

112. Parl FF, Wetherall NT, Halter S, Schuffman S, Mitchell WN: Comparison of histochemical and biochemical assays for estrogen receptors in human breast cancer cell lines. *Cancer Res* 44: 415–422, 1984

113. Holdaway IM, Bowdich: Variation in receptor status between primary and metastatic breast cancer. *Cancer* 52: 479–485, 1983

114. Allegra JC, Barlock A, Huff KK, Lippman ME: Changes in multiple or sequential estrogen receptor determinations in breast cancer. *Cancer* 45: 792–794, 1980

115. Hawkins RA, Roberts MM, Forrest APM: Oestrogen receptors and breast cancer: current status. *Br J Surg* 67: 153–169, 1980

116. Thomas-Morvan C, Carayon P, Schlumberger M, Vignal A, Tubiana M: Thyrotrophin stimulation of adenylcyclase and iodine uptake in human differentiated cancer. *Acta Endocrinologica* 101: 25–31, 1982

117. Seligmann M, Vogler LB, Preudhomme JL, Guglielmi P, Brouer JC: Immunological phenotypes of human leukemias of the B-cell lineage. *Blood Cells* 7: 237–246, 1981

118. Warnke RA, Weiss LM: Practical approach to the immunodiagnosis of lymphomas emphasizing differential diagnosis. *Cancer Surveys* 4: 349–358, 1985

119. Lemerle J: The treatment of B-cell non Hodgkin's malignant lymphomas in Europe. Recent and on-going studies. In: *Burkitt's Lymphomas*, Lenoir G, O'Donnor G, Olweny CL (edit). Lyon: IARC, 1985, pp 383–398

120. Bernard A, Boumsell L, Patte C, Lemerle J: Leukemia versus lymphoma in children: a worthless question? *Med Ped Oncol*, 1986 (in press)

121. Mirro J, Zipf TF, Pui CH, Kitchingman G, Williams D, Melvin S, Murphy SB, Stass S: Acute mixed lineage leukemia: clinicopathologic correlations and prognostic significance. *Blood* 66: 1115–1123, 1985

122. Sachs L: Normal development programmes in myeloid leukemia: regulatory proteins in the control of growth and differentiation. *Cancer Surveys* 1: 321–342, 1982

123. MacKillop WJ, Ciampi A, Till JE, Buick RN: A stem cell model of human tumor growth: implication for tumor cell clonogenic assays. *J Nat Cancer Inst* 70: 9–16, 1983

124. Imura H: Ectopic hormone production viewed as an abnormality in regulation of gene expression. *Adv Cancer Res* 33: 39–75, 1980

125. Seeger RC, Brodeur GC, Sather H, Dalton A, Siegel SE, Wong KY, Hammond D: Association of multiple copies of the N-myc oncogene with rapid progression neuroblastomas. *New England J Med* 313: 1111–1116, 1985

126. Riou G, Benois M, Torjman I, Dutronquay V, Orth G: Présence de génome de papillome virus et amplification des oncogènes C-Myc et C-Ha-Ras dans les cancers envahissants du col de l'utérus. *C R Acad Sc* (Paris) 299: 575-580, 1984

127. Riou G, Barrois M, Dutronquay V, Orth G: Presence of papilloma virus DNA sequences. Amplification of c-myc and c-Ha-ras oncogenes and enhanced expression of c-myc in carcinomas of the uterine cervix. In: *Papilloma Viruses: Molecular and Clinical Aspects*. UCLA Symposium on molecular and cellular biology. New Series 32. New York: Alan Liss, 1985, pp 47–56

128. Terrier P, Douc-Rasy S, Schlumberger M, Fragu P, Tubiana M, Caillou B, Travagli JP, Riou G: Enhanced expression of the C-myc oncogene in a case of anaplastic carcinoma of the thyroid gland. *Proc Symp thyroid Cancer,* Montpellier, 1985, Excerpta Medical Congress Series, pp 287–288

129. Cleary ML, Sklar J: DNA rearrangements in non-Hodgkin's lymphomas. *Cancer Surveys* 4: 331–348, 1985

8. Histopathology and its prognostic significance

J.D. CRISSMAN and R.J. ZARBO

During the past few years, considerable information on histologic features in tumor grading has resulted from the rapidly expanding armamentarium of tissue- and tumor-associated antibodies. The following discussion will examine newly developing concepts in histopathology which have a bearing on the prognosis of the cancer patient. It is restricted to consideration of tumor grading, tumor invasion and vascular invasion.

Tumor grading

In the last few years, polyclonal and monoclonal antibodies have become available for identification of cellular constituents indicating differentiation. Antibodies are now used for identification of the intermediate filaments present in the cytoplasm of both normal and neoplastic cells, although aberrant expression is common in some neoplasms. Antibodies directed against each of the five specific classes of intermediate filaments are used to subclassify malignant neoplasms and this approach may provide a future immunologic subclassification of human cancer [1].

The origin of the neoplasm is often reflected by the type of intermediate filament content. Examples of this are astrocytomas which express the intermediate filament glial fibrillary acidic protein, and epithelial neoplasms which express one of the many keratin peptides [2]. Neoplasms of mesenchymal origin express the intermediate filament vimentin, but a number of epithelial neoplasms also develop co-expression of this intermediate filament [3]. Undifferentiated muscle tumors can be defined by content of desmin (a muscle-specific intermediate filament) and neurofilaments are commonly expressed in neuroendocrine neoplasms. The characterization of a cell's intermediate filament content may allow a more accurate identification of neoplasms which are otherwise too poorly differentiated to allow accurate subclassification.

Although there is now available an increasing list of antibodies for identification of cellular features indicative of differentiation, many of these immunologic techniques require special fixation for optimum antigen preservation. In some instances, frozen sections are required for the demonstration of fixation-sensitive antigens, and in other instances, fixation with mercuric-based fixatives or alcohol can be used. It has been shown that the majority of the aldehydes, particularly formaldehyde and glutaraldehyde, often cause cross-linking or 'masking' which does not allow antigen recognition by the specific antibody [4].

Traditionally, the histopathologist reports on the characteristics of a neoplasm, with emphasis on the cell type, possible organ of origin and degree of differentiation or tumor grade. Both nuclear characteristics and cytologic features are considered in the determination of tumor grade, but in addition, the architectural organization of the tumor tissue is a major consideration. Ideally, all of these features should be included in deciding the degree of differentiation or tumor grade.

Well differentiated tumors are likely to behave in a more indolent or less aggressive fashion, while neoplasms that are poorly differentiated will behave in a more aggressive fashion. Poorly differentiated tumors invade more widely with a greater propensity for vascular space invasion and metastasis to lymph nodes and/ or distant sites. Thus, Broders observed that cytoplasmic differentiation reflected by keratin formation was a valuable index in estimating tumor behavior in squamous cell carcinoma [5]. Later he included nuclear pleomorphism in his grading schema, and subsequently the presence of nucleoli, mitoses and other factors, have been integrated into the traditional grading system now applied by most histopathologists.

In general, the more closely a neoplasm resembles the tissue of origin, the better the differentiation or grade and this observation applies to squamous cell carcinomas where keratinization is an indicator of tumor differentiation. But the interrelationship of the cells to the pattern of keratin expression is also important. Malignant neoplasms such as verrucous carcinoma, that tend to produce keratin only on the tumor surface, represent the most differentiated form of squamous cell carcinoma. This well differentiated type of squamous cell carcinoma invades with broad well demarcated tumor-host borders, is not capable of invading vascular spaces and does not metastasize [6].

In most squamous cell carcinomas, the pattern of keratinization is less well organized, and other distributions of keratinization occur. Extracellular keratin pearls formed within the tumor represent an abortive attempt at surface maturation. Single cells with intracellular keratinization also represent a less successful attempt at differentiation.

Similar observations can be made for adenocarcinomas. Those neoplasms which form glands, particularly glands excreting substances normally produced by the tissue of origin, represent the best differentiated adenocarcinomas. Breast adenocarcinomas that commonly invade as cords of malignant cells are a good example. When these cords form a readily identifiable lumen, this represents

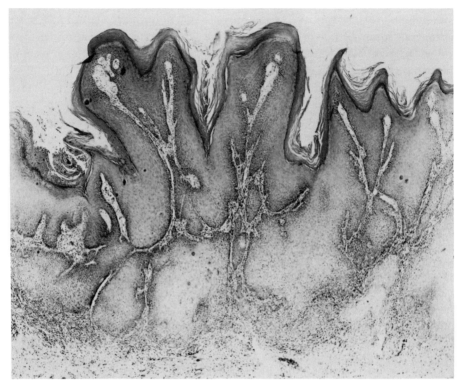

Figure 1. Verrucous carcinoma is an extremely well differentiated carcinoma that invades as broad blunt pegs of cells.

better differentiation, while cords of single cells without identifiable lumen reflect a lesser degree of differentiation [7].

Similar observations apply to sarcomas. Sarcomas that express cytoplasmic features which allow recognition of mesenchymal origin are the best differentiated (Fig. 2). For example, evidence of cytoplasmic differentiation in liposarcoma, fibrosarcoma and leiomyosarcoma includes mature-appearing fat, collagen production or abundant smooth muscle, respectively [8]. Many of these sarcomas can be graded by assessing not only the histologic subtype, but cellular pleomorphism, degree of cellularity, mitotic activity, presence and pattern of necrosis [8, 9] (Fig. 3). However, some sarcomas such as rhabdomyosarcoma, angiosarcomas, Ewing's and synovial sarcoma are aggressive neoplasms and can not reproducibly be graded [8].

Nuclear alterations in malignant tumor cells can be assessed independently of cytoplasmic maturation and growth pattern, and are helpful in evaluating the degree of tumor differentiation [10]. Neoplasms which display variation in nuclear size and staining, and do not closely resemble normal tissue nuclei are

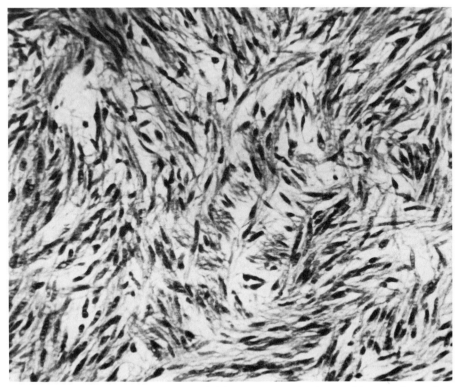

Figure 2. A well differentiated or low grade leiomyosarcoma closely resembles smooth muscle in cellularity, cytoplasmic and nuclear features.

considered less differentiated [5]. These nuclear characteristics are commonly associated with anaplastic neoplasms with more aggressive behavior.

Some of the increase in nuclear staining reflects abnormal or aneuploid numbers of chromosomes within the malignant neoplasm [11, 12]. The association of DNA aneuploidy with malignant tumors has been verified in Feulgen-stained tissue sections using absorption spectrophotometry [13]. With the advent of flow cytometry and the increased ability to produce single cell suspensions [14] or nuclear preparations [15] of solid tumors, many malignant tumors have been shown to contain aneuploid cell populations [11, 12]. Numerous clinical studies of a variety of solid tumors and leukemia/lymphomas have concluded that neoplasms with abnormal or aneuploid DNA content behave in a more aggressive fashion than do tumors with a normal or diploid DNA content [16, 17,18] (see chapter 7).

Frequency of mitoses in histological sections has also been valuable in some neoplasms in estimating biological behavior. This is best established for uterine leiomyosarcomas and is the basis for determining their malignant potential [19].

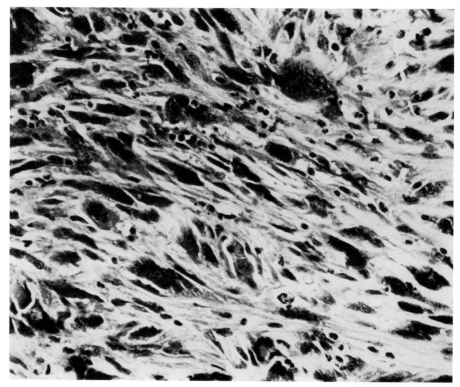

Figure 3. In contrast, a high grade leiomyosarcoma exhibits increased cellularity, marked nuclear pleomorphism and numerous atypical mitoses.

The presence of mitotic figures is also essential for the diagnosis of malignancy in nerve sheath tumors [20].

It is recognized that increased numbers of mitotic figures usually reflect (but imperfectly correlate with) the tumor doubling time or the replicating cycle of individual tumor cells. The frequency of tumor cell division has been studied by incubating slices of tissue with tritiated thymidine [21, 22]. The thymidine labelling index (TLI), like the mitotic index, is related to the rate of cell proliferation and for breast carcinoma there is a significant correlation between the TLI and the likelihood of relapse [23, 24, 25] (see chapter 7).

In flow cytometric DNA analysis [26], the DNA histogram will demonstrate the cellular kinetics as well as the modal DNA content. Estimates of the number or proportion of cells in the synthesis phase (S-phase) results in a quantitative assessment of the tumor's proliferative capacity, a parameter that is often poorly estimated by conventional histopathologic observation [27].

In the case of breast cancer, tumors with lower DNA ploidy values tend to be histologically low grade and estrogen receptor positive, whereas those with higher

DNA ploidy values are more anaplastic and usually estrogen receptor negative [28]. The percent of cells in S-phase is significantly higher in poorly differentiated ductal carcinomas, medullary carcinomas and recurrent tumor or metastasis, as well as in estrogen receptor negative tumors [29]. Multivariate regression analysis does not show aneuploidy to be an independent prognostic factor in predicting a poor prognosis, as it is related to other aggressive histologic features in breast cancer.

Tumor invasion

Tumor invasion is a characteristic of malignancy and is commonly associated with a lack of differentiation or high grade tumors [30, 31]. Although there are obvious exceptions, highly invasive tumors are usually highly metastatic. One exception is basal cell carcinoma, an invasive malignant neoplasm that rarely metastasizes. Although widely invasive, basal cell carcinomas do not appear to infiltrate vascular structures, and invariably have readily identifiable circumferential basement membrane at the host stroma-tumor interface [32]. The latter characteristic is shared only with benign or non-invasive neoplasms. Basement membrane does occur in many invasive carcinomas, but it is usually patchy in its distribution [33] and found only in well differentiated portions of the tumor [34]. It is unlikely that a neoplasm actively producing well formed basement membrane would simultaneously degrade vascular basement membrane and gain access to vascular spaces.

Proliferative indices of malignant tumors tend to be closely related to tumor invasion, so that neoplasms with rapid rates of proliferation and tumor doubling times are usually highly metastatic [35, 36], although invasiveness appears to depend on protein synthesis and not on DNA synthesis [37]. Rapidly proliferating tumor cells have an increased capacity to detach from the main body of the tumor [38]. The latter feature would readily allow invasion as small aggregates of tumor or as single cells, a histologic feature associated with blood and lymph vessel invasion [39].

A characteristic of malignant cells is to invade vascular spaces, leading to metastasis and death. The recent isolation of a tumor-produced autocrine factor that increases tumor motility and invasion has advanced our understanding of the functional characteristics associated with tumor cell invasion [40]. Nevertheless, knowledge of the critical steps in tumor progression is poor [41], and although individual tumor cell motility may be extremely important in tumors that invade as single cells, it has yet to be proved applicable to neoplasms which grow in the cohesive pattern characteristic of many human carcinomas [42]. These cohesive aggregates of tumor may invade by cell proliferation, creating expansion pressures and forcing the tumor through host stroma.

Spread of malignant neoplasms includes both local invasion (which itself can occasionally cause organ failure and host death) and invasion of vascular spaces leading to metastases. The former complication depends on the location of the primary tumor, and the organ or tissue susceptibility to local destruction. The latter is initiated by tumor invasion of the vascular spaces which is the initial step toward successful completion of the metastatic cascade (see chapter 9).

A number of investigators have attempted to identify basement membrane-degrading enzymes secreted by invading tumors, and although several reports have correlated enzyme expression with malignant potential [43], the role of these enzymes is not clear. The first enzyme to receive serious attention was plasminogen activator (PA), but subsequent studies have failed to show a clear-cut role for PA in tumor invasion [44]. Probably the most convincing data has been on a collagenase specific for type IV collagen, an intrinsic component of basement membranes. This has been shown to be present in increased amounts in malignant tumors, and the amount and expression of collagenase IV appears to correlate with malignant potential in several tumor models [43]. In addition, heparinases have also been correlated with metastatic potential in a number of murine tumor models and may also play a role in some, if not all, invasive tumors [45].

Another enzyme which has been demonstrated in increased amounts in many tumors is a cysteine proteinase similar to cathepsin B [46]. Not only is it increased in numerous murine tumors, but studies of human tumor explants have shown increased production by carcinomas compared to benign neoplasms [47]. It may play an important role in tumor cell invasion.

While tumors that are most successful in achieving access to vascular spaces are those which are highly invasive, it has also been shown that tumors with a high degree of differentiation (low grade histologically) are less likely to result in metastasis. Squamous cell carcinomas growing in organized cords or aggregates are less likely to gain access to vascular structures [39] (Fig. 4 and 5). Again, adenocarcinomas that form readily indentifiable tubules, such as those occuring in the breast, are also less likely to result in distant metastasis [48, 49] (Fig. 6).

Poorly differentiated adenocarcinomas on the other hand, are more apt to metastasize. Thus, nasopharyngeal carcinomas which are poorly differentiated (sometimes referred to as lymphoepithelioma) are examples of a neoplasm that often grows as dissociated single cells [50]. and commonly have microscopic primaries but widespread metastases at the time of diagnosis. Similarly, poorly differentiated adenocarcinomas of the breast that grow as non-cohesive single cells without evidence of tubule formation commonly have the highest frequency of metastasis [51, 49].

To sum up, it appears that the pattern of invasion, in conjunction with the degree of tumor organization or differentiation, are strong predictors of lymphatic or blood vascular invasion. Tumors which infiltrate the adjacent host stroma as single cells or small irregular cords of cells appear to have the greatest tendency to invade small vascular spaces and to the subsequent development of metastasis. This has been confirmed for a number of human tumors, including breast [30,

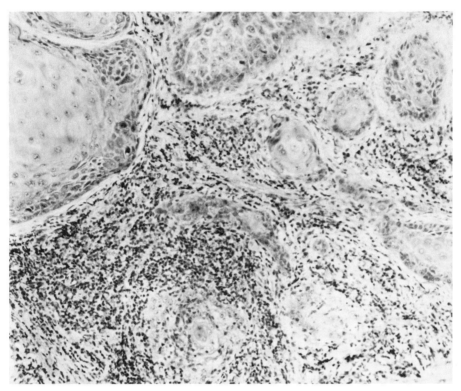

Figure 4. Large, blunt, circumscribed invasive nests characterize this well differentiated squamous cell carcinoma. This pattern of invasion is least likely to attain vascular invasion.

31, 51], colon [52], stomach [53, 54], urinary bladder [55, 56], uterine cervix [57, 58], larynx [59] and tonsil [39].

Vascular invasion

It was noted above that neoplasms which infiltrate in relatively small irregular cords or as single cells are more commonly associated with vascular space penetration. Distinguishing lymphatic from blood capillary spaces is nearly impossible in routine tissue sections. Blood capillaries are completely surrounded by an identifiable basement membrane, and special staining by either anti-laminin or type IV collagen antibodies will demonstrate it [60]. While some lymphatic capillary equivalents may show some fragments, or be partially surrounded by basement membrane, small lymphatic vascular structures usually have an incomplete basement membrane [61, 62].

The presence of malignant tumor in vascular spaces is associated with a poor prognosis. This has been demonstrated for tumors of the breast [30, 31, 51],

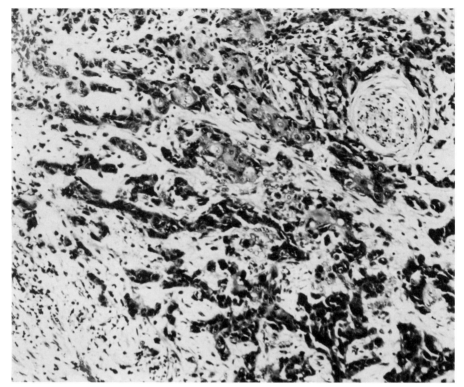

Figure 5. In contrast, this poorly differentiated squamous cell carcinoma invades as irregular narrow cords and single cells. Vascular invasion is seen more often with this pattern of invasion. Note the perineural invasion.

stomach [63], tonsil [39], urinary bladder [64], uterine cervix [65, 66], and colon [67, 68]. It is assumed that invasion of vascular spaces leads to an increased frequency of successful metastasis, either in regional lymph nodes or distant sites.

However, while invasion and successful penetration of vascular spaces represents completion of several of the initial steps required in the metastatic cascade [69, 70], penetration of vascular spaces is not necessarily followed by clinical metastasis [71]. In many animal models there is daily release of large numbers of tumor cells into the vascular system [72] and there are numerous reports of circulating tumor cells in human disease [73]. Despite these findings, a number of the animal models and patient studies have failed to demonstrate the development of distant metastasis, even in the face of large numbers of circulating tumor cells [74, 75].

These observations are important in the interpretation of vascular space involvement in histological sections. If one calculates the geometry of tissue sections used in the evaluation of both experimental and human tumors, it is evident that

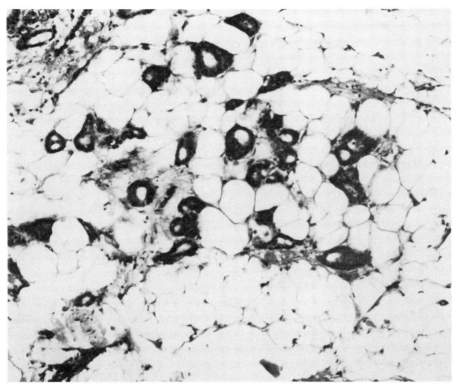

Figure 6. Well formed infiltrative tubules characterize the well differentiated tubular carcinoma of breast that demonstrates a low metastatic potential.

the actual plane of section represents a small portion of the total tumor-host interface [76]. Therefore, the identification of unequivocal vascular space invasion in a section implies that it is a relatively prominent feature inthe tumor being examined. Although there is extensive proliferation of blood vascular spaces within the tumor itself, blood or lymphatic vascular penetration is best identified at the edge of the growing tumor.

In some tumors (in our experience, mostly in breast cancer) extensive vascular space tumour is prominent (Fig. 7). This is commonly associated with extensive lymphatic metastasis, and secondary lymphatic obstruction and dilatation which makes the space between the endothelial-lined lymphatic and the tumor thrombus more prominent. Extensive vascular space tumor suggests that large volumes of tumor cells are likely to be released into either the lymphatic or blood circulation.

Tumor growth in large veins is said to be an indicator of poor prognosis [68], and the larger the aggregates of tumor cells released into the circulation, the more likely they are to successfully establish metastases [77]. This may explain why tumor growth involving large veins is associated with a high frequency of

120

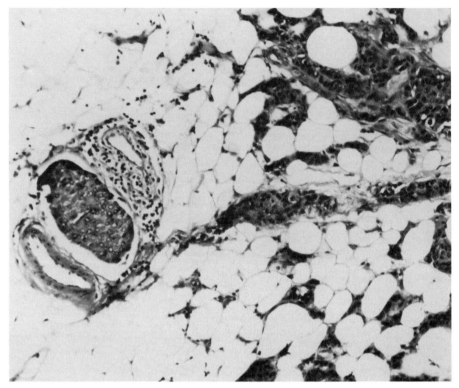

Figure 7. A lymphatic tumor embolus is present in this poorly differentiated ductal carcinoma of breast that invades as small non-cohesive aggregates.

metastases, while vascular space involvement by tumor does not necessarily emply successful distant metastasis, either in regional lymph nodes or distant systemic sites [71, 78].

References

1. Miettinsen M, Lehto VP, Virtanen I: Antibodies to intermediate filament proteins in the diagnosis and classification of human tumors. *Ultrastruct Pathol* 7: 83–107, 1984
2. Sun TT, Eichner R, Nelson WG, Tseng SCG, Weiss RA, Jarvinen M, Woodcock-Mitchell J: Keratin classes: molecular markers for different types of epithelial differentiation. *J Invest Dermatol* 81: 109S–115S, 1983
3. Gould VE: The coexpression of distinct classes of intermediate filaments in human neoplasms. *Arch Pathol Lab Med* 109: 984–989, 1985
4. Battifora H, Kopinski M: The influence of protease digestion and duration of fixation of the immunostaining of keratins. A comparison of formalin and ethanol fixation. *J Histochem Cytochem*. In press
5. Broders AC: Carcinoma: Grading and practical application. *Arch Pathol* 2: 376–381, 1926

6. McDonald JS, Crissman JD, Gluckman JL: Verrucous carcinoma of the oral cavity. *Head Neck Surg* 5: 22–29, 1982

7. Azzopardi JG, Chepick OF, Hartmann WH, Jafarey NA, Llombart-Bosch A, Ozzello L, Rilke F, Sasano N, Sobin LN, Sommers SC, Stalsberg H, Sugar J, Williams AO: The World Health Organization histological typing of breast tumors-Second Edition. *Am J Clin Pathol* 78: 805–816, 1982

8. Russell WO, Cohen J, Enzinger F, Hajdu SI, Heise H, Martin RG, Meissner W, Miller WT, Schmitz RL, Suit HD: A clinical and pathological staging system for soft tissue sarcomas. *Cancer* 40: 1562–1570, 1977

9. Costa J, Wesley RA, Glatstein E, Rosenberg SA: The grading of soft tissue sarcomas. Results of a clinicohistopathologic correlation in a series of 163 cases. *Cancer* 53: 530–541, 1984

10. Black, MM, Speer FD, Opler SR: Structural representations of tumor host relationships in mammary carcinoma. Biologic and prognostic significance. *Am J Clin Pathol* 26: 252–265, 1956

11. Barlogie B, Drewinko B, Schumann J, Gohde W, Dosik G, Latreille J, Johnston DA, Freireich EJ: Cellular DNA content as a marker of neoplasia in man. *Am J Med* 69: 195–203, 1980

12. Friedlander ML, Hedley DW, Taylor IW: Clinical and biological significance of aneuploidy in human tumors. *J Clin Pathol* 37: 961–974, 1984

13. Sandritter W, Carl M, Ritter W: Cytophotometric measurements of the DNA-content of human malignant tumors by means of the Feulgen reaction. *Acta Cytol* 10: 26–30, 1966

14. Waymouth C: Methods for obtaining cells in suspension from animal tissues. Chapter 1. In: *Cell Separation: Methods and Selected Applications*, Academic Press, NYC, 1982, pp. 1–29

15. Vindelov LL, Christensen IJ, Nissen NI: A detergent-trypsin method for the preparation of nuclei for flow cytometric DNA analysis. *Cytometry* 3: 323–327, 1983

16. Wolley RC, Schreiber K, Koss LG, Karas M, Sherman A: DNA distribution in human colon carcinomas and its relationship to clinical behavior. *J Natl Cancer Inst* 69: 15–22, 1982

17. Olszewski W, Darzynkiewicz Z, Rosen PP, Schwartz MK, Melamed MR: Flow cytometry of breast carcinoma. I. Relation of DNA ploidy level to histology and estrogen receptor. *Cancer* 48: 980–984, 1981

18. Braylan RC, Benson NA, Nourse VA: Cellular DNA of human neoplastic B-cells measured by flow cytometry. *Cancer Res* 44: 5010–5016, 1984

19. Taylor HB, Norris HJ: Mesenchymal tumors of the uterus. IV. Diagnosis and prognosis of leiomyosarcomas. *Arch Path* 82: 40–44, 1966

20. Trojanowski JQ, Kleinman GM, Proppe KH: Malignant tumors of nerve sheath origin. *Cancer* 46: 1202–1212, 1980

21. Meyer JS, Bauer WC, Rao BR: Subpopulations of breast carcinoma defined by S-phase fraction, morphology and estrogen content. *Lab Invest* 39: 225–235, 1978

22. Meyer JS: Cell kinetic measurements of human tumors. *Human Pathol* 13: 874–877, 1982

23. Tubiana M, Pejovic MJ, Renaud A, Contesso G, Chavandra N, Gioanni J, Malaise EP: Kinetic parameters and the course of the disease in breast cancer. *Cancer* 47: 937–943, 1981

24. Gentili C, Sonfilippo O, Silvestrini R: Cell proliferation and its relationship to clinical features and relapse in breast cancers. *Cancer* 48: 974–979, 1981

25. Meyer JS, Friedman E, McCrate M, Bauer WC: Prediction of early course of breast carcinoma by thymidine labeling. *Cancer* 51: 1879–1886, 1983

26. Frankfurt OS, Greco WR, Slocum HK, Arbuck SG, Gamarra M, Pavelic ZP, Rustum YM: Proliferative characteristics of primary and metastatic human solid tumors by DNA flow cytometry. *Cytometry* 5: 629–635, 1984

27. McDivitt RW, Stone KR, Craig RB, Meyer JS: A comparison of human breast cancer cell kinetics measured by flow cytometry and thymidine labeling. *Lab Invest* 52: 287–291, 1985

28. Olszewski W, Darzynkiewicz Z, Rosen PP, Schwartz MK, Melamed MR: Flow cytometry of breast carcinoma: I. Relation of DNA ploidy level to histology and estrogen receptor. *Cancer* 48: 980-984, 1981

122

29. Moran RE, Black MM, Alpert L, Straus MJ: Correlation of cell cycle kinetics, hormone receptors, histopathology and nodal status in human breast cancer. *Cancer* 54: 1586–1590, 1984

30. Baak JPA, Kurver PHJ, De Snoo-Niewlaat AJE, De Graef S, Makkink B, Boon ME: Prognostic indicators in breast cancer. *Histopathol* 6: 327–339, 1982

31. Sharkey FE: Biological meaning of stage and grade in human breast cancer: review and hypothesis. *Breast Cancer Res Treat* 2: 299–322, 1982

32. Cam Y, Bellon G, Poulin G, Caron Y, Birembaut P: Distribution of type IV collagen in benign and malignant epithelial proliferations. *Invasion Metast* 4: 61–71, 1984

33. Bosman FT, Havenith M, Cleutjens JPM: Basement membranes in cancer. *Ultrastruct Pathol* 8: 291–304, 1985

34. Sakr WA, Zarbo RJ, Jacobs JR, Crissman JD: Distribution of basement membrane in squamous cell carcinoma of the head and neck. *Am J Surg Pathol.* In Press

35. Glucksmann A: The relation of radiosensitivity and radiocurability to the histology of tumour tissue. *Br J Radiol* 21: 559–566, 1948

36. McDivitt RW, Stone KR, Craig RB, Palmer JO, Meyer JS, Bauer WC: A proposed classification of breast cancer based on kinetics information. *Cancer* 57: 269–276, 1986

37. Thorgeirsson VP, Tvrpeenniemi-Hujanen T, Neckers LM, Johnson DW, Liotta LA: Protein synthesis but not DNA synthesis is required for tumor cell invasion *in vitro. Invasion Met* 4: 73–83, 1984

38. Weiss L: Studies on cellular adhesion in tissue culture. VII. Surface activity and cell detachment. *Exp Cell Res* 33: 277–288, 1964

39. Crissman JD, Liu WY, Gluckman JL, Cummings G: Prognostic value of histopathologic parameters in squamous cell carcinoma of the oropharynx. *Cancer* 54: 2295–3001, 1984

40. Liotta LA, Mandler R, Murano G, Katz DA, Gordon RK, Chiang PK, Schiffmann E: Tumor cell autocrine motility factor. *Cell Biol.* In Press

41. Liotta LA, Rao CN, Barsky SH: Tumor invasion and the extracellular matrix. *Lab Invest* 49: 636–649, 1983

42. Gershman H: Three-dimensional models for the study of invasion and mestastasis. Chapter 14. In: *Tumor Invasion and Metastasis*, LA Liotta and IR Hart, Eds., Martinus Nijhoff, Boston, 1982, pp. 231–266

43. Liotta LA, Tryggvason K, Garbisa S, Hart I, Foltz CM, Shafie S: Metastatic potential correlates with enzymatic degradation of basement membrane collagen. *Nature* 284: 67–68, 1980

44. Goldfarb RH: Proteases in tumor invasion and metastases. Chapter 22. In: *Tumor Invasion and Metastasis*, LA Liotta and IR Hart, Eds., Martinus-Nijhoff, The Hague/Boston/London, 1982, pp. 375–390.

45. NaKajima M, Irimura T: DiFerrante N, Nicolson GL: Metastatic melanoma cell heparinase. *J Biol Chem* 259: 2283–2290, 1984

46. Sloane BF, Honn KV: Cysteine proteinases and metastasis. *Cancer Met Rev* 3: 249–263, 1984

47. Poole AR, Tiltman KJ, Recklies AD, Stoker TAM: Differences in secretion of the proteinase cathepsin B at the edges of human breast carcinomas and fibroadenomas. *Nature* (London) 273: 545–547, 1980

48. Cooper HS, Patchefsky AS, Krall RA: Tubular carcinoma of the breast. *Cancer* 42: 2334–2342, 1978

49. Parl FF, DuPont WD: A retrospective cohort study of histologic risk factors in breast cancer patients. *Cancer* 50: 2410–2416, 1982

50. Shanmugaratnam K, Chan SH, de-The G, Goh JEH, Khor TH, Simons MJ, Tye CY: Histopathology of nasopharyngeal carcinoma. *Cancer* 44: 1029–1044, 1979

51. Nealon TF Jr, Nkongho A, Grossi C, Gillooley J: Pathologic identification of poor prognosis stage I $(T_1N_0M_0)$ cancer of the breast. *Ann Surg* 190: 129–132, 1979

52. Spratt JS, Spjut HJ: Prevalence and prognosis of individual clinical and pathologic variables associated with colorectal carcinoma. *Cancer* 20: 1976–1985, 1967

53. Urban CH, McNeer G: The relation of the morphology of gastric carcinoma to long and short term survival. *Cancer* 12: 1158–1162, 1959

54. Steiner PE, Maimon SN, Palmer WL, Kirsner JB: Gastric cancer: Morphologic factors in five-year survival after gastrectomy. *Am J Pathol* 24: 947–969, 1948

55. Austen G, Friedell GH: Observations on local growth patterns of bladder cancer. *J Urol* 93: 224–229, 1965

56. Soto EA, Friedell GH, Tiltman AJ: Bladder carcinoma as seen in giant histologic sections. *Cancer* 39: 447–455, 1977

57. Beecham JB, Halvorsen T, Kolbenstvedt A: Histologic classification, lymph node metastases and patient survival in stage Ib cervical carcinoma. *Gynecol Oncol* 6: 95–105, 1978

58. Baltzer J, Lohe KJ, Kopeke W, Zander J: Histologic criteria for prognosis in patients with operated squamous cell carcinoma of the cervix. *Gynecol Oncol* 13: 184–194, 1982

59. McGavran MH, Bauer WC, Ogura JH: The incidence of cervical lymph node metastases from epidermoid carcinoma of the larynx and their relationship to certain characteristics of the primary tumor. *Cancer* 14: 55–66, 1961

60. Barsky SH, Baker A, Siegal GP, Togo S, Liotta LA: Use of anti-basement membrane antibodies to distinguish blood vessel capillaries from lymphatic capillaries. *Am J Surg Pathol* 7: 667–677, 1983

61. Bettelhein R, Mitchell D, Gusterson BA: Immunocytochemistry in the identification of vascular invasion in breast cancer. *J Clin Pathol* 37: 364–366, 1984

62. Casley-Smith JR: Lymph and lymphatics. *Microcirculation* 1: 423–468, 1977

63. Kodama Y, Inokuchi K, Soejima K: Growth patterns and prognosis in early gastric carcinoma. *Cancer* 51: 320–326, 1983

64. Bell JT, Burney SW, Friedell GH: Blood vessel invasion in human bladder cancer. *J Urol* 105: 675–678, 1971

65. Zander J, Baltzer J, Lohe KJ, Ober KG, Kaufmann C: Carcinoma of the cervix: An attempt to individualize treatment. *Am J Obstet Gynecol* 139: 752–759, 1981

66. Stendahl V, Ecklund G, Willen R: Prognosis of invasive squamous cell carcinoma of the uterine cervix: A comparative study of the predictive values of clinical staging Ib-III and a histopathologic malignancy grading system. *Int J Gynecol Pathol* 2: 42–54, 1983

67. Copeland EM, Miller LD, Jones RS: Prognostic factors in carcinoma of the colon and rectum. *Am J Surg* 116: 875–881, 1968

68. Talbot IC, Ritchie S, Leighton M, Hughes AO, Bussey HJH, Morson BC: Invasion of veins by carcinoma of the rectum: Method of detection, histologic features and significance. *Histopathol* 5: 141–163, 1981

69. Sugarbaker EV: Some characteristics of metastasis in man. *Am J Pathol* 97: 623–632, 1979

70. Carter RL: Some aspects of the metastatic process. *J Clin Pathol* 35: 1041–1049, 1982

71. Sedlis A, Sall S, Tsukada Y, Park R, Mangan C, Shingleton H, Blessing JA: Microinvasive carcinoma of the uterine cervix: A clinicopathologic study. *Am J Obstet Gynecol* 133: 64–74, 1979

72. Butler TP, Gullino PM: Quantitation of cell shedding into efferent blood of mammary adenocarcinoma. *Cancer Res* 35: 512–516, 1975

73. Engell HC: Cancer cells in the circulating blood. *Acta Chir Scand Supp* 201: 1–70, 1955

74. Weiss L: Metastatic inefficiency. Chapter 6. In: *Tumor Invasion and Metastasis*. LA Liotta and IR Hart, Eds, Martinus-Nijhoff, The Hague/Boston/London, 1982, pp. 81–98

75. Tarin D, Price JE, Kettlewell MGW, Souter RG, Vass ACR, Crossley B: Mechanisms of human tumor metastasis studied in patients with peritoneovenous shunts. *Cancer Res* 44: 3584–3592, 1984

76. Wilkinson E.J., Hause L: Probability in lymph node sectioning. *Cancer* 33: 1269–1274, 1974

77. Liotta LA, Kleinerman J, Saidel GM: The significance of hematogenous tumor cell clumps in the metastatic process. *Cancer Res* 36: 889–894, 1976

78. Roche WD, Norris HJ: Microinvasive carcinoma of the cervix. The significance of lymphatic invasion and confluent patterns of stromal growth. *Cancer* 36: 180–186, 1975

9. Pointers to metastasis

E.J. ORMEROD and I.R. HART

Introduction

The formation of a secondary tumour deposit requires that cells released from the tumour survive a series of complex interactions with various host defences of both a specific and non-specific nature. These interactions can be divided into a sequence of discrete steps. Disseminating cells must (1) invade locally and penetrate lymphatics or small blood vessels; (2) detach from the invasive front, to be released either as individual cells or as small emboli into these channels; (3) passage throughout the body surviving both the trauma of this event and the potentially lethal confrontations with specific and non-specific immune mechanisms; (4) arrest either at the walls of minor blood vessels or within the lymph nodes; (5) extravasate, presumably utilising the same mechanisms that are used during the process of invasion and intravasation and (6) grow progressively at the distant site to give rise to a metastasis which may itself subsequently metastasize [1–5].

Weiss [6] has pointed out that while the popular view of metastasis is of a remorseless, efficient process, in reality this is not the case. Rather, metastasis is an inefficient process where few of the cells released into the circulation survive to form distant metastases [6]. This inefficiency has been demonstrated not only in experimental tumour systems [7] but also in spontaneous human cancers. Tarin [8] for example, showed that patients implanted with peritoneo-venous shunts to relieve ascites resulting from ovarian carcinoma, released millions of viable neoplastic cells into the circulation, but frequently failed to develop any evidence of metastatic disease even over extended time periods.

The inefficiency of the metastatic process coupled with the observation that cancer cell populations are heterogeneous for a variety of phenotypes [9–11] have led to the idea that pre-existing metastatic subpopulations within the original primary tumour give rise to metastases [12–14]. This hypothesis suggests that metastasis is a predetermined, nonrandom event and, as an obvious corollary, that attempts to identify tumour cell properties associated with metastasis should compare cancer cell populations of varying metastatic potentials.

There has been considerable controversy over the idea that neoplasms contain a subpopulation of stable metastatic variants [5, 15, 16]. At present, no cellular properties have been identified which automatically characterise a cell, or group of cells, as belonging to a metastatic subpopulation, and the view of metastasis as a selective or non-random event remains to be proven. Nonetheless, the acceptance of this concept by a large number of workers has led to considerable research aimed at identifying such properties. Some aspects of this more recent work will be considered below under the following headings:
– Oncogenes and tumour metastasis
– Immunological modulation of tumour spread
– Patterns of metastasis
– Implications for clinical treatment

Oncogenes and tumour metastasis

One line of research linking cellular oncogenes with neoplasia was the discovery that the acutely transforming animal retroviruses contained oncogenes unrelated to essential virion genes, but having close homology with sequences in normal cells from which they probably arose through rare transductions by retroviruses without onc genes [17, 18]. These cellular homologues of viral onc genes have been termed proto-oncogenes (c-onc) and, since they are harboured by all vertebrate cells, one of the critical steps in carcinogenesis may be the activation of a cellular proto-oncogene into an oncogene [18].

There are a number of ways this oncogenic potential could be achieved. For example, there is the possibility that a dosage effect is involved, so that increased production of the appropriate gene product may be sufficient for neoplastic conversion. Alternatively, or concomitantly, activation could result from the translocation of the chromosomal locus carrying the proto-oncogene to a new chromosomal site, where expression could be affected by its juxtaposition to different genes. Finally, it is possible that structural alterations, resulting from mutations in the proto-oncogenes, bring about conversion to the activated oncogenes.

Evidence has accumulated that many of these mechanisms may have occurred in tumour material [19–21]. The evidence that proto-oncogenes play a crucial role in the development of neoplasia is largely circumstantial. Nevertheless, the likely role of some of the cellular oncogenes in tumour development has been confirmed in recent experiments, where the introduction of these genes into transgenic mice has resulted in the subsequent development of characteristic tumours [22, 23].

The second line of investigation to link cellular oncogenes with neoplasia has resulted from DNA transfection studies. Genomic DNA from a variety of human and animal tumours, when transfected into an immortalised murine fibroblast line NIH/3T3, has produced full morphological transformation of some of the recipient NIH/3T3 cells, and endowed them with the capacity to form progressively growing tumours in recipient mice [24, 25]. In most instances, the genes responsible for the transforming capacity of these tumours have proved to be the cellular homologues of the ras oncogenes [26, 27]. Activation of these genes is generally a consequence of somatic point mutations at codon 12 or 61 of the encoded ras gene product, resulting in a single amino acid substitution [28].

There are a few reports in the literature which suggest that cellular oncogenes may also play a role in metastasis. In the most direct approach to examining the effect of cellular oncogenes on metastatic behaviour, benign or 'normal' cell lines have been transfected with genomic DNA from metastatic human tumours or with cloned oncogenes, and the subsequent metastatic behaviour of these lines has been examined [29–32]. The results are still rather confusing.

Thorigeirsson et al. [30] showed that, in contrast to parent or spontaneously transformed cells, NIH/3T3 cells transfected with DNA from malignant tumours produced experimental and spontaneous metastases in nude mice. In subsequent studies, this group showed that this effect was attributable solely to the presence of the activated T24 ras-Ha gene [31]. They also found that normal early-passage rat fibroblasts transformed by a recombinant construct of the T24 oncogene, linked to a Moloney sarcoma virus long terminal repeat fragment containing the viral enhancers [33], were also fully metastatic in nude mice [31]. This finding raises the question of how a single transforming gene induces the complex process of metastasis. Does the gene act in additive fashion to add growth capacity to cells already expressing all the necessary gene products for metastasis? Does the integrated oncogene induce genetic instability in recipient cells, allowing the generation of metastatic variants as a secondary consequence of transformation? Does the ras gene switch on a cascade of cellular gene products allowing the cell to complete all the steps in the metastatic sequence? [31].

The results obtained with the NIH/3T3 cells could in part be explained by the observations of Greig et al. [32] who found that normal untransfected NIH/3T3 cells are able to express both tumourigenic and metastatic properties, suggesting that the activated c-Ha-ras oncogene merely accelerated the appearance of metastases [32]. Bernstein and Weinberg [34] also found that NIH/3T3 cells transfected with the activated ras-Ha oncogene were metastatic in immunoincompetent nude mice but, in contrast to the results of Greig et al. [32], failed to get any tumours or metastases to develop in these animals from the injection of untransformed cells. Acquisition of metastatic activity in immunocompetent NFS/NCR mice by these cells resulted from the transfer of a discrete human DNA fragment, obtained from a human metastatic tumour, which was shown to be unrelated to the known ras oncogenes [24].

With the exception of the early-passage rat embryo fibroblasts used by Muschel and co-workers [31], all these studies have utilised NIH/3T3 cells as recipient cells. Recently, Vousden et al. [35] have managed to enhance the metastatic activity of a mouse mammary carcinoma by transfecting cells with a construct containing the activated ras-Ha gene linked to a gene encoding for resistance to a neomycin-like antibiotic, allowing the selection of transfected cells. Another approach to transfection, which has been used to analyse the likely involvement of cellular oncogenes in the metastatic behaviour of experimental tumours, has been the examination of the expression or activation of such genes in variants of defined metastatic activity isolated from the same parental tumour [36–38].

In biopsies of human cancer, the analysis of alterations in the expression of cellular oncogenes during the course of tumour progression and in the acquisition of malignancy has provided similarly equivocal results. Examination of RNA from premalignant polyps and tumours of the colorectum showed significant elevation of expression of the ras-related oncogenes as compared to normal colorectal mucosa [39], but identification of the p21 ras oncogene product with monoclonal antibodies showed that the presence of the protein was not useful in identifying cells at different stages of carcinogenesis [40]. Furthermore, no direct relationship was evident between elevated levels of ras-related RNA and conventional staging criteria and clinical outcome [41].

Gallick et al. [42], using immunoprecipitation of p21 ras products from material recovered from primary and metastatic colon tumours actually showed that all of nine metastases had considerably reduced p21-ras expression irrespective of the site of metastasis. In almost direct contrast to these results, monoclonal antibodies generated by utilising a synthetic peptide (reflecting amino acid positions 10–17) of the human T-24 ras gene as an immunogen [43], have been used to show an apparent correlation between p21-ras expression and depth of penetration of primary colon tumours [44].

Alterations of ras and myc oncogenes have been reported in more than one-third of human solid tumours, and apparent allelic deletions of these oncogenes appear to be correlated with progression and metastasis of carcinomas and sarcomas [45]. However, perhaps the best example of correlation between changes in cellular oncogenes and acquisition of aggression or metastatic activity is provided by the cellular genes homologous to the v-myc oncogene. In a variety of cancers, amplification of c-myc has occurred in advanced, widespread tumours or in aggressive primary neoplasms [45]. In small cell lung carcinoma(SSLC) amplification of c-myc appears to be associated with an extremely malignant variant cell type [46]. More recent reports show that the N-myc gene may also be amplified in cell lines derived from these aggressive tumours [47, 48].

Amplification of the N-myc gene is often detected in neuroblastomas or neuroblastoma-derived cell lines [49, 50] and the presence of amplification appears to correlate with tumour stage, in that low-stage patients with good prognoses showed no evidence of amplification, whereas this alteration was present in approximately half the poor-prognosis patients with stage 3 and 4 disease [51]. In summary, although at present there is very little direct support for an association between acquisition of metastatic capacity and alterations in cellular oncogene expression, this uncertainty may reflect the small number of studies completed to date.

Immunological modulation of tumour spread

The role of the immune system in the limitation of tumour development is still uncertain and is likely to depend on the mode of tumour induction. Nevertheless, metastasizing single cells or small groups of cells are highly likely to interact with a variety of host immune effector cells. The fact that metastasis occurs only after the primary tumour has developed and allowed for priming of the immune response, further increases the likelihood that this process is susceptible to immune modulation. Indeed, the lung-colonizing capacity of murine tumours can be influenced markedly by either the immune status of recipient animals or the immunogenicity of the injected cells [52]. Recent investigations have concentrated on changes in the immunogenic status of the metastatic cells, and whether the expression of metastatic capacity is a consequence of escape from immune surveillance.

The major histocompatibility complex (MHC) is a large genetic region that regulates many of the activities of immune cells. Within the MHC, the class 1 genes include the transplantation antigens, originally identified on the basis of their role as targets for graft rejection [53]. In man, the genes for the class 1 antigens map to the HLA-A -B and -C regions of the MHC, whereas in the mouse, these genes map to the H-2 or T1a regions of the MHC where the polymorphic histocompatibility antigens H-2K, D and L are products of the H-2 loci [53]. The histocompatibility antigens are cell surface glycoproteins, distributed widely on nearly all cell types, and these antigens play an obligatory role in targeting the attack of cytolytic T lymphocytes which only recognise antigens of virally infected or neoplastic cells as 'foreign' in association with such class 1 molecules.

The finding that certain malignant tumours have reduced or undetectable levels of class 1 antigens has raised the possibility that this may have been the reason for their escape from putative immune surveillance mechanisms allowing them to avoid being killed by cytolytic T-cells during dissemination [54, 55]. Experimental studies on murine tumours have in part confirmed this hypothesis, but have also shown that this view is likely to be somewhat simplistic. Transfection of H-2 genes into cells of metastatic and non-metastatic clones lacking MHC-encoded H-2K genes has been used to restore expression of H-2K antigens. *De novo* expression of H2-K has been shown to cause a profound decrease in the metastatic capacity of the malignant clone in immunocompetent recipient mice, while the behavioural traits of these cells in immunologically impaired mice remained unaltered [56]. This situation is compatible with the idea that an inverse relationship exists between malignancy and expression of MHC class 1 molecules.

However, in a series of studies Feldman and his colleagues [57–60] have shown that the opposite relationship may occur. In the T10 sarcoma and the 3LL Lewis lung carcinoma, metastatic activity appears to be associated with expression of H-2D region molecules [59, 60]. These results suggest that the H-2D and H-2K encoded antigens differ in their immunogenic effect: the H-2D region molecules may have preferentially brought about the induction of suppressor cells, whereas the H-2K region antigens elicited a strong immune response [60].

In addition, in the Lewis lung carcinoma expression of the metastatic phenotype brought about by exposure of these cells to 5-azacytidine has been accompanied by enhanced expression of a glycoprotein showing strong homology to MHC class 1 antigen [61]. These results make it clear that escape of disseminating cells from MHC class 1-mediated immune surveillance might be the consequence of either loss of class 1 antigens, with no cytotoxic T-lymphocyte recognition, or the enhancement or activation of class 1 antigen expression leading to an attenuated immune response [53].

Unfortunately, mouse tumours express a variety of antigens, such as viral antigens, which in conjunction with class 1 antigens may bring about elimination of the cells for reasons totally unconnected with their neoplastic or metastatic nature. Because of this, the question of whether MHC class 1 antigen expression plays a fundamental role in regulating tumour spread is more likely to be solved by the study of material isolated from primary and secondary tumours of cancer patients. Using this approach, deficiencies in expression of class 1 histocompatibility antigens have been demonstrated in a number of cell lines derived from human cancers [62–65], though differences between primary and metastatic cancers are not always evident [66].

Natural killer (NK) cells (non-adherent, non-phagocytic spontaneously cytotoxic effector cells) are also thought to play a pivotal role in regulating metastatic spread [67–69]. It has recently been proposed that NK cells, in contrast to T-lymphocytes, may recognise the lack, rather than the presence, of cell surface molecules [70]. In the light of the above discussion regarding MHC antigen expression, it is interesting that a common feature of many NK cell targets is the absence or reduced expression of class 1 molecules [67]. Indeed, H-2 negative B16 cells have been shown to exhibit reduced pulmonary colonization relative to their parental counterparts, and this deficiency was attributable to their increased elimination by natural killer cells [71]. As Karre [72] has pointed out, such a mechanism would predict for increased H-2 expression during tumour progression, a finding which is compatible with the published data on mouse tumours, if the increased expression of D-end encoded alleles is considered [57–60].

In summary, the nature of the immune response in limiting metastasis is complex, and while animal model systems can be used to demonstrate the role of adaptive and non-adaptive immunity in modulating tumour dissemination, the relevance of these results to cancer spread in man is uncertain. We need to continue analysis of fresh human material from primary and secondary tumours from the same patient, using monoclonal antibodies to class 1 products of specific alleles for immunohistological staining or combined with FACS analysis.

Tumour dormancy

Recurrence of overt neoplastic disease many years after the removal or successful treatment of the primary tumour suggests that neoplastic cells can persist for long periods in a clinically healthy host. Although evidence for this recurrence is based upon similarities in histological appearance of the original and recurrent tumours, it does not rule out the possibility of a second transformation event. It is however more likely that the neoplastic cells have maintained themselves in a clinically quiescent state throughout the remission period, and two major mechanisms are proposed in the control of tumour dormancy [73, 74].

First, the proliferative capacity of the neoplastic cells might be inhibited as a consequence of unfavourable physiological conditions such as sequestration of cells at an avascular site [75], or the lack of specific growth-promoting substances such as hormones [76]. Fisher and Fisher [77] showed that trauma to rat livers known to contain Walker 256 carcinoma cells led to development of tumours within a few weeks, whereas control, non-traumatized animals failed to develop lesions. It is possible that an increase in the concentration of mitogenic substances (such as platelet-derived growth factor) could be responsible for the growth stimulation of the tumour cells. Alternatively, the enhanced vascularisation that accompanies wound healing could bring about such growth stimulation, since the proliferative rate of tumour cells is related to vascularity [78]. In this view, the emergence of cells from the dormant state would be attributable to changes in the microenvironment causing cells to move out of the G_O phase and back into the cell replication cycle.

The second mechanism proposed for maintaining the dormant state is regulation by immunological restraint and certainly in experimental animals, an immunosuppressive regime can bring about the emergence of overt tumours previously maintained as dormant metastases [79]. In this view, the neoplastic cells continue cycling, but the size of the tumour is restricted because a balance is maintained between cell division and cell death. Such a balance need not necessarily be as 'fine' as would at first seem indicated, since in order that the tumour be considered dormant it need only be undetectable; a situation which might allow for quite wide fluctuations in cell number. Movement from the latent state could then result from impairment of immune function in the host, allowing the proliferation of previously checked cells. Alternatively, it could result from the production of mutant cells which are able to escape from immune surveillance through, for example, alterations in MHC class 1 antigen expression.

Pattern of metastases

Clinical observations have established that malignant tumours of a defined histological type frequently metastasize preferentially to specific organs [5], and similar observations apply in experimental animal tumors. In spite of a substantial amount of work on experimental systems, we have advanced little beyond Paget [80] in understanding the exact mechanisms responsible for preferential metastatic development.

Three general explanations have been proffered to explain non-random metastatic patterns; (1) that gross disease is a consequence of mechanistic factors alone, so that site specificity is a direct consequence of the anatomical location of the primary tumour; (2) that disseminating cells are spread throughout the body but only develop into obvious growths in response to some characteristics of the organ microenvironment, the so-called 'seed-and-soil' hypothesis; (3) that secondary tumour development is a reflection of cell-cell recognition leading to specific adhesion to endothelial cells, or basement membrane components, in particular organs [81, 82].

Weiss [5] concluded that the mechanical hypothesis could account satisfactorily for the majority of early metastatic patterns, but was insufficient to account for the manifestations of later stage disease. Sugarbaker [83] similarly pointed out that results supportive of the mechanical hypothesis were obtained primarily from patients with early stage tumours of low or moderate metastatic capacity, whereas evidence for the 'seed-and-soil' hypothesis has been generated from autopsy material (representing a later stage of the disease), or from studies with highly aggressive metastatic tumours where widespread dissemination is achieved early in tumour development. The observations with peritoneovenous shunts are an example of data which are consistent with the 'seed-and-soil' hypothesis [8, 84]. Considerable experimental effort has recently been directed towards investigating whether metastatic development is a consequence of specific growth ('seed-and-soil') or specific entrapment (cellular recognition).

Cell-cell recognition and specific arrest

Lymphocytes recirculate continuously between the lymphoid organs via both the blood and lymph vasculature [85]. This migration is not a random process but is regular to maintain the integrity and cellular composition of the various lymphoid organs. Entrance of lymphocytes into Peyer's patches and lymph nodes is a consequence of specific interactions between these circulating cells and the endothelial cells lining post-capillary high endothelial venules [85, 86]. This specificity of binding can be demonstrated by incubating lymphocytes on fresh frozen sections of mesenteric lymph nodes [87].

Using this assay it has been shown that populations of cells that home poorly *in vivo* bind poorly *in vitro*, whereas cells that home well *in vivo* after intravenous injection are able to bind well to tissue sections *in vivo* [87]. It is therefore possible that the patterns of organ-specific colonization exhibited by murine tumours subsequent to intravenous injection [88, 89] could be the consequence of similar affinities. This theory is supported by recent work which has shown that two murine tumour lines bind preferentially to cryostat sections of the tissues that they colonize *in vivo* [90], and that *in vitro* selection for organ-specific adherence was associated with increased ability to colonize that organ following re-injection into recipient mice [91].

Using a monoclonal antibody which recognises a cell-surface molecule involved in the specific homing of lymphocytes [85], it has proved possible to detect hybrid β-galactosidase complementary DNA (cDNA) fusion proteins [92]. Analysis of three independent cDNA clones isolated using this antibody screening technique has shown that each encodes the protein, ubiquitin [92, 93]. The amino acid sequence of purified lymphocyte-homing-receptor has shown the presence of two amino termini, one of which corresponds exactly to the amino terminus of ubiquitin, suggesting that this protein may play an important role in cell-cell interactions and adhesions [93].

Could such an approach be utilized to isolate genes encoding for recognition molecules on the surface of tumour cells? The demonstration that monoclonal antibodies can be generated against murine melanoma cells which inhibit their adhesion *in vitro* and block lung colonization *in vivo* [94] suggests that such an approach is indeed feasible. The relevance of the work with lymphocytes may be that it has shown that specific regions of blood vessels do contain and express receptors for circulating cells, but there still is no definitive proof that metastatic patterns of even those murine tumours exhibiting preferential binding to organs *in vitro* [90] are in fact due to specific recognition mechanisms [82].

Differential growth

The corner stone of the 'seed and soil' hypothesis is that the environment of certain organs is conducive to the growth of sequestered cells of specific tumour types or, conversely, that these same environments may exert an inhibitory effect on the proliferation of tumour cells which fail to colonise such organs. In the past, attempts to mimic this type of control over proliferative responses, using extracts from a variety of organs, have failed to establish correlations with metastatic patterns [82]. Recently however, it has been reported that such correlations may be detected for certain tumours [95].

The association between organ environment and clinically manifest tumour development may be suggested by recent work demonstrating a link between oncogenes and growth factors. It has been recognised for some time that transformed cells require fewer exogenous growth factors for efficient proliferation than do their normal counterparts [96]. This finding led to the proposition that transformation might be a consequence of the endogenous production and secretion of polypeptide growth factors which, through the expression of cell surface receptors for that factor, could induce cellular proliferation [97]. This process has been termed autocrine stimulation [89].

Oncogenes may confer growth factor autonomy on malignant cells through at least two possible mechanisms [99]. First, the demonstration [100, 101] that the sis oncogene encodes a protein, p^{28}-sis, that is virtually identical to platelet derived growth factor (PDGF) suggested that constitutive expression of a growth factor might be one way in which oncogenes could produce proliferative autonomy in transformed cells. Second, it is possible that changes in the growth factor receptor itself may result in growth stimulation, even in the absence of exogenous, or intrinsically produced, growth factors.

Thus, the finding that the product of the v-erb-B oncogene represents a truncated version of the epidermal growth factor (EGF) receptor, provided evidence that malfunctioning receptors could act to produce mitogenic responses [102]. Subsequent to this confirmation of a direct link between a growth factor receptor and an oncogene product [102], it was shown that the fms oncogene is an altered version of the normal gene coding for the CSF-1 receptor on mononuclear phagocytes [103], and that cDNA of human oestrogen receptor from MCF-7 cells (for which oestrogens are mitogenic) shows extensive homology with the v-erb A oncogene [104].

What is the significance of these findings in determining the location of secondary tumour growth? Since disseminated cancer cells travel either as individual cells or as small emboli, their subsequent growth at distant sites is likely to be dependent on autocrine, rather than paracrine, stimulation. If metastasis is indeed a selective process, is it possible that the cells which give rise to metastases do so because they are best able to respond to autocrine proliferation? Certainly a recent report has indicated that metastasis in breast carcinoma appears to be associated with the presence of the EGF receptor [105].

The microenvironment of the organ might either provide polypeptide growth factors or modulate expression of growth factor receptors. This possibility has been hinted at by Neal *et al.* [106] who found that in transitional cell carcinoma of the bladder, staining for the EGF receptor was associated with poor differentiation and invasion. These authors suggest that the demonstration in human tumours of a receptor for a growth factor which is found in high levels in the local environment (EGF being present at high concentration in the urine) could have important implications if such receptors could be shown to be functional [106]. Also, in the light of the report linking the oestrogen receptor with the v-erb-A oncogene [104], it could be of significance that oestrogen receptor status of breast cancers may be correlated with specific metastatic patterns [107]. Further information will emerge both as a result of experimental studies and the use of monoclonal antibodies to stain sections from human tumor material [105, 106].

Implications for clinical treatment

In a recent review [108] Poste set out the problems in treatment that arise as a direct consequence of the biology of metastasis. First, the heterogeneous nature of tumours may ensure that populations of cells with different susceptibilities to anti-neoplastic agents exist within the tumour [108]. Additionally, the suggestion that metastatic tumour cell subpopulations are able to generate variants at appreciably higher frequencies than normal or benign cells [109] makes it theoretically possible that metastases might be more able to generate drug resistant populations, thus forestalling conventional treatment.

Second, the pharmacokinetics of systemically administered drugs may have varying effects on the response of tumour deposits depending on their locations within the body. For example, animal studies have shown that pulmonary metastatic tumour nodules are more sensitive to a number of anti-neoplastic drugs than are the primary subcutaneous or muscle tumours [110–112]. This sensitivity to chemotherapy may be a consequence of the more rapid growth and better vascularisation of metastases as compared to the primary tumour, since in man, metastases tend to grow more readily than do primaries and particularly in the case of lung metastases, may grow at an exponential rate. However, there are also reports in animal models of improved response to chemotherapy by pulmonary metastases which have shown slower doubling times than the primary tumour [122]. Thus, faster growth rates might not always be a prerequisite for obtaining better responses.

Sometimes too, the anatomical situation of the secondary tumour will not favour the achievement of optimal drug concentrations. For example, metastases to the brain may be protected from multi-agent chemotherapy by the inability of these agents to cross the blood-brain barrier.

When the mechanisms of tumour progression and tumour heterogeneity are considered, there is the theoretical possibility that drugs used to treat cancer may actually facilitate movement from the benign to the malignant state [113]. Nowell [114] proposed that this progression was due to genetic alterations, and resulted from the inherently greater genetic instability of neoplastic cells as compared to their normal counterparts. In the natural course of events, progression would result from innate host/tumour cell interactions. However, external factors such as treatment could modify this development and, since many anti-neoplastic drugs are mutagenic [115, 116], chemotherapy might lead to the facilitation of the process [113]. In model systems, the lung-colonizing capacity of human and murine tumours can be enhanced significantly by pre-treating neoplastic cells with 5-azacytidine [117], hydroxyurea [118] and methotrexate [119].

While we have, as yet, no firm evidence that such treatments actually do enhance aggression, these studies show that under specific conditions it is possible to increase the metastatic capacity of tumour cells by prior exposure to commonly used antineoplastic agents. This phenomenon conceivably could account for the lack of therapeutic gain obtained in chemotherapy of solid malignancies in spite of improvements in supportive care [120].

Many proposed treatments, such as stimulation of NK cell activity or blocking of cellular adhesion by administration of specific antibodies or anticoagulants [108], suffer from the fundamental drawback that they are targeted to a step in the metastatic process that has probably occurred by the time treatment can be initiated. It has been said that 50% of patients with solid malignancies already have established metastases at the time of presentation [121], underlining the fact that the requirement for treatment of disseminated cancer is an agent which attacks established growths in distant locations. Experimental studies in mice [122] and autopsy data from man [123] show that metastases can metastasize, suggesting that the types of treatment cited above could only have a supplementary role in preventing the extension of this cascade or inhibiting possible iatrogenic spread, but they are unlikely to eradicate already established metastases.

Immunotherapy of cancer has attempted for many years to generate cells capable of discriminating between normal and neoplastic cells and killing the neoplastic cells. Recently, Rosenberg has reduced pulmonary and hepatic metastatic nodules in mice by injecting lymphokine-activated killer cells plus recombinant interleukin-2 (RIL-2) into tumour bearing animals [124, 125], although high doses of RIL-2 alone also constituted successful therapy [126]. These techniques have now been transferred to the clinic where early results look promising [127].

Fidler and co-workers have had similar success in treating established metastases in mice using liposome-encapsulated macrophage-activating agents [128–130]. These compounds activate macrophages to the tumouricidal state, and the use of liposomes ensures their targeting to the phagocytic cells [131]. This treatment has not yet been examined in a clinical trial.

The use of monoclonal antibodies would also seem to hold great promise for treatment. However, like systemically delivered drugs, the localisation of antibodies will be affected by the permeability and quantity of tumour blood vessels, a characteristic that may vary with the nature of the colonized organ. Furthermore, the epitope recognised by the antibody will be expressed by only a percentage of the cells forming a heterogeneous tumour. In fact, qualitative and quantitative differences in antigen expression have been detected both within primary tumours and between metastases and their primary tumours [108]. While the use of a panel of monoclonal antibodies might circumvent this problem, the number of antigens expressed by cells within a metastatic deposit could be almost limitless.

To avoid the problems associated with cellular heterogeneity, one could link the monoclonal antibody to a radioisotope capable of producing cytotoxicity within a limited field. Such a technique has however the limitation that damage to normal tissues, such as liver and spleen, following non-specific uptake could represent a significant impediment to therapy [132]. Nevertheless, Lenhard *et al.* [133] using an ^{131}I-linked antiferritin antibody, have achieved partial remission of disease in 40% of 38 patients suffering from advanced progressive Hodgkin's disease.

Conclusion

Conventional therapy has found disseminated disease to be refractory to cure. Newer approaches, based upon an appreciation of the biology of metastatic spread, are beginning to show signs of promise which hopefully, may be fulfilled in the next decade.

References

1. Fidler IJ, Hart IR: Principles of cancer biology: cancer metastasis. In: *Cancer Principles and Practice of Oncology*. DeVita VT, Hellman S, Rosenberg SA, (eds). Lippincott, Philadelphia, Vol. 1, pp 113–124, 1985
2. Fidler IJ, Hart IR: Biological diversity in metastatic neoplasms: origins and implications. *Science* 217: 998–1003, 1982
3. Fidler IJ, Gersten DM, Hart IR: The biology of cancer invasion and metastasis. *Adv Cancer Res* 28: 149–250, 1978
4. Poste G, Fidler IJ: The pathogenesis of cancer metastasis. *Nature* 283: 139–146, 1980
5. Weiss L: *Principles of Metastasis*. Weiss L (ed) London, Academic Press, 1985
6. Weiss L: Random and nonrandom processes in metastasis and metastatic inefficiency. *Inv Met* 3: 193–207, 1983
7. Butler TP, Gullino PM: Quantitation of cell shedding into efferent blood of mammary adenocarcinoma. *Cancer Res* 35: 512–516, 1975
8. Tarin D, Vass AC, Kettlewell MG, Price JE: Absence of metastatic sequelae during long-term treatment of malignant ascites by peritoneo-venous shunting. A clinico-pathological report. *Inv Met* 4: 1–12, 1984
9. Hart IR, Fidler IJ: The implications of tumor heterogeneity for studies on the biology of cancer metastasis. *Biochim Biophys Acta* 651: 37–50, 1981
10. Poste G, Greig RG: On the genesis and regulation of cellular heterogeneity in malignant tumors. *Inv Met* 2: 137–176, 1982
11. Fidler IJ: Tumor heterogeneity and the biology of cancer invasion and metastasis. *Cancer Res* 38: 2651–2660, 1978
12. Fidler IJ, Kripke ML: Metastasis results from preexisting variant cells within a malignant tumor. *Science* 197: 893–395, 1977

13. Kripke ML, Gruys E, Fidler IJ: Metastatic heterogeneity of cells from an ultraviolet-light-induced murine fibrosarcoma of recent origin. *Cancer Res* 38: 2962–2967, 1978

14. Talmadge JE and Fidler IJ: Enhanced metastatic potential of tumor cells harvested from spontaneous metastases of heterogeneous murine tumors. *J Nat Cancer Inst* 69: 975–980, 1982

15. Alexander P: The biology of metastases. *Cancer Topics* 4: 116–117, 1984

16. Weiss L, Holmes JC, Ward PM: Do metastases arise from pre-existing subpopulations of cancer cells. *Br J Cancer* 47: 81–89, 1983

17. Deusberg PH: Retroviral transforming genes in normal cells? *Nature* 304: 219–226, 1983

18. Hunter T: Oncogenes and proto-oncogenes: how do they differ? *J Nat Cancer Inst* 73: 773–785, 1984

19. Klein G, Klein E: Evolution of tumours and the impact of molecular oncology. *Nature* 315: 190–195, 1985

20. Cooper GM: Activation of transforming genes in neoplasms. *Br J Cancer* 50: 137–142, 1984

21. Bishop JM: Cellular oncogenes and retroviruses. *Ann Rev Biochem* 52: 301–354, 1983

22. Hanahan D: Heritable formation of pancreatic β-cell tumours in transgenic mice expressing recombinant insulin-simian virus 40 oncogenes. *Nature* 315: 115–122, 1985

23. Adams JM, Harris AW, Pinkert CA, Corcoran LM, Alexander WS, Cory S, Palmiter RD, Brinster RL: The c-myc oncogene driven by immunoglobulin enhancers induces lymphoid malignancy in transgenic mice. *Nature* 318: 533–538, 1985

24. Shi C, Padhy LC, Murray M, Weinberg RA: Transforming genes of carcinomas and neuroblastomas introduced into mouse fibroblasts. *Nature* 290: 261–264, 1981

25. Hopkins N, Besmer P, DeLeo AB, Law LW: High-frequency cotransfer of the transformed phenotype and a tumor-specific transplantation antigen by DNA from the 3-methylcholanthrene-induced Meth A sarcoma of Balb/c mice. *Proc Natl Acad Sci USA*. 78: 7555–7559, 1981

26. Parada LF, Tabin CJ, Shih C, Weinberg RA: Human EJ bladder carcinoma oncogene is homologue of Harvey sarcoma virus ras gene. *Nature* 297: 474–478, 1982

27. Der CJ, Krontiris TG, Cooper GM: Transforming genes of human bladder and lung carcinoma cell lines are homologous to the ras genes of Harvey and Kirsten sarcoma viruses. *Proc Natl Acad Sci USA* 79: 3637–3640, 1982

28. Balmain A: Transforming ras oncogenes and multistage carcinogenesis. *Br J Cancer* 51: 1–7, 1985

29. Bondy GP, Wilson S, Chambers AF: Experimental metastatic activity of H-ras transformed NIH 3T3 cells. *Cancer Res* 45: 6005–6009, 1985

30. Thorgeirsson UP, Turpeenniemi-Hijanen T, Williams JE, Westin EH, Heilman CA, Talmadge JE and Liotta LA: NIH/3T3 cells transfected with human tumor DNA containing activated ras oncogenes express the metastatic phenotype in nude mice. *Mol Cell Biol* 5: 259–262, 1985

31. Muschel RJ, Williams JE, Lowy DR and Liotta LA: Harvey ras induction of metastatic potential depends upon oncogene activation and the type of recipient cell. *Am J Path* 121: 1–8, 1985

32. Greig RG, Koestler TP, Trainer DL, Corwin SP, Miles L, Kline T, Sweet R, Yokoyama S, Poste G: Tumorigenic and metastatic properties of 'normal' and ras-transfected NIH/3T3 cells. *Proc Natl Acad Sci USA* 82: 3698–3701, 1985

33. Spandidos DA, Wilkie NM: Malignant transformation of early passage rodent cells by a single mutated human oncogene. *Nature* 310: 469–475, 1984

34. Bernstein SC, Weinberg RA: Expression of the metastatic phenotype in cells transfected with human metastatic DNA. *Proc Natl Acad Sci USA* 82: 1726–1730, 1985

35. Eccles SA, Marshall C, Vousden K, Purvies H: Enhanced metastatic capacity of mouse mammary carcinoma cells transfected with H-ras. *Treat ment of metastasis: Problems and prospects*: Abstract, 1984

36. Kris RM, Avivi A, Bar-Eli M, Alon Y, Carmi P, Schlessinger J, Raz A: Expression of Ki-ras oncogene in tumor cell variants exhibiting different metastatic capabilities. *Int J Cancer* 35: 227–230, 1985

138

37. Vousden KH, Marshall CJ: Three different activated ras genes in mouse tumours; evidence for oncogene activation during progression of a mouse lymphoma. *EMBO J* 3: 913–917, 1984

38. Yuhki N, Hamada J-I, Kuzumaki N, Takeichi N, Kobayashi H: Metastatic ability and expression of c-fos oncogene in cell clones of a spontaneous rat mammary tumor. *Jpn J Cancer Res* 77: 9–12, 1986

39. Spandidos DA, Kerr IB: Elevated expression of the human ras oncogene family in premalignant and malignant tumours of the colorectum. *Br J Cancer* 49: 681–688, 1984

40. Kerr IB, Lee FD, Quintamilla M, Balmain A: Immunocytochemical demonstration of p21 ras family oncogene product in normal mucosa and in premalignant and malignant tumours of the colorectum. *Br J Cancer* 52: 695–700, 1985

41. Kerr IB, Spandidos DA, Finlay IG, Lee FD, McArdle CS: The relation of ras family oncogene expression to conventional staging criteria and clinical outcome in colorectal carcinoma. *Br J Cancer* 53: 231–236, 1986

42. Gallick GE, Kurzrock R, Kloetzer WS, Arlinghans RB, Gutterman JU: Expression of p21^{ras} in fresh primary and metastatic human colorectal tumors. *Proc Natl Acad Sci USA* 82: 1795–1799, 1985

43. Horan Hand P, Thor A, Wunderlich D, Muraro R, Caruso A, Schlom J: Monoclonal antibodies of predefined specificity detect activated gene expression in human mammary and colon carcinomas. *Proc Natl Acad Sci USA* 81: 5227–5231, 1984

44. Thor A, Hand PH, Wunderlich D, Caruso A, Muraro R, Schlom J: Monoclonal antibodies define differential ras gene expression in malignant and benign colonic disease. *Nature* 311: 562–565, 1984

45. Yokata J, Tsunetsugu-Yokota Y, Battifora H, Le Feure C, Cline MJ: Alterations of myc, myb and ras^{Ha} proto-oncogenes in cancers are frequent and show clinical correlation. *Science* 231: 261–265, 1986

46. Little CD, Nau MM, Carney DN, Gazdar AF and Minna JD: Amplification and expression of the c-myc oncogene in human lung cancer cell lines. *Nature* 306: 194–196, 1983

47. Nau MM, Brooks BJ, Carney DN, Gazdar AF, Battey JF, Sausville EA, MInna JD: Human small-cell lung cancers show amplification and expression of the N-myc gene. *Proc Natl Acad Sci USA* 83: 1092–1096, 1986

48. Nau MM, Brooks BJ, Battery J, Sausville E, Gazdar AF, Kirsch IR, McBride OW, Bertness V, Hollis GF, Minna JD: L-myc, a new myc-related gene amplified and expressed in human small cell lung cancer. *Nature* 318: 69–73, 1985

49. Kohl NE, Gee CE, Alt FW: Activated expression of the N-myc gene in human neuroblastomas and related tumors. *Science* 226: 1335–1337, 1984

50. Schwab M, Ellison J, Busch M, Rosenau W, Varmus HE, Bishop JM: Enhanced expression of the human gene N-myc consequent to amplification of DNA may contribute to malignant progression of neuroblastoma. *Proc Natl Acad Sci USA* 81: 4940–4944, 1984

51. Brodeur GM, Seeger RC, Schwab M, Varmus HE, Bishop JM: Amplification of N-myc in untreated human neuroblastomas correlates with advanced disease stage. *Science* 224: 1121–1123, 1984

52. Fidler IJ, Kripke ML: Tumor cell antigenicity, host immunity and cancer mestastasis. *Cancer Immunol Immunother* 7: 201–205, 1980

53. Goodenow RS, Vogel JM, Linsk RL: Histocompatibility antigens on murine tumours. *Science* 230: 777–783, 1985

54. Travers PJ, Arklie JL, Trowsdale J, Patillo RA, Bodmer WF: Lack of expression of HLA-ABC antigens in choriocarcinoma and other human tumor cell lines. *Natl Cancer Inst Monogr* 60: 175–180, 1982

55. Doyle A, Martin W. John, Funa K, Gazdar A, Carney D, Martin SE, Linnoila I, Cuttitta F, Mulshine J, Bunn P, Minna J: Markedly decreased expression of class I histocompatibility antigens, protein and mRNA in human small-cell lung cancer. *J Exp Med* 161: 1135–1151, 1985

56. Wallich R, Balbuc N, Hammerling GL, Katzav S, Segal S, Feldman M: Abrogation of metastatic properties of tumour cells by de novo expression of H-2K antigen following H-2 gene transfection. *Nature* 315: 301–305, 1985

57. Isakov N, Katzav S, Feldman M, Segal S: Loss of expression of transplantation antigens encoded by the H-2K locus on Lewis lung carcinoma cells and its relevance to the tumor's metastatic properties. *J Natl Cancer Inst* 71: 139–145, 1983

58. Katzav S, de Baetselier PD, Tartakovsky B, Feldman M, Segal S: Alterations in major histocompatibility complex phenotypes of mouse cloned T10 sarcoma cells: association with shifts from non metastatic to metastatic cells. *J Natl Cancer Inst* 71: 317–324, 1983

59. Eisenbach L, Hollander N, Greenfeld L, Yakor H, Sega S and Feldman M: The differential expression of H-2K versus H-2D antigens, distinguishing high-metastatic from low-metastatic clones, is correlated with the immunogenic properties of the tumor cells. *Int J Cancer* 34: 567–573, 1984

60. Katzav S, Segal S, Feldman M: Immunoselection in vivo of H-2D phenotypic variants from a metastatic clone of sarcoma cells results in cell lines of altered metastatic competence. *Int J Cancer* 33: 407–415, 1984

61. Olsson L: Identification of a gene and its product associated with metastatic activity. *Fed Proc* 44: 5414A, 1985

62. Lampson La, Fisher CA, Whelan JP: Striking paucity of HLA-A, B, C and 2-microglobulin on human neuroblastoma cell lines. *J Immunol* 130: 2471–2478, 1983

63. Trowsdale J, Travers P, Bodmer WF, Patillo RA: Expression of HLA-A, -B and -C and beta 2-microglobulin antigens in human choriocarcinoma cell lines. *J Exp Med* 152 (Suppl): 11–17, 1980

64. Arce-Gomez B, Jones EA, Banstable CJ, Solomon E, Bodmer WF: The genetic control of HLA-A and B antigens in somatic cell hybrids: requirement for beta 2 microglobulin. *Tissue Antigens* 11: 96–112, 1977

65. Ruiter DJ, Bergman W, Welvoat K, Scheffer E, van Vloten WA, Ruso C, Ferrone S: Immunohistochemical analysis of malignant melanomas and nevocellular nevi with monoclonal antibodies to distinct monomorphic determinants of HLA antigens. *Cancer Res* 44: 3930–3935, 1984

66. Taramelli D, Fossati G, Mazzocchi A, Delia D, Ferrone S, Parmiani G: Class I and II HLA and melanoma-associated antigen expression and modulation on melanoma cells isolated from primary and metastatic lesions. *Cander Res* 46: 433–439, 1986

67. Moore M: Editorial. Natural immunity to tumours – theoretical predictions and biological observations. *Br J Cancer* 52: 147–151, 1985

68. Barlozzari T, Leonhardt J, Wiltrout RH, Herberman RB, Reynolds CW: Direct evidence for the role of LGL in the inhibition of experimental tumor metastases. *J Immunol* 134: 2783–2789, 1985

69. Hanna N, Burton RC: Definitive evidence that natural killer (NK) cells inhibit experimental tumor metastasis in vivo. *J Immunol* 127: 1754–1758, 1981

70. Karre K: Role of target histocompatibility antigens in regulation of natural killer cell activity – a reevaluation and a hypothesis. In: *Mechanisms of Cytotoxicity by Natural Killer Cells*, Herbeman RB and Callewaert D (eds) Academic Press, Orlando, pp 81–92, 1985

71. Taniguchi K, Karre K, Klein G: Lung colonisation and metastasis by disseminated B16 melanoma cells: H-2 associated control at the level of the host and the tumor cell. *Int J Cancer* 36: 503–510, 1983

72. Karre K, Ljunggren HG, Piontek G, Kiessling R: Selective rejection of H-2-deficient lymphoma variants suggests alternative immune defence strategy. *Nature* 319: 675–678, 1986

73. Alexander P: Dormant metastases – studies in experimental animals. *J Pathol* 141: 379–383, 1984

74. Wheelock EF, Brodovsky HS: Dormant cancer. In: *Prolonged Arrest of Cancer*, Stoll BA (ed) John Wiley, NY, pp 87–103

75. Brem S, Brem H, Folkman J, Finkelstein D, Patz A: Prolonged tumor dormancy by prevention of neovascularization in the vitreous. *Cancer Res* 36: 2807–2812, 1976

76. Noble RL, Hoover L: A classification of transplantable tumors in Nb rats controlled by estrogen from dormancy to autonomy. *Cancer Res* 35: 2935–2941, 1975

77. Fisher B, Fisher ER: Experimental studies of factors influencing hepatic metastases. II. Effects of partial hepatectomy. *Cancer* 12: 929–932, 1959

78. Tannock IF: The relation between cell proliferation and the vascular system in a transplanted mouse mammary tumour. *Br J Cancer* 22: 258–273, 1968

79. Vousden KH, Eccles SA, Purvies H, Marshall CJ: Enhanced spontaneous metastasis of mouse carcinoma cells transfected with an activated C-Ha-ras 1 gene. *Int J Cancer* 37: 427–433, 1986

80. Paget S: The distribution of secondary growth in cancer of the breast. *Lancet* 1: 571–573, 1889

81. Weiss L, Voit A, Lane WW: Metastatic patterns in patients with carcinomas of the lower oesophagus and upper rectum. *Inv Met* 4: 47–60, 1984

82. Hart IR: 'Seed and soil' revisited: mechanisms of site-specific metastasis. *Cancer Met Rev* 1: 5–17, 1982

83. Sugarbaker EV: Patterns of metastasis in human malignancies. In: *Cancer Biology Reviews*, Marchalonis JJ, Hanna MG, Fidler IJ (eds) Vol. 2. Marcel Dekker, New York, 1980

84. Tarin D, Price JE, Kettlewell MGW, Souter RG, Vass ACR, Crossley B: Mechanisms of human tumor metastasis studied in patients with peritoneovenous shunts. *Cancer Res* 44: 3584–3592, 1984

85. Gallatin WM, Weissman IL, Butcher EC: A cell-surface molecule involved in organ-specific homing of lymphocytes. *Nature* 304: 30–34, 1983

86. Stamper HB, Woodruff JJ: Lymphocyte homing into lymph nodes: in vitro demonstration of the selective affinity of recirculating lymphocytes for high-endothelial venules. *J Exp Med* 144: 828–833, 1976

87. Burcher EC, Scollay R, Weissman IL: Lymphocyte adherence to high endothelial venules: Characterisation of a modified *in vitro* assay, and examination of the binding of syngeneic and allogeneic lymphocyte populations. *J Immunol* 123: 1996–2003, 1979

88. Nicolson GL: Cancer metastasis organ colonization and the cell surface properties of malignant cells. *Biochim Biophys Acta* 695: 113–176, 1982

89. Hart IR, Talmadge JE, Fidler IJ: Metastatic behaviour of a murine reticulum cell sarcoma exhibiting organ-specific growth. *Cancer Res* 41: 1281–1287, 1981

90. Netland PA, Zetter BR: Organ-specific adhesion of metastatic tumor cells in vitro. *Science* 224: 113–115, 1984

91. Netland PA, Zetter BR: Metastatic potential of B16 melanoma cells after in vitro selection for organ-specific adherence. *J Cell Biol* 100: 720–724, 1985

92. St. John T, Gallatin WM, Siegelman M, Smith HT, Fried VA, Weissman IL: Expression cloning of a lymphocyte homing receptor cDNA: ubiquitin is the reactive species. *Science* 231: 845–850, 1986

93. Siegelman M, Bond MW, Gallatin WM, St. John T, Smith HT, Fried VA, Weissman IL: Cell surface molecule associated with lymphocyte homing is a ubiquitinated branched-chain glycoprotein. *Science* 231: 823–829, 1986

94. Vollmers HP, Birchmeier W: Monoclonal antibodies that prevent adhesion of B16 melanoma cells and reduce metastases in mice: Crossreaction with human tumor cells. *Proc Natl Acad Sci USA* 80: 6863–6867, 1983

95. Horak E, Darling D, Tarin D: Analysis of organ-specific effects on metastatic tumour formation. *J Natl Cancer Inst*. In press

96. Sporn MB, Roberts AB: Autocrine growth factors and cancer. *Nature* 313: 745–747, 1985

97. Todaro GJ, De Larco JE: Growth factors produced by sarcoma virus-transformed cells. *Cancer Res* 38: 4147–4154, 1978

98. Sporn MB, Todaro GE: Autocrine secretion and malignant transformation of cells. *New Eng J Med* 303: 878–880, 1980

99. Weinberg RA: The action of oncogenes in the cytoplasm and nucleus. *Science* 230: 770–776, 1985

100. Waterfield MD, Scrace GT, Whittle N, Stroobant P, Johnsson A, Wasteson A, Westermark B, Heldin C, Huang J, Deuel TF: Platelet-derived growth factor is structurally related to the putative transforming protein p28^{sis} of simian sarcoma virus. *Nature* 304: 35–39, 1983

101. Doolittle RF: Angiotensinogen is related to the antitrypsin-antithrombin-ovalbumin family. *Science* 222: 417–419, 1983

102. Downward J, Yarden Y, Mayes E, Scrace G, Totty N, Stockwell P, Ullrich A, Schlessinger J, Waterfield MD: Close similarity of epidermal growth factor receptor and v-erb-B oncogene protein sequences. *Nature* 307: 521–527, 1984

103. Sherr CJ, Rettenmier CW, Sacca R, Roussel MF, Look At, Stanley ER: The c-fms proto-oncogene product is related to the receptor for the mononuclear phagocyte growth factor, CSF-1. *Cell* 41: 665–676, 1985

104. Green S, Walter P, Kumar V, Krust A, Bornert J, Argos P, Chambon P: Human oestrogen receptor cDNA: sequence, expression and homology to v-erb A. *Nature* 320: 134–139, 1986

105. Sainsbury JRC, Farndon JR, Sherbert GV, Harris AL: Epidermal-growth-factor receptors and oestrogen receptors in human bladder cancer. *Lancet* 1: 364–366, 1985

106. Neal DE, Marsh C, Bennett MK, Abel PD, Hall RR, Sainsbury JRC, Harris AL: Epidermal-growth-factor receptors in human bladder cancer: comparison of invasive and superficial tumours. *Lancet* 1: 366–368, 1985

107. Stewart JF, King RJB, Sexton SA, Millis RR, Rubens RD, Hayward JL: Oestrogen receptors, sites of metastatic disease and survival in recurrent breast cancer. *Europ J Cancer* 17: 449–453, 1981

108. Poste G: Pathogenesis of metastatic disease: implications for current therapy and for the development of new therapeutic strategies. *Cancer Treat Rep* 70: 183–199, 1986

109. Cifone MA, Fidler IJ: Increasing metastatic potential is associated with increasing genetic instability of clones isolated from murine neoplasms. *Proc Natl Acad Sci USA* 78: 6949–6952, 1981

110. Donelli MG, Colombo T, Broggini M, Garattini S: Differential distribution of antitumour agents in primary and secondary tumours. *Cancer Treat Rep* 61: 1319–1324, 1977

111. Donelli MG, Colombo T, Dagnino G, Madonna M, Garattini S: Is better drug availability in secondary neoplasms responsible for better response to chemotherapy? *Eur J Cancer* 17: 201–209, 1981

110. Smith KA, Begg AC, Denekamp J: Differences in chemosensitivity between subcutaneous and pulmonary tumours. *Eur J Cancer Clin Oncol* 21: 249–256, 1985

113. Kerbel RS, Davis AJS: Facilitation of tumour progression by cancer therapy. *Lancet* II: 977–978, 1982

114. Nowell P: The clonal evolution of tumor cell populations. *Science* 194: 23–28, 1976

115. Benedict WF, Baker MS, Haroun L, Choi E, Ames BN: Mutagenicity of cancer chemotherapeutic agents in the salmonella/microsome test. *Cancer Res* 37: 2209–2213, 1979

116. Singh B, Gupta RS: Mutagenic responses of thirteen anticancer drugs on mutation induction at multiple genetic loci and on sister chromatid exchanges in Chinese hamster ovary cells. *Cancer Res* 43: 577–584, 1983

117. Ormerod EJ, Everett CA, Hart IR: Enhanced experimental metastatic capacity of a human tumor line following treatment with 5-azacytidine. *Cancer Res* 46: 884–890, 1986

118. McMillan TJ, Rao J, Hart IR: Enhancement of experimental metastasis by pretreatment of tumor cells with hydroxyurea. *Int J Cancer* 38: 61–65, 1986

119. McMillan TJ, Hart IR: The enhancement of experimental metastatic capcity of a murine melanoma by pre-treatment with anticancer drugs. *Clin Exp Met.* In press

120. Feinstein AR, Sosin DM, Wells CK: The Will Rogers Phenomenon: stage migration and new diagnostic techniques as a source of misleading statistics for survival in cancer. *New Eng J Med* 312: 1604–1608, 1985

121. Schabel FM: Concepts for systemic treatment of micrometastases. *Cancer* 35: 15–24, 1975

122. Hart IR, Fidler IJ: Role of organ selectivity in the determination of metastatic patterns of B16 melanoma. *Cancer Res* 40: 2281–2287, 1980

123. Viadana E, Bross IDJ, Pickren JW: Cascade spread of blood-borne metastases in solid and non-solid cancers of humans. In: *Pulmonary Metastasis.* Weiss L and Gilbert HA (eds), Hall, Boston, Mass, pp 142–167, 1978

124. Mule JJ, Shu S, Schwarz SL, Rosenberg SA: Adoptive immunotherapy of established pulmonary mestastases with LAK cells and recombinant interleukin-2. *Science* 225: 1487–1489, 1984

125. Rosenberg SA, Mule JJ, Spiess PJ, Reichert CM, Schwarz SL: Regression of established pulmonary metastases and subcutaneous tumor mediated by the systemic administration of high-dose recombinant interleukin 2. *J Exp Med* 161: 1169–1188, 1985

126. La Freniere R, Rosenberg SA: Successful immunotherapy of murine experimental hepatic metastases with lymphokine-activated killer cells and recombinant interleukin 2. *Cancer Res* 45: 3735–3741, 1985

127. Rosenberg SA: Combined modality therapy of cancer – what is it and when does it work. *New Eng J Med* 1512–1514, 1985

128. Fidler IJ: Therapy of spontaneous metastases by intravenous injection of liposomes containing lymphokines. *Science* 208: 1469–1471

129. Fidler IJ, Sone S, Fogler WE, Barnes ZL: Eradication of spontaneous metastases and activation of alveolar macrophages by intravenous injection of liposomes containing muramyl dipeptide. *Proc Natl Acad Sci USA* 78: 1680–1684, 1981

130. Xu ZL, BUcana CD, Fidler IJ: In vitro activation of murine kupffer cells by lymphokines or endotoxins to lyse syngeneic tumor cells. *Am J Path* 117: 372–379

131. Schroit AJ, Hart IR, Madsen J, Fidler IJ: Selective delivery of drug encpasulated in liposomes: natural targeting to macrophages involved in various disease states. *J Biol Response Modifiers* 2: 97–100, 1983

132. Oldham RK, Smalley RV: Biologicals and biological response modifiers. In: *Cancer Principles and Practice of Oncology.* Devita VT, Hellman S, Rosenberg SA (eds) Philadelphia, Vol. 1. pp 2223–2245, 1985

133. Lenhard RE, Order SE, Spunberg JJ, Asbell SO, Leibel SA: Isotopic immunoglobulin: a new systemic therapy for advanced Hodgkin's disease. *J Clin Oncol* 3: 1296–1300, 1985

10. Oncofetal and functional antigens in tissue

M.R. SCHWARTZ and W.B. PANKO

Introduction

Tumor markers is a term generally applied to products or of non-neoplastic tissue in response to tumors. Other terms that have been used include tumor-associated antigens, biomarkers, and cell markers. As no universal tumor marker and no tumor-specific antigen has yet been identified, we prefer to call these markers specific gene products or genes, depending on their type. At the present time, most markers we recognize are specific gene products which may be subclassified in several ways. Most tumor-related specific gene products are hormone receptors such as estrogen receptor, hormones such as calcitonin or human chorionic gonadotrophin, enzymes such as prostatic acid phosphatase or neuron specific enolase, and oncofetal antigens such as carcinoembryonic antigen or α fetoprotein.

A specific gene product may provide us with information about the biologic character of tumors in several ways:
- The presence of a marker which is normally present in tissue may indicate that tumor is better differentiated than one that lacks the marker. This is illustrated by the presence of estrogen receptor in breast carcinoma.
- The presence of a marker or specific gene product such as α fetoprotein which is not normally present in non-neoplastic tissue may indicate a loss or normal characteristics by the tumor.
- The presence of a normal but ectopic specific gene product, such as human chorionic gonadotrophin in gastric carcinoma may also indicate a loss of normal characteristics by a tumor.
- The presence of a normal specific gene product under inappropriate conditions, such as casein in breast carcinoma, may also indicate a loss of control mechanisms by a tumor.

Regardless of what specific gene products may tell us about cell lineage, they can be useful in predicting tumor behavior. The presence of these markers in the serum can be useful in monitoring response to therapy and detecting preclinical recurrence of tumor. Many specific gene products can be measured in blood or body fluids. However, the level of a specific marker in serum will depend on access of the marker to the circulation, rate of clearance, hepatic and renal function, hydration of the host, amount of production by the tumor, and amount of tumor. For these reasons, and because some markers cannot be measured in blood or other body fluids (e.g., estrogen receptor in blood), there has been an increasing interest in the identification of various specific gene products in tissue.

The presence or absence of any specific gene product must be interpreted with caution with respect to the implications it may have for prognosis. Thus, if tissue studies do not demonstrate any of the specific gene product of interest, whereas the serum does, this may be due to inadequate tissue sampling of a heterogeneous neoplasm, insensitive identification techniques, or loss of antigenic marker during processing. The reverse may also apply. Again, the presence or absence of a specific gene product does not yield any information about the host's response to the tumor.

There any many tumor markers or specific gene products and it is more useful to discuss a few in depth rather than present an encyclopedic list. The markers selected are those of current interest and the subject of more investigations. These include the oncofetal antigens, carcinoembryonic antigen and α fetoprotein; human chorionic gonadotrophin and other placental proteins; and blood group antigens.

Carcinoembryonic antigen

Carcinoembryonic antigen (CEA) was first described by Gold and Freedman in 1965 [1–2]. They described tumor-specific antigens in adenocarcinoma of the colon which they could not identify in normal colon. Because these and identical antigens were subsequently identified in other endodermally-derived, malignant neoplasms of the gastrointestinal tract and pancreas, as well as in fetal gut, pancreas, and liver between two and six months of gestation, CEA was intitially thought to be a specific marker of gastrointestinal tumors. However, it has subsequently been identified, predominantly by immunohistochemical methods, also in a variety of normal adult and malignant tissues, including normal colonic mucosa, colon in chronic ulcerative colitis, medullary carcinoma of the thyroid, germ cell tumors, cystosarcoma phylloides, and carcinomas of the breast, lung, kidney, urinary bladder, cervix, endometrium, and ovary.

CEA is a glycoprotein having a molecular weight of about 180,000 daltons. It has become apparent over the past twenty years that there are a number of substances found in normal tissues and neoplasms which cross-react with many available CEA antibodies because of shared antigenic determinants [3]. These substances include nonspecific cross-reacting antigen (NCA), NCA-2, normal fetal antigens-1 and -2, normal fetal cross-reacting antigen, and biliary glycoprotein I. The diverse specificities of various CEA antisera and the presence of these cross-reacting antigens in the tested tissue are partially responsible for the variation in results between studies of CEA in tissue. Many investigators have not used CEA antisera absorbed to decrease cross reaction with these related glycoproteins and glycolipids.

ABO(H) blood group substances are biochemically similar to CEA and may also cross-react with antibodies to CEA. This raises questions about the reported frequency of CEA in various normal and neoplastic tissues. For example, Nap et al. [4] found that immunoeroxidase staining for CEA disappeared in normal lung, liver, stomach, and spleen, as well as in four of nine previously positive breast carcinomas (but not in normal colon and colon carcinoma) after absorbing commercial CEA antisera with nonspecific cross-reacting antigen from white blood cells.

Although serial plasma CEA levels in patients with colorectal carcinoma are widely accepted as useful in monitoring for tumor recurrence and response to treatment in metastatic disease, there is lack of agreement as to the utility of assessing tissue CEA in this or any other type or carcinoma. Using primarily immunohistochemical techniques, CEA has been localized in 70–100% of large bowel adenocarcinomas, as well as in normal or nonneoplastic colonic mucosa, although in a smaller number of studies and always with a lesser number of cells staining to a lesser degree. Au et al. [5], using an immunoperoxidase technique and commercial polyclonal CEA antiserum not further absorbed, found no staining of normal colonic mucosa and positive staining of all forty colorectal carcinomas tested. As half of the patients survived more than five years and the other half died of their carcinoma within five years, Au et al. concluded that, in the absence of techniques for quantitative evaluation, presence or absence of tissue CEA was not of prognostic value.

There are contradictory findings in studies of the relationship of tissue CEA to histologic grade in large bowel carcinomas. Some investigators find significantly less tissue CEA in well differentiated carcinomas, others find less in poorly differentiated carcinomas, and still others find no significant relationship at all [6–8].

Several investigators have suggested that immunohistochemical staining of a large bowel adenocarcinoma for CEA may predict the usefulness of serial plasma CEA determinations for monitoring disease recurrence or progression. Using radioimmunoassay for measurement of CEA content in extracts of colorectal carcinomas, Wagener et al. [9] found that, although there was no significant correlation between tumor CEA concentration and plasma CEA, high plasma CEA levels were rarely associated with low tumor CEA content. Thus, in general, significant CEA production by the carcinoma appeared to be required for elevation of the plasma CEA level.

Goslin et al. [10] immunocytochemically examined poorly differentiated colorectal carcinomas from seventeen patients. All of the patients with negative CEA staining of their primary or metastatic tumor had normal preoperative plasma CEA levels, and none manifested elevated CEA plasma levels postoperatively despite development of metastatic disease in all. On the other hand, all patients with positive staining of their primary tumor, who had been operated on for cure and who subsequently relapsed, developed elevated CEA plasma levels before clinical detection of their recurrence.

Midiri *et al.* [8] found that eight of thirty-eight (21%) patients with elevated preoperative plasma CEA had negative immunocytochemical staining for CEA. Four of these patients were found to have elevated CEA due to liver or other disease not related to the carcinoma, illustrating that elevated plasma CEA in the face of negative tissue staining does not necessarily imply undetected metastases or technical problems with the staining. Of nineteen patients with normal preoperative plasma CEA levels, eleven (58%) had carcinomas which stained positively.

What can we conclude from these studies? Given the very high frequency of immunohistochemically detectable CEA in colorecal adenocarcinomas, the difficulties in quantitation of immunohistochemical stains, and the heterogeneity of antibodies, the presence or absence of stainable CEA does not appear to provide reliable prognostic information about survival. While a few small studies suggest that the presence of stainable tissue CEA will predict the usefulness of postoperative CEA serum levels, the numbers in the studies are small and the results among studies conflicting. We do not feel that routine staining of primary colorectal carcinomas for selection of patients to be followed with serial CEA levels is warranted at this time.

There are conflicting results and conclusions from studies of tissue CEA in other organs. Based on results similar to their earlier ones about colorectal carcinoma, Goslin *et al.* [10] reported that the presence of immunocytochemically detectable CEA in small cell carcinoma of the lung predicted the usefulness of serial plasma CEA levels in monitoring response to therapy and prediction of relapse. Elevated plasma CEA appeared to be associated with tumor CEA production as measured by positive staining, although the correlation was not perfect.

After evaluating patients who underwent radical surgery for all types of lung carcinoma except well differentiated squamous cell carcinoma, Ford *et al.* [11] found, in contrast to Goslin *et al.* [12], that immunocytochemical staining was not of value in selecting patients for serial CEA monitoring nor was it of prognostic value. They attributed this to the overall high frequency of positive staining (78%), with frequencies similar in patients with low and high pre- and postoperative serum CEA levels.

There has been considerable attention directed at CEA in breast carcinoma as a possible predictor of biologic behavior. The results of the studies are conflicting, with broad variance among described relationships between CEA and a number of clinical, pathologic, and. biochemical parameters. The percentage of CEA positive breast carcinomas varies from 1.6% to over 90% and CEA has been identified infrequently in normal or fibrocystic breast tissue. Shousha et al. [13] in a retrospective immunohistochemical study found that patients with CEA positive carcinomas had significantly lower five and ten year survival rates than patients with CEA negative carcinomas. There was no significant relationship between presence of tumor CEA and histologic type. A similar type of study using a more specific antiserum [14] found an apparent relationship between histologic differentiation and presence of CEA, with poorly differentiated carcinomas having the lowest incidence of CEA.

Smith et al. [15] using an immunocytochemical technique found no relationship between the presence or absence of stainable CEA in the primary carcinoma and recurrence-free survival. However, the CEA status of the axillary lymph nodes was significantly related to recurrence and prognosis. Schwartz et al. [16] found no relationship between tumor CEA content and tumor size, histologic type, degree of differentiation, estrogen or progesterone receptor content, axillary lymph node status, patient age, menstrual status, or race. There was a statistically significant relationship between cytosol CEA content and postsurgical treatment-pathologic stage, with carcinomas from patients in combined stages III-IV having significantly higher CEA content than those from patients in combined stages I-II disease.

Mansour et al. [17] in a prospective immunoperoxidase study of patients with stages I and II breast carcinoma found only 68% concordance between tissue and preoperative plasma CEA. A significantly greater proportion of CEA positive carcinomas were stage II rather than stage I.

Several recent studies of breast carcinoma have not found a relationship between prognosis and a number of tumor markers, including CEA [18–19]. Using the methodology of Mansour et al. [17], the Eastern Cooperative Oncology Group (ECOG) evaluated immunohistochemical staining of CEA in breast carcinomas of postmenopausal node-positive women. This cooperative group did not find any correlation between presence of tissue CEA and disease-free interval [20].

α Fetoprotein

α fetoprotein (AFP) is normally synthesized in the yolk sac, liver, and, to a lesser extent, gastrointestinal tract of the embryo and fetus. Malignant neoplasms arising from the liver, i.e., hepatocellular carcinoma and hepatoblastoma, and those containing yolk sac elements are commonly associated with AFP production. AFP has also been identified in occasional gastrointestinal tract carcinomas, rare lung carcinomas, some hepatic metastases, and germ cell tumors other than yolk sac tumors.

Interest in recent years has focused on AFP in germ cell tumors, particularly those of testicular origin. AFP has been identified in testicular, ovarian, and extragonadal yolk sac tumors by virtually all investigators. Except for one questionable case report, pure seminomas are not associated with AFP production. While some investigators have identified AFP only in yolk sac elements, others have demonstrated AFP in approximately 50–75% of embryonal carcinomas and in a smaller proportion of epithelial teratomatous components [21–24]. Some of the variation may be due to differences in distinction between yolk sac tumors and embryonal carcinoma among various investigators or to the difficulty in localizing AFP and problems of reproducibility with most AFP antisera.

Morinaga *et al.* [24] demonstrated good correlation between results of radioimmunoassay of tissue extracts and immunoperoxidase stains for HCG and AFP, i.e., tissues negative by RIA did not stain and vice versa. There are few good studies correlating serum levels and tissue localization of AFP and HCG. In many of the studies, serum levels were obtained in many laboratories making comparison difficult, and in other studies only postoperative levels drawn at variable intervals were available. Using an immunoperoxidase technique, Kurman *et al.* [21] demonstrated AFP in testicular germ cell tumors of eight of thirteen patients (53%) with elevated serum AFP. Tumors which stained positively for AFP occurred more frequently, although not exclusively, in patients with higher levels of serum AFP. Mostofi [25], studying 300 testicular tumors for AFP and HCG by immunoperoxidase, also noted a correlation between the level of the marker in serum or urine and the quantity of cells staining in tissue sections.

While the presence of AFP has not been shown to be an independent predictor of prognosis [26], some believe that the demonstration of AFP (or HCG) in testicular germ cell tumors indicates the likely elevation of the marker when the tumor metastasizes [27]. Conversely, one would not expect elevated serum AFP levels with metastases from a primary which stained negatively.

Human chorionic gonadotrophin and other placental proteins

While human chorionic gonadotrophin (HCG) is normally produced in the placenta, it has been found in the serum, urine, and tissue of patients with a variety of trophoblastic and nontrophoblastic malignant neoplasms. There have been a number of hypotheses as to why ectopic production of HCG by non-trophoblastic tumors occurs. These include recruitment of uncommitted cells, derepression of genes, and random mutation. HCG-like material has been described in normal spermatozoa, testis, liver, colon, pituitary, plasma, and fetal liver and kidney [28]. If HCG is produced in normal tissue, than derepression of genes in malignant neoplasms would be quantitatively, rather than qualitatively, different from normal. The possibility exists, of course, that the HCG assays are detecting cross-reacting antigens.

Most of the studies of placental proteins in tumors have focused on testicular germ cell tumors. While β-HCG and AFP are generally accepted as useful serum markers in the followup of patients with these tumors, the significance of these markers in tissue is less clear. β-HCG is almost universally identified in choriocarcinomas and choriocarcinomatous components of mixed germ cell tumors. β-HCG has been localized immunohistochemically predominantly in the syncytiotrophoblast, with lesser amounts in the trophoblast. Using immunohistochemical techniques, various investigators have reported finding β-HCG in 40-70% of nonseminomatous testicular germ cell tumors, the vast majority of which are not choriocarcinomas. Embryonal carcinomas frequently contain cells which stain positively for β-HCG, whereas yolk sac tumors do much less frequently, and teratomatous components of germ cell tumors still more rarely [21–24]. In these nonchoriocarcinomatous tumors, β-HCG is almost always localized in syncytiotrophoblastic giant cells or in tumor giant cells, and only rarely in mononuclear tumor cells. While earlier studies suggested that the presence of β-HCG positive cells in testicular non-seminomatous germ cell tumors adversely affected prognosis, later studies have not found their presence to be of prognostic significance [26, 29–30].

There has been considerable speculation on the significance of detectable β-HCG in testicular seminomas. β-HCG has been identified immunocytochemically in 3–23% of seminomas [21–24, 31]. In addition to differences in antisera and techniques, some of the variation may be related to the number of sections examined. β-HCG in seminomas is localized in syncytiotrophoblastic giant cells (or occasionally in tumor giant cells) which may be infrequent, and therefore missed if a number of sections are not examined. Not all of the syncytiotrophoblastic giant cells will stain with antisera against β-HCG. Problems of correlating tissue and serum β-HCG in individual patients have been discussed above (see AFP discussion). The proportion of patients with seminoma presenting with elevated serum β-HCG is similar to the proposition of seminomas with stainable β-HCG. The elevated serum β-HCG in patients with allegedly pure seminomas has been attributed to the syncytiotrophoblastic giant cells producing β-HCG. The possibility does of course exist that an elevated serum β-HCG in a patient with apparently pure seminoma may be due to an occult focus of nonseminomatous tumor.

While some investigators have concluded that pure seminomas with β-HCG-positive cells have a worse prognosis [32], most have not found their presence to adversely affect prognosis [31, 33]. This generally concurs with conclusions reached relative to the presence of syncytiotrophoblastic giant cells *per se* in seminomas.

Other placental proteins including pregnancy-specific-β-1-glycoprotein (SP-1), placental protein five (PP5), and placental lactogen have been studied in testicular germ cell tumors to a lesser extent than β-HCG . They have been found in choriocarcinomas where they appear to be localized immunocytochemically primarily to syncytiotrophoblastic giant cells with occasional localization to other multinucleated or uninucleated giant cells [22, 30–31]. The presence of these additional placental proteins has not been shown to be related to prognosis [30–31].

The data on β-HCG in tumors from other organs is much less substantial. β-HCG has been found, primarily in immunocytochemical studies, in a variety of nontesticular germ cell tumors, including ovarian and extragonadal germ cell tumors, hepatoblastomas, and carcinomas of the lung, breast, stomach, colon, and ovary. Other placental proteins have also been identified in a variety of nongerm cell neoplasms [28, 34]. In a retrospective immunoperoxidase study of breast carcinomas, Horne *et al.* [35] found SP-1, HCG, and placental lactogen in 76%, 60%, and 82% of the cases, respectively. While there was no prognostic significance related to the presence or absence of HCG, patients with carcinomas negative for placental lactogen survived significantly longer than those with positive carcinomas. The relationship between longer survival and absence of the marker was stronger for SP-1.

Several recent studies have been unable to demonstrate a relationship between prognosis and a number of tumor markers, including placental proteins. In a collaborative retrospective immunoperoxidase study of multiple tumor markers in 233 cases of invasive breast carcinoma, Lee *et al.* [18] identified β-HCG, placental lactogen, SP-A, α-lactalbumin, and CEA in 18%, 30%, 56%, 56%, and 79% of the carcinomas, respectively. There was no significant relationship between any of these markers and a number of clinical, pathologic, and epidemiologic parameters. Futhermore, none of the markers alone or in combination were useful in assessing prognosis, with the expression of none being significantly related to likelihood of recurrence, interval before recurrence, or presence of metastases. In another immunoperoxidase study of multiple markers in breast carcinoma, Barry *et al.* [19] were also not able to demonstrate a relationship between prognosis and a number of tumor markers, including CEA, casein, secretory component of IgA, α-lactalbumin, SP-1, and placental lactogen.

Kuhajda *et al.* [36–37] have demonstrated a significant correlation between immunocytochemically detected pregnancy-associated plasma protein (PAPP-A) in primary breast carcinomas and early recurrence (within two years of mastectomy) in stage I and II disease. In patients with stage II breast carcinoma, these investigators found that staining for SP-1 was not significantly correlated with early recurrence while staining for PP5 was but was not independent of PAPP-A positivity. None of the other many clinical and pathologic features examined correlated with early recurrence in this study. In patients with stage I carcinoma, PAPP-A positivity and estrogen receptor status were independent predictors of early recurrence. PAPP-A, like SP-1 and PP5, is normally found in the placenta. These proteins apparently have local immunosuppressive and anti-coagulative effects. It has been suggested that production of PAPP-A by the carcinoma may locally alter the coagulation system, thus allowing neoplastic cells to enter and travel within vessels to produce metastases [37].

Blood group antigens

ABO(H) blood group antigens are glycosamines which are attached to the surface membranes of red blood cells, endothelial cells, and a variety of epithelial cells including those of lung, cervix, breast, gastrointestinal tract, kidney, and urinary bladder. Expression of blood groop antigens is altered in neoplasms. The most common finding is decrease or loss of ABO(H) expression, although in some tumors blood group antigens re-emerge in locations where they cannot be detected in normal adult tissue, such as in distal colon and rectum.

Much of the interest in ABO(H) blood group antigens in tissue has focused on transitional cell carcinomas of the urinary bladder. While earlier studies were performed using the specific red blood cell adherence test, more recently immunoperoxidase techniques have been used employing anti-A and anti-B antisera and the lectin Ulex europaeus as an anti-O(H antigen) reagent. Wiley *et al.* [38] using an immunoperoxidase technique to detect blood group antigens A and B in transitional cell carcinomas demonstrated that the presence of these antigens was significantly related to histologic grade and clinical course. In their study, all carcinomas which stained positively were noninvasive stage 0 tumors, and all but one of these was grade I or II. In contrast, over half of the blood group antigen negative carcinomas were invasive and over half were grade III. Of those patients with adequate follow-up, none with blood group antigen positive tumors developed invasive carcinoma, whereas most with blood group antigen negative tumors either presented with invasive carcinoma or developed it at a later date.

These findings agree with those of most other investigators, who have reported that the absence of ABO(H) blood group antigens in transitional cell carcinoma correlates with higher histologic grade, higher stage, greater incidence of recurrence, and greater incidence of subsequently developing invasive carcinoma in initially noninvasive tumors. However, not all studies are in agreement. For example, Nakatsu *et al.* [39] using immunoperoxidase techniques to study ABO(H) antigens in transitional cell carcinomas of the bladder found that the absence of blood group antigens did not correlate with subsequent intravesical recurrences.

The T blood group antigen or Thomas-Friedenreich antigen is the precursor of the blood group MN system. It is normally present in a masked state on the surface of red blood cells covered with a terminal sialic acid. Whereas many investigators have not identified this antigen in normal epithelial tissue, some have identified it in a variety of normal organs, such as large bowel and breast, more often after unmasking of the antigen by neuraminidase digestion. The T antigen has been detected much more frequently in malignant neoplasms.

The lectin, peanut agglutinin binds to the major determinant of the T antigen, β-D-galactose(1–3)-N-acetyl-D-galactosamine. This lectin has been used in immunocytochemical studies to localize the T antigen in histologic sections. Using this method without neuraminidase digestion, Coon *et al.* [40] detected T antigen in

152

28% of low grade and 67% of high grade transitional cell carcinomas of the urinary bladder. Cryptic T antigen could be identified after digestion in most of the T-antigen negative, low grade transitional cell carcinomas but in only one T-antigen negative, high grade tumor. There was a statistically significant correlation between T-antigen status and histologic grade, tumor recurrence, and subsequent invasion. Low grade carcinomas which were T-antigen positive or cryptic T-antigen negative had a significantly increased incidence of subsequent invasion.

Cooper [41] demonstrated peanut lectin binding in six of fifteen cases of normal colonic epithelium and in an additional eight after neuraminidase digestion. Twenty-six of thirty-three (79%) rectosigmoid carcinomas bound peanut lectin, and all but one of the seven initially negative carcinomas showed positive staining after neuraminidase treatment. Cooper found no correlation between tumor stage and T antigen status as identified by peanut lectin binding.

The peanut lectin may apparently bind to antigens other than the T antigen. Klein et al. [42] identified peanut lectin binding in normal and malignant breast tissue. In most cases, there was concurrence and similar distribution between staining with peanut lectin and with monoclonal antibodies against milk fat globule membrane, leading the authors to conclude that the peanut lectin receptor in breast is a constituent of a milk protein. Staining with peanut lectin was reported to be related to some degree with histologic differentiation. There was good correlation between results of peanut lectin binding and steroid hormone content. The majority of estrogen and progesterone receptorpositive carcinomas showed positive lectin binding, whereas only a few estrogen and progesterone receptor negative carcinomas did. Over 75% of patients with breast carcinomas having greater than 10% peanut lectin binding tumor cells responded to endocrine therapy, whereas only about 14% of patients having less than 10% such cells responded.

Polyclonal and monoclonal antibodies to T antigen as well as to Tn antigen, the immediate precursor of T, have also been used in immunohistochemical studies. Anti-Tn does not generally react with normal tissue. However, most carcinomas express both T and Tn antigen identifiable by these antibodies [43]. Studies are in progress looking at Tn as a predictor of agressiveness of a carcinoma.

Conclusion

It is difficult to draw many conclusions from most of the studies which have been done to date. There is a great heterogeneity of techniques and results. Many of the reported studies are of a small number of patients and/or tumors, with total cases per study not infrequently 20–30. Futhermore, many of the studies are retrospective and thus subject to all the problems of retrospective studies.

Most of the current studies of tumor markers in tissue, other than steroid receptors, have been done using immunocytochemical techniques and polyclonal antibodies. While one of the advantages of immunocytochemistry is that the cells presumably containing the antigen of interest can be visualized, there are numerous problems with this technique, many of which relate to the differences among the various studies. Many of the differences among studies are attributable to the following factors:

- One of the causes of heterogeneity among studies is the variable definition of positive, e.g., in one study positive might be defined as at least 20% of the cells staining positively, whereas in another study positive might be defined as at least 50% of the cells being stained.
- The varying specificities and binding properties of the primary antisera are an important source of heterogeneity among studies. This is exemplified by studies of CEA, where differences in antibody specificity and cross-reactivity to normal glycoproteins has lead to very conflicting data. Much of the present work has been done with polyclonal antibodies which have variable sensitivity and specificity and for which there is a limited supply of any one preparation.
- It is difficult to standardize the reagents.

The development of monoclonal antibodies promises to provide an unlimited supply of homogeneous reagents of reproducible specificity and sensitivity. However, the use of monoclonal antibodies will not abolish the heterogeneity among studies as there are diverse specificities among these antibodies. This is mainly due to the fact that each monoclonal antibody detects only one antigenic determinant on a molecule, but these are not the same from antibody to antibody. Furthermore, while cross-reactions are reduced in frequency with the use of monoclonal antibodies, they are not eliminated, as monoclonal antibodies may recognize a common determinant present on different molecules.

Other sources of differences among the immunocytochemical studies are differing immunocytochemical techniques and technical problems. Proper tissue processing is crucial. Autolysis, improper fixation, and excess heat will all result in destruction of antigen. Digestion of tissue sections, antibody titer, duration of incubation, and staining reagents can all affect the results. A major problem with most of the current immunocytochemical studies is the lack of reproducible quantification. This, added to the factors discussed above, makes it very difficult to make reliable comparisons between studies or reach definite conclusions about individual studies.

References

1. Gold P, Freedman SO: Demonstration of tumor-specific antigens in human colonic carcinomata by immunological tolerance and absorption techniques. *J Exp Med* 121: 439–462, 1965

2. Gold P, Freedman SO: Specific carcinoembryonic antigens of the human digestive system. *J Exp Med* 122: 467–481, 1965

3. Burtin P: The carcinoembryonic antigen of the digestive system (CEA) and the antigens cross-reacting with it. *Ann Immunol* (Paris) 129: 185–198, 1978

4. Nap M, ten Hoor KA, Fleuren GJ: Cross-reactivity with normal antigens in commercial anti-CEA sera, used for immunohistology. The need for tissue controls and absorptions. *Am J Clin Pathol* 79: 25–31, 1983

5. Au FC, Stein BS, Gennaro AR, Tyson RR: Tissue CEA in colorectal carcinoma. *Dis Colon Rectum* 27: 16–18, 1984

6. Rognum T, Elgjo K, Brandtzaeg P *et al.*: Plasma carcinoembryonic antigen concentrations and immunohistochemical patterns of epithelial marker antigens in patients with large bowel carcinoma. *J Clin Pathol* 35: 922–933, 1982

7. O'Brien MJ, Zamcheck N, Burke B *et al.*: Immunocytochemical localization of carcinoembryonic antigen in benign and malignant colorectal tissues. Assessment of diagnostic value. *Am J Clin Pathol* 75: 283–290, 1981

8. Midiri G, Amanti C, Benedetti M *et al.*: CEA tissue staining in colorectal cancer patients. A way to improve the usefulness of serial serum CEA evaluation. *Cancer* 55: 2624–2629, 1985

9. Wagener C, Muller-Wallraf R, Groner J, Breuer H: Plasma concentration of carcinoembryonic antigen: Correlation with immunohistochemical and radioimmunological tumor parameters. In: *Carcino-embryonic Proteins*, Vol. II, Lehmann FG (ed). Amsterdam: Elsevier/North-Holland Biomedical Press, 1979, pp 833–839

10. Goslin R, O'Brien MJ, Steele G *et al.*: Correlation of plasma CEA and CEA tissue staining in poorly differentiated colorectal carcinoma. *Am J Med* 71: 246–253, 1981

11. Ford CHJ, Stokes HJ, Newman CE: Carcinoembryonic antigen and prognosis after radical surgery for lung cancer. Immunocytochemical localization and serum levels. *Br J Cancer* 44: 145–153, 1981

12. Goslin RH, O'Brien MJ, Skarin AT *et al.*: Immunocytochemical staining for CEA in small cell carcinoma of lung predicts clinical usefulness of the plasma assay. *Cancer* 52: 301–306, 1983

13. Shousha S, Lyssiotis T, Godfrey VM, Scheuer PJ: Carcinoembryonic antigen in breast-cancer tissue: a useful prognostic indicator. *Br Med J* 1: 777–779, 1978

14. Walker RA: Demonstration of carcinoembryonic antigen in human breast carcinomas by the immunoperoxidase technique. *J Clin Pathol* 33: 356–360, 1980

15. Smith R, Howell A, Minawa A, Morrison JM: The clinical value of immunohistochemically demonstrable CEA in breast cancer: A possible method of selecting patients for adjuvant therapy. *Br J Cancer* 46: 757–764, 1982

16. Schwartz MR, Randolph RL, Panko WB: Carcinoembryonic antigen and steroid receptors in the cytosol of carcinoma of the breast. Relationship to pathologic and clinical features. *Cancer* 55: 2464–2471, 1985

17. Mansour EG, Hastert M, Park CH *et al.*: Tissue and plasma carcinoembryonic antigen in early breast cancer: A prognostic factor. *Cancer* 51: 1243–1248, 1983

18. Lee AK, Rosen PP, DeLellis RA *et al.*: Tumor marker expression in breast carcinomas and relationship to prognosis. An immunohistochemical study. *Am J Clin Pathol* 84: 687–696, 1985

19. Barry JD, Koch TJ, Cohen C *et al.*: Correlation of immunohistochemical markers with patient prognosis in breast carcinoma: A quantitative study. *Am J Clin Pathol* 82: 582–585, 1984

20. Gilchrist KW, Kalish L, Gould VE, *et al.*: Immunostaining for carcinoembryonic antigen does not discriminate for early recurrence in breast cancer. The ECOG experience. *Cancer* 56: 351–355, 1985

21. Kurman RJ, Scardino PT, McIntire R, *et al.*: Cellular localization of alpha-fetoprotein and human chorionic gonadotropin in germ cell tumors of the testis using an indirect immunoperoxidase technique. A new approach to classification utilizing tumor markers. *Cancer* 40: 2136–2151, 1977

22. Jacobsen GK, Jacobsen M, Clausen PP: Distribution of tumor-associated antigens in the various histologic components of germ cell tumors of the testis. *Am J Surg Pathol* 5: 257–266, 1981

23. Wittekind C, Wichman T, Von Kleist S: Immunohistological localization of AFP and HCG in uniformly classified testis tumors. *Anticancer Research* 3: 327–333, 1983

24. Morinaga S, Ojima M, Sasano N: Human chorionic gonadotropin and alpha-fetoprotein in testicular germ cell tumors. An immunohistochemical study in comparison with tissue concentration. *Cancer* 52: 1281–1289, 1983

25. Mostofi FK: Pathology of germ cell tumors of testis. A progress report. *Cancer* 456: 1735–1754, 1980

26. Kramer SA, Wold LE, Gilchrist GS, *et al.*: Yolk sac carcinoma: An immunohistochemical and clinicopathologic review. *J Urol* 131: 315–318, 1984

27. Heyderman E: Advances in pathology and immunocytochemistry. *J Royal Soc Med* (Suppl No 6) Vol 78: 9–18, 1985

28. Heyderman E, Chapman DV, Richardson TC *et al.*: Human chorionic gonadotropin and human placental lactogen in extragonadal tumors. An immunoperoxidase study of ten non-germ cell neoplasms. *Cancer* 56: 2674–2682, 1985

29. Raghavan D, Peckham MJ, Heyderman E *et al.*: Prognostic factors in clinical stage I non-seminomatous germ-cell tumours of the testis. *Br J Cancer* 45: 167–173, 1982

30. Masters JWR, Parkinson MC, Miller ID, Horne CHW: The prevalence and prognostic significance of trophoblastic proteins in testicular teratoma. *Diagnostic Histopathology* 6: 247–252, 1983

31. Steffens J, Friedmann W, Nagel R: Immunohistochemical and radioimmunological determination of B-HCG and pregnancy-specific B1-protein in seminomas. *Urol Int* 40: 72–75, 1985

32. Morgan DAL, Caillud JM, Bellet D, Eschwege F: Gonadotrophin-producing seminoma: A distinct category of germ cell neoplasm. *Clin Radiol* 33: 149–153, 1982

33. Javadpour N: Human chorionic gonadotropin in seminoma (Commentary). *J Urol* 131: 407, 1984

34. Ito H, Tahara E: Human chorionic gonadotropin in human gastric carcinoma. A retrospective immunohistochemical study. *Acta Pathol Jpn* 33: 287–296, 1983

35. Horne CHW, Reid IN, Milne GD: Prognostic significance of inappropriate production of pregnancy proteins by breast cancers. *Lancet* 1: 279–282, 1982

36. Kuhajda FP, Abeloff MD, Eggleston JC: Pregnancy-associated plasma protein A: A clinically significant predictor of early recurrence in Stage II breast carcinoma. *Hum Path* 16: 228–235, 1985

37. Kuhajda FP, Eggleston JC: Pregnancy-associated plasma protein A. A clinically significant predictor of early recurrence in Stage I breast carcinoma is independent of estrogen receptor status. *Am J Pathol* 121: 342–348, 1985

38. Wiley EL, Mendelsohn G, Droller MJ, Eggleston JC: Immunoperoxidase detection of carcinoembryonic antigen and blood group substances in papillary transitional cell carcinoma of the bladder. *J Urol* 128: 276–280, 1982

39. Nakatsu H, Kobayashi I, Onishi Y *et al.*: ABO(H) blood group antigens and carcinoembryonic antigens as indicators of malignant potential in patients with transitional cell carcinoma of the bladder. *J Urol* 131: 252–257, 1984

40. Coon JS, Weinstein RS, Summers JL: Blood group precursor T-antigen expression in human urinary bladder carcinoma. *Am J Clin Pathol* 77: 692–699, 1982

41. Cooper HS: Peanut lectin-binding sites in large bowel carcinoma. *Lab Invest* 47: 383–390, 1982

42. Klein PJ, Vierbuchen M, Fisher J *et al.*: The significance of lectin receptors for the evaluation of hormone dependence in breast cancer. *J Steroid Biochem* 19: 839–844, 1983

43. Springer GF, Taylor CR, Howard D *et al.*: Tn, a carcinoma-associated antigen, reacts with anti-Tn of normal human sera. *Cancer* 55: 561–569, 1985

11. Factors in resistance to chemotherapy cure

L. LEVIN, J.F. HARRIS and A.F. CHAMBERS

This chapter considers mechanisms of resistance and also the ways of overcoming resistance to chemotherapy in the cancer patient. First it will consider 'apparent' drug resistance which arises when an otherwise effective drug is unable to reach the tumor cells in sufficiently high concentration. Second, it will discuss biological aspects of true drug resistance, emphasizing the genetic development of drug resistant cells [see Table 1].

Apparent resistance to chemotherapy

A number of factors can lead to failure of a drug to reach tumor cells in sufficiently high concentration to be cytotoxic. Thus, bioavailability may be affected by absorption (for drugs given orally), by factors affecting drug activation (e.g., conversion of cyclophosphamide to phosphoramine mustard by hepatic microsomes), protein binding, or drug delivery to the tumor site. As most cytotoxic drugs are administered intravenously and impaired drug activation is uncommon, the most important reason for apparent drug resistance is impaired drug delivery to the tumor site in sufficiently high concentration.

Anatomical site

Inability of cytotoxic drugs to reach the tumor site is illustrated in the case of tumors of the central nervous system. In this situation, the tumor is in an anatomically sequestered site, and drug delivery is impeded by physiological barriers such as tight junctions between endothelial cells in the CNS capillaries. It is controversial whether this blood brain barrier is intact in malignant brain tumors [1], but nevertheless, there is considerable evidence that it represents an obstacle to drug delivery. It is not uncommon to see tumor regression in extraneural sites while there is concomitant increase in the size of brain metastases.

Successful imaging of cerebral mestastases by contrast medium only after disrupting the blood brain barrier by an intracarotid mannitol infusion [2] also implies a pre-existing impediment to drug delivery (overcome in the case of leptomeningeal metastases by administering the drug intrathecally). Osmotic disruption of the blood brain barrier [2] may thus offer a new approach to the treatment of CNS tumors with cytotoxic drugs. An alternative is the use of drugs such as BCNU which are able to cross the blood brain barrier.

Dose intensity considerations

For most chemosensitive tumors, the dose response curve is steep, and relatively small reductions in dose may be associated with a markedly reduced clinical response which may inappropriately be attributed to true drug resistance. Higher doses of cytotoxic drugs may improve response rates, but this is often associated with unacceptable toxicity. Regional arterial perfusion has been used in an attempt to increase tumor drug concentration and intracarotid and intrahepatic infusions of cytotoxic drugs have been tested respectively in the treatment of brain tumors and hepatic metastasis from colorectal cancer. While some studies report improved response rates, the results of randomly controlled prospective studies are needed.

Enhanced cytotoxicity may result from increasing the concentration of drug per unit time by continuous intravenous infusion, and recent technical advances in venous access and ambulatory portable pumps have made infusional chemotherapy a practical reality. Not only has this approach enhanced the antitumor effect

Table 1. Factors affecting drug resistance

---

1. Apparent resistance:
   Anatomical site of tumor
   Pharmacological
      Bio-availability
      Dose intensity
      Drug scheduling
      Route of administration – e.g., regional arterial perfusion, intraperitoneal delivery
   Extracellular matrix
      Tumor vessel formation
      Matrix diffusability

2. Cellular mechanisms (Predominantly genetically mediated)
   Cell membrane diffusibility influencing drug influx and efflux
   Drug activation and catabolism
   Target enzyme changes
   Cellular repair capacity
   Growth fraction

---

of drugs such as vindesine and 5-fluorouracil [3, 4] but it has also led to reduced toxicity, allowing for larger cumulative doses of drug to be administered [4, 6].

Intratumoral drug delivery

The ability of the drug to reach individual cells depends both on the degree of vascularization within the tumor and on the position of individual tumor cells relative to capillaries. Tumor vascularization is influenced by tumor angiogenesis factor, produced by tumor cells early in tumor growth, resulting in capillary endothelial cell proliferation [7]. The resulting vessel formation will influence the ability of both nutrients and oxygen, on the one hand, and chemotherapeutic agents, on the other, to reach tumor cells.

The position of a tumor cell relative to capillaries, influences not only diffusion of drug but also the metabolic and cell cycle status of individual cells. The farther a cell is from a capillary, the lower the nutrient, oxygen and drug concentrations around the cell will be, assuming uninterrupted diffusion out from the capillary. These concentrations will be even lower if diffusion is slowed or blocked by, for example, tumor cell contacts or extracellular matrix components.

The three dimensional architecture of solid tumors has been modelled experimentally by the use of multicellular spheroids [8, 9]. Spheroids grown *in vitro* demonstrate a number of features observed also in solid tumors *in vivo*: they have an outer layer of well-oxygenated dividing cells; they have an inner layer of poorly-oxygenated viable but cell cycle arrested cells; and they have a central core of necrotic cells. The position of a cell in a spheroid and the degree of hypoxia have been shown in many systems to markedly affect its sensitivity to a variety of drugs [9–11]. Cells that are hypoxic and slowly (or non-) cycling, may be apparently resistant to drug treatment, and if spared by the chemotherapy, will regenerate.

Spheroids have also been used to model the distribution of various drugs, by diffusion or other means, to various portions of a solid tumor through the use of radio-labelled or fluorescent drugs [9, 12]. Experimental studies have clearly shown that effective drug concentration can vary grossly within a spheroid. Furthermore, individual drugs have been shown to have different abilities to penetrate into spheroids, so that for example, 5-fluorouracil (5FU) rapidly reaches all cells in some spheroids while vinblastine penetrates very poorly into spheroids of the same tumor cell types [13].

Such variability is expected to apply in solid tumors as well. For example, limited penetration into solid tumor tissue may be one of the factors influencing resistance to Adriamycin [14, 15] and relative hypoxemia interferes with the cytotoxic activity of Adriamycin [16]. The use of electron-affinic sensitizers such as misonidazole may facilitate the cytotoxic action action of chemotherapeutic agents in a hypoxemic environment [17].

Biological perspective of drug resistance

The *in vitro* identification of drug-resistant mutants has stimulated studies of mechanisms to explain drug resistance. Furthermore, recent advances in recombinant DNA and monoclonal antibody technologies are providing powerful tools for the investigation of drug resistance at the molecular level. This section will consider some somatic cell genetic concepts which are proving to be useful in elucidating such mechanisms.

Many studies indicate that the development of drug resistant, variant cells has a genetic basis, resulting from, for example, point mutations, deletions, and amplifications. Changes in a variety of gene products can influence sensitivity to chemotherapy.

While the eukaryotic genome was once considered to be static, we now realize that the genomes of both normal and tumor cells can undergo major changes. Thus, in normal development, immunoglobulin production by B lymphocytes represents a gene product created from a set of rearranged DNA sequences [18].

During tumorigenesis, a variety of genomic changes have been described including changes in chromosome number, chromosome translocations and deletions, gene amplification, and gene modification by methylation [19–23]. These changes at the DNA level may modulate gene activity and thus change cell phenotype (see chapter 9). Nowell proposed that, during tumor progression, cells with increasingly malignant phenotypes (including drug resistance) arise, due to genetic instability of tumor cells [24, 25]. Selective pressures in the host environment encourage the growth of the more malignant cells. In this view, genetic change and instability are central to tumor progression. In his review of progression Foulds concluded that stochastic or random chance variation is evident at all stages of tumor development [26].

Goldie and Coldman [27–30] have extended this reasoning to the generation of drug-resistant mutants within a tumor using the somatic mutation analysis of Luria and Delbruck [31]. The basis of their mathematical model is that mutants are generated by a spontaneous random process, and their model places primary emphasis on the mutation rate. As a tumor grows, the odds will increase for the occurrence of drug-resistant mutations. There is a critical tumor population size at which the likelihood of a mutation rapidly approaches certainty. Fig. 1 outlines the Luria-Delbruck analysis, and illustrates the rapid development of drug-resistant, mutant cells as the tumor grows beyond the critical size. This shows how both tumor size and mutation rate can determine the success or failure of chemotherapy in this model.

Recent work has attempted to make estimates of rates of generation of drug-resistant cells in tumors. A comparison of mutation rates for different mechanisms of drug resistance in experimental systems is summarized by Ling *et al.* in a review of quantitative genetic analysis of tumor progression [32]. Rates reported range from 10^{-3} for mutations involving gene amplification to 5×10^{-8}

160

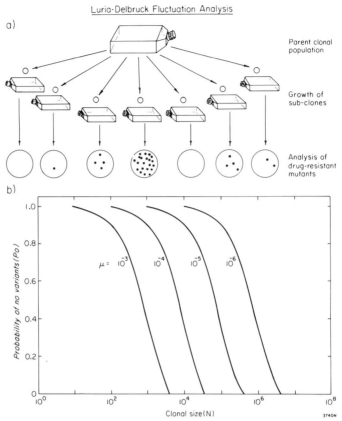

Figure 1. Luria-Delbruck Fluctuation Analysis. a) Diagram of a fluctuation test to detect the spontaneous generation of drug-resistant mutants. A typical feature of this type of experiment is the large variation in the occurrence of drug-resistant mutants in parallel clonal populations grown to the same population size, with some clones having no mutants and others having many. This variation arises due to the random nature of mutant generation, with some clonal populations developing mutants at various points during their growth, and others by chance developing no mutants. The *rate* of generation (μ) of such mutants can be calculated, knowing the clonal population size (N), as summarized by Ling *et al.* [32]. b) The relationship between mutation rate (μ) and the probability of a clonal population of cells remaining drug-sensitive (i.e., having no variants), as the total number of cells (N) in the population increases. The steep slopes of these curves indicate that small increases in population size have dramatic effects on the probability of development of drug-resistant mutants. The mutation rate determines the critical population size at which drug resistance is likely to develop, with higher mutation rates (e.g, 10^{-3}) resulting in the development of drug-resistance in very small populations, and lower mutation rates (e.g., 10^{-6}) permitting growth to much larger population sizes before drug-resistant mutants are likely to arise.

Reprinted, with permission, from Ling *et al.* [32].

for point mutations in a gene product. It is apparent that subclinical tumors (less than 10^7 cells) could already have developed drug-resistant mutants involving amplification of genes. In advanced tumor cells, large scale gene amplification has been observed both as aberrant, homogeneously-staining regions of chromosomes or as extrachromosal, nuclear bodies called double-minutes [22, 33].

Some mechanisms of drug resistance

In the past, the mechanism of drug resistance was examined biochemically to identify relevant target enzymes. More recently, somatic cell genetic concepts of mutation theory have been applied but in fact, both views of resistance are complementary. While biochemical definition of relevant target enzymes helps to provide information for design of new drugs or refinements to existing drugs, the somatic cell genetic approach has demonstrated how cellular mutation, resulting in altered quantity or structure of a target molecule, can radically change cellular responsiveness to a cytotoxic drug.

Membrane permeability

For chemotherapeutic agents to be effective, they must first enter the tumor cell, and target molecules that hinder or enhance the entry of drugs into cells may have a profound influence on the effectiveness of chemotherapy. Many drugs become concentrated within cells during a period of a few minutes, largely due to strong binding to intracellular targets [34]. Several studies indicate that drug influx across the plasma membrane occurs by an unmediated diffusion process, and that efflux occurs by an energy dependent, wide-spectrum system [34].

The biochemical and physical properties of cell membranes that mediate drug transport are not clear. One genetic approach to investigation involves the characterization of membrane mutants of *in vitro* grown cell lines that are selected to be resistant to particular drugs. This approach has recognized a plasma membrane component, P-glycoprotein (a glycoprotein of molecular size approximately 170 KD) that is associated with a multi-drug resistant phenotype [34–38]. This molecule is found at low levels in normal cells and at much higher levels in cells that are resistant to a variety of non-cross-reactive drugs. While first identified in *in vitro* grown cells, high levels of P-glycoprotein have also been identified in human tumor samples [38, 39]. It is not yet possible to explain how the P-glycoprotein might modulate pleiotropic membrane transport, but the c-DNA and monoclonal antibody probes have been developed and will be used to analyze this question further [40, 41].

It appears that the P-glycoprotein is part of a gene family [38] and that members of this family may be differentially amplified. It is reasonable to speculate, therefore, that amplification of the P-glycoprotein gene underlies the over-expression of P-glycoprotein associated with at least some cases of multi-drug resistance. The definition of normal function of P-glycoprotein is a crucial issue. As differential expression of P-glycoprotein may be an important regulatory point for the control of normal cell membrane permeability, this may also be an important factor in the modulation of drug susceptibility of tumors showing differentiation. Another important issue is whether P-glycoprotein is expressed by the 'stem' cells rather than by the bulk of differentiated cells. Such techniques may help to identify potential target molecules that can modulate tumor cell sensitivity to chemotherapeutic drugs, and offer the potential of exploiting this knowledge clinically to overcome resistance to chemotherapy [38].

Enhanced drug efflux is another important mechanism which may be responsible for resistance to drugs such as anthracyclines, vinca alkaloids and methotrexate [42–47], as the cytotoxic effects of a drug may be influenced by its intracellular accumulation and retention. While impaired drug efflux is poorly inderstood, attempts have been made to enhance drug retention using various maneuvers. Probenecid, for example, inhibits the efflux of methotrexate from murine tumor cells *in vitro* [46] and quinidine inhibits the efflux of vincristine and Adriamycin from drug resistant tumor lines [48] with resulting increased cytotoxicity.

Calcium channel blockers and calmodulin inhibitors have also been found to impede the efflux of vincristine and Adriamycin from drug-resistant tumor cells [49–53]. Intracellular levels of vincristine may be increased ten-fold in vincristine-resistant P388 leukemia cells by exposing them to various calcium channel blockers [49]. Furthermore, the concurrent administration of verapamil with vincristine to mice bearing vincristine-resistant P388 leukemia produces an enhanced chemotherapeutic effect. Enhanced cytotoxicity by calcium channel blockers seems to preferentially affect tumor cells, with little added toxicity to normal cells [54, 55].

Precise mechanisms by which calcium channel blockers maintain intracellular levels of cytotoxic drugs are not fully understood. Efflux of antitumor agents may be controlled by the calcium-calmodulin complex and, indeed, calmodulin inhibitors such as chlomiprimine potentiate the effect of vincristine in vincristine-resistant tumor bearing mice [56]. The efficacy of calcium channel blockers to enhance intracellular Adriamycin levels appears to be dependent on the presence of extracellular calcium, and has been shown to produce pronounced G2/M block [51]. Whatever mechanism is involved, influences on the cell membrane also appear to be important and may account for the pleiotropic effect of this multiple drug resistant phenomenon which is shared with the P-glycoprotein observations (vide supra). Studies are looking into the concomitant use of calcium channel blockers and calmodulin inhibitos with cytotoxic drugs, in an attempt to overcome multiple drug resistance.

Target enzymes, drug activation and catabolism

One approach both to the design of chemotherapeutic agents and to strategies for

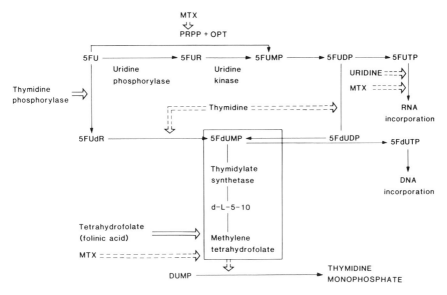

Figure 2. Metabolism of 5-Fluorouracil (5-FU) to demonstrate possible inhibition and enhancement of cytotoxic effect. A decrease in activating enzymes may lead to drug resistance. For further explanation see text.
Double solid arrow = enhancing effect.
Double dotted line arrow = inhibiting effect.
PRPP = phosphoribosyl pyrophosphate.
MTX = Methotrexate.
OPT = orotic acid phosphoribosyl transferase.

overcoming drug resistance has been the analysis of metabolic pathways at risk for attack by cytotoxic drugs. One of the best studied, the biochemical pathway for fluoropyrimidines, is outlined in Fig. 2. The cytotoxic effect of these compounds occurs by inhibition of thymidylate synthetase, incorporation into RNA and incorporation into DNA by activation to 5-FdUMP, 5-FUTP and 5-FdUTP, respectively. The mutation or modulation by differentiation of the activities of the key enzymes shown in Fig. 2 may result in decreased activation and consequent drug resistance.

Combination drug therapies have been examined for the fluoropyrimidines. Manipulation of the intracellular concentration of cytotoxic intermediates by both cytotoxic and normal compounds may result in increased drug efficacy. Prior treatment with methotrexate may both enhance and inhibit the effects of 5-FU [see Fig. 2]. In preliminary studies using sequential methotrexate and 5-FU in patients with advanced colorectal carcinoma, improved clinical responses have not been shown to date, although the results of phase III studies are awaited [57, 58].

The therapeutic index of 5-FU may be improved by giving this drug in combination with thymidine [59]. This effect is thought to be brought about by encouraging incorporation of 5-FU metabolites into RNA rather than into DNA (see Fig. 2).

Thymidylate synthetase plays an important role in resistance to 5-FU and methotrexate. Gene amplification of thymidylate synthetase appears responsible for development of resistance to this combination of drugs [60]. Qualitative changes in the enzyme thymidylate synthetase with decreased affinity for 5-dUMP has also been identified in resistant cell lines [61].

The salvage enzymes of purine and pyrimidine bases are key sites of mutational and differentiation modulation of cytotoxic effect. Resistance to drugs such as 6-mercaptopurine, 6-thioguanine and ara-C commonly arises due to decreased activity of the activating kinase. Responsiveness to these drugs often depends on the degree to which the tumor cell uses nucleotide salvage pathways relative to *de novo* synthesis pathways. Furthermore, cell lines resistant to 6-mercaptopurine or 6-thioguanine because of deficiency in an enzyme of the salvage pathway, must resort to *de novo* purine synthesis and this may then enhance sensitivity to drugs such as methotrexate and azaserine [62, 63].

In addition to biochemical activation, drug catabolism has also been identified as a mechanism responsible for drug resistance. For example, ara-C deamination by deoxycytidine deaminase to the less active arabinosile uracil has been reported as a mechanism for resistance to this drug [64]. Ara-C is normally activated by deoxycytidine kinase and the finding that deoxycytidine deaminase activity was higher than deoxycytidine kinase activity in solid tumor biopsies [65] may be one of the reasons why solid tumors are generally not responsive to this drug.

Another example of a target enzyme at risk in chemotherapy is dihydrofolate reductase (DHFR) which is inhibited by the drug methotrexate, which binds tightly to DHFR. Somatic cell genetic analyses of drug-resistant mutants have revealed that methotrexate resistance can arise from both qualitative and quantitative changes in the DHFR gene [66, 67]. Gene amplification at the DHFR locus has been well described in *in vitro* culture systems [33, 66], as have mutations in the DHFR gene resulting in a structurally altered enzyme [67].

In the analysis of human tumors, both qualitative and quantitative changes have also been observed. Clinical resistance to methotrexate in previously-treated patients appears to be associated with 2-4-fold amplification in gene copy number [68–70]. Methotrexate-resistant human promyelocytic leukemia cells have a 20-fold increase in dihydrofolate reductase activity compared with sensitive cells and yet this activity is not associated with an increase in dihydrofolate reductase protein [71]. In this system the increased dihydrofolate reductase specific activity was found to be associated with an alteration in the structure of this enzyme; it was not possible however to assess whether these altered properties occurred as a result of post-translational alterations in the enzyme [72].

Cellular repair and misrepair of drug induced lesions

The ability of tumor cells to overcome drug-induced DNA damage is probably an important mechanism for resistance to cytotoxic drugs such as alkylating agents. DNA repair is a major factor in resistance to alkylating agents in mouse ascites tumors [73] and in several strains of Dunning rat tumor [74], although the repair enzymes have not been isolated and characterized.

Rapid repair from DNA damage inflicted by Adriamycin on P388 murine leukemia cells was found to be characteristic of an Adriamycin-resistant line when compared with an Adriamycin-sensitive line [75]. It may be possible to overcome this kind of resistance by using drugs which inhibit repair of DNA strand breaks. Ara-C for example prevents DNA strand break repair in L1210 murine leukemia cells [76] and pretreatment of human HeLa cells with ara-C prevents DNA repair following x-ray-induced DNA damage [77].

Mutator genes may be important in the generation of drug-resistant cells. The mutator phenotype suggests that increased mutation rates may accelerate the progression rate of tumor cells surviving chemotherapy. This is a specialized prediction of Nowell's hypothesis discussed above. In tissue culture, Chinese hamster ovary cells were obtained, by serial selection in FUdR and methotrexate, with higher rate of mutation at unrelated genetic loci [78]. This mutator phenotype results from a mutation of CTP synthetase that changes the nucleotide pool concentrations [79]. Additional mutator phenotypes in cell mutants of T-lymphosarcoma cell lines are associated with changes in the M1 subunit of ribonucleoside diphosphate reductase and deficiency in deoxycytidylate deaminase [80].

The role of cell kinetics in chemotherapy

Not all chemotherapeutic failures can be attributed to the development of genetically drug-resistant cells. There are cases, for example, where chemotherapy is initially successful, but relapse occurs, and is again treatable with the same chemotherapeutic agent. This situation may arise due to considerations outlined earlier, such as the failure of the first course of chemotherapy to reach all tumor cells or an initial treatment with an insufficient dose. However, another explanation is that the tumor cells that were not killed by the initial treatment were in non-cycling state or in a non-responsive phase of the cell division cycle.

Chemotherapeutic agents are generally considered to be most effective against cycling cells, and many agents are known to kill cells preferentially in a particular phase of the cell cycle. Certainly the effects of chemotherapy on normal cells are seen in those population of normal cells with a high division fraction, namely cells of the bone marrow and gut epithelia. It is therefore apparent that the fraction of a cell population passing through a drug-responsive phase during the time of drug treatment will markedly affect the maximum proportion of the cell population that can be killed by that drug treatment. This consideration has in the past led to (i) attempts to characterize various tumors on the basis of cell cycle time, proportion of cycling cells, and relative times spent in each portion of the cell cycle; (ii) attempts to alter drug scheduling in patients or in experimental animal models to accomodate these cell cycle data [81–83].

The usefulness of cell cycle considerations in drug scheduling has been hampered by the observation that not all cells in a tumor are necessarily cycling. Some cells may be in a quiescent G_0 state (or arrested at some other point in the cell cycle), and may well be spared no matter what scheduling scheme is use. This concept has recently been considered by Alexander [84] with respect especially to acute myelocytic leukemia. Such quiescent cells could lead to metastatic disease appearing long after an apparent cure.

A number of factors influence the kinetic properties of a given tumor. For example, some tumor types, such as small cell lung cancer, are exceptionally fast growing, while others, such as thyroid carcinoma, grow much more slowly. Tumors with a large population of quiescent cells will be more difficult to treat with chemotherapeutic agents that require actively cycling cells for their cytotoxic activity. Furthermore, the growth kinetics of hormone-responsive tumors can be influenced by host hormone levels, which in turn will influence their sensitivity to chemotherapy. During tumor progression, selection for more aggressively growing tumor cells may occur, which in theory should make them more sensitive to cell cycle-dependent chemotherapy.

Finally, the architecture of a tumor can markedly influence growth properties, with cells at the periphery of a tumor growing actively, and cells toward the center tending to be quiescent (and thus unharmed by chemotherapeutic agents that preferentially kill cycling cells). The use of multicellular spheroidsin modelling the cell cycle kinetics of solid tumors and the generation of quiescent, apparently drug-resistant cells has been reviewed recently [8]. By whatever means they arise, quiescent cells that are non-responsive to chemotherapeutic agents can result in drug resistance and failure of chemotherapy.

Conclusion

The dose response relationship for most cytotoxic drugs is very steep. Since drug delivery is determined by the anatomical site of the tumor, dose intensity, drug scheduling and the extracellular milieu (including tumor blood vessel formation and matrix diffusability), all these factors need to be considered before attributing drug resistance to intracellular mechanisms.

Cellular resistance mechanisms are predominantly genetically-mediated and occur either *de novo*, or during tumorigenesis as a result of high mutation rates which are characteristic of most tumors. This can give rise to changes in cell membrane permeability, drug activation and catabolism, qualitative and quantitative changes in target enzyme production and cellular repair capability following sublethal damage inflicted by cytotoxic drugs. Furthermore, the growth fraction determines response to chemotherapy and while this may be characteristic of certain tumor types, it is often unpredictable and may also be a genetically-determined function of tumor growth.

Various mechanisms for possible intervention to overcome drug resistance have been discussed. While drug resistance is multifactorial and cross resistance to a variety of drugs is common, advances in research may identify ways of intercepting common mechanisms for the apparently heterogeneous phenomenon of drug resistance. The expression of P-glycoprotein in drug resistant cells offers particular promise in this regard.

References

1. Vick NA, Khandekar JD, Bigner DD: Chemotherapy of brain tumors: the 'blood-brain barrier' is not a factor. *Arch Neurol* 34: 523–526, 1977
2. Neuwelt EA, Frenkel EP, Diehl J, Vu LH, Rapoport S, Hill S: Reversible osmotic blood-brain barrier disruption in humans: implications for the chemotherapy of malignant brain tumors. *Neurosurg* 7: 44–52, 1980
3. Bodey GP, Yap HY, Yap BS: Continuous infusion vindesine in solid tumors. *Cancer Treat Rev* 7: 39–45, 1980
4. Seifert P, Baker LH, Reed ML *et al.*: Comparison of continuously infused 5-fluorouracil with bolus injection in treatment of patients with colorectal adenocarcinoma. *Cancer* 36: 123–128, 1975
5. Legha SS, Benjamin RS, Mackay B: Reduction of doxorubicin cardiotoxicity by prolonged continuous intravenous infusion. *Ann Intern Med*: 133–139, 1982
6. Cooper KR, Hung WK: Prospective study of pulmonary toxicity of continuously infused bleomycin. *Cancer Treat Rep* 65: 419–425, 1981
7. Folkman J: How is blood vessel growth regulated in normal and neoplastic tissue? *Cancer Res* 46: 467–473, 1986
8. Sutherland RM, Durand RE: Growth and cellular characteristics of multicell spheroids. *Recent Results in Cancer Research* 95: 24–49, 1984
9. Nederman T, Twentyman P: Spheroids for studies of drug effects. *Recent Results in Cancer Research* 95: 84–102, 1984
10. Olive PL: Different sensitivity to cytotoxic agents of internal and external cells of spheroids composed of thioguanine-resistant and sensitive cells. *Br J Cancer* 43: 85–92, 1981
11. Nederman T: Effects of vinblastine and 5-fluorouracil on human glioma and thyroid cancer cells in monolayers and spheroids. *Cancer Res* 44: 254–258, 1984
12. Olive PL, Chaplin DJ, Durand RE: Pharmacokinetics, binding and distribution of Hoechst 33342 in spheroids and murine tumors. *Br J Cancer* 52: 739–746, 1985
13. Nederman T, Carlsson J, Malmqvist M: Penetration of substances into tumor tissue – a methodological study on cellular spheroids. *In Vitro* 17: 290–298, 1981
14. Sutherland RM, Eddy HA, Bareham B, Reich K, Vanantwerp D: Resistance to Adriamycin in multicellular spheroids. *Int J Radiat Oncol Biol Phys* 5: 1225–1230, 1979
15. Ozols RF, Locker G, Doroshaw J, Grotzinger K, Myers CE, Young RC: Adriamycin pharmakokinetics and tissue penetration in murine ovarian cancer. *Cancer Res* 39: 3209–3214, 1979
16. Tannock I, Response of aerobic and hypoxic cells in a solid tumor to Adriamycin and cyclophosphamide and interaction of the drugs with radiation. *Cancer Res* 42: 4921–4926, 1982

168

17. Brown JM: Clinical perspectives for the use of new hypoxic cell sensitizers. *Int J Radiat Oncol Biol Phys* 8: 1491–1497, 1982.
18. Leder P: The genetics of antibody diversity. *Sci American* 246: 71–83, 1982
19. Gilbert F: Chromosomes, genes and cancer: a classification of chromosome abnormalities in cancer. *J Natl Cancer Inst* 71: 1107–1114, 1983
20. Honey NK, Shows TB: The tumor phenotype and the human gene map. *Cancer Genet Cytogenet* 10: 287–310, 1983
21. Yunis JJ: The chromosomal basis of human neoplasia. *Science* 221: 227–236, 1983
22. Alitalo K: Amplification of cellular oncogenes in cancer cells. *Medical Biology* 62: 304–317, 1984
23. Jones PA, DNA methylation and cancer. *Cancer Res* 46: 461–466, 1986
24. Nowell PC: The clonal evolution of tumor cell populations. *Science* 194: 23–28, 1976
25. Nowell PC: Mechanisms of tumor progression. *Cancer Res* 46: 2203–2207, 1986
26. Foulds L: *Neoplastic Development*, Academic Press, London, 1975
27. Goldie JH, Coldman AJ: A mathematical model for relating the drug sensitivity of tumors to their spontaneous mutation rate. *Cancer Treat Rep* 63:: 1727–1733, 1979
28. Goldie JH, Coldman AJ, Gudauskas GA: Rationale for the use of alternating non-cross-resistant chemotherapy. *Cancer Treat Rep* 66: 439–449, 1982
29. Goldie JH, Coldman AJ: Quantitative model for multiple levels of drug resistance in clinical tumors. *Cancer Treat Rep* 67: 923–931, 1983
30. Goldie JH, Coldman AJ: The genetic origin of drug resistance in neoplasms: implications for systemic therapy. *Cancer Res* 44: 3643–3653, 1984
31. Luria SE, Delbruck M: Mutations of bacteria from virus sensitivity to virus resistance. *Genetics* 28: 491–511, 1943
32. Ling V, Chambers AF, Harris JF, Hill RP: Quantitative genetic analysis of tumor progression. *Cancer Metastatsis Rev* 4: 173–194, 1985
33. Schimke RT: *Gene Amplification*. Cold Spring Harbor Laboratory, New York, 1982
34. Riordan JR, Ling V: Genetic and biochemical characterization of multidrug resistance. *Pharmacol Ther* 28: 51–75, 1985
35. Ling V: Genetic basis of drug resistance in mammalian cells. In: *Drug and Hormone Resistance in Neoplasia*. Bruchovsky N, Goldie JH (ed). CRC Press, Miami 1982, 1–19
36. Kartner N, Riordan JR, Ling V: Cell surface P-glycoprotein associated with multidrug resistance in mammalian cell lines. *Science* 221: 1285–1288, 1984
37. Ling V: Multidrug resistance and chemotherapy. *Head and Neck Cancer* 1: 393–395, 1985
38. Gerlach JH, Kartner N, Bell DR, Ling V: Multidrug resistance. *Cancer Surveys*, 5: 25–46, 1986
39. Bell DR, Gerlach JH, Kartner N, Buick RN, Ling V: Detection of P-Glycoprotein in ovarian cancer: a molecular marker associated with multidrug resistance. *J Clin Oncol* 3: 311–315, 1985
40. Riordan JR, Deuchars K, Kartner N, Alon N, Trent J, Ling V: Amplification of P-glycoprotein genes in multidrug resistant to mammalian cell lines. *Nature* 316: 817–819, 1985
41. Kartner N, Evernden-Porelle D, Bradley G, Ling V: Detection of P-glycoprotein in multidrug resistant cell lines by monoclonal antibodies. *Nature* 316: 820–823, 1985
42. Dan K: Active outward transport of daunomycin in resistant Ehrlich ascites tumor cells. *Biochem Biophys Acta* 323: 466–483, 1973
43. Inaba M, Kobayashi H, Sakurai Y, Johnson RK: Active efflux of daunomycin and Adriamycin in sensitive and resistant sublines of P388 leukemia. *Cancer Res* 39: 2200–2203, 1979
44. Skovsgaard T: Mechanisms of cross-resistance between vincristine and daunorubicin in Ehrlich ascites tumor cells. *Cancer Res* 38: 4722–4727, 1978
45. Beck WT: Vinca alkaloid-resistant phenotype in cultured human leukemic lymphoblasts. *Cancer Treat Rep* 67: 875–882, 1983
46. Sirotnak FM, Moccio DM, Young CW: Increased accumulation of methotrexate by murine tumor cells in vitro in the presence of probenecid which is mediated by a preferential inhibition of efflux. *Cancer Res* 41: 966–970, 1981

47. Henderson GB, Zeveley EM: Transport routes utilized by L1210 cells for the influx and efflux of methotrexate. *J Biol Chem* 259: 1526–1531, 1984

48. Tsuruo T, Iida H, Kitatoni Y, Yokoto K, Tsukayashi S, Sakurai Y: Effects of quinidine and related compounds on cytotoxicity and cellular accumulation of vincristine and Adriamycin in drug-resistant tumor cells. *Cancer Res* 44: 4303–4307, 1984

49. Tsuruo T, Iida H, Tsukayashi S, Sakurai Y: Overcoming of vincristine resistance in P388 leukemia in vivo and in vitro through enhanced cytotoxicity of vincristine and vinblastine by verapamil. *Cancer Res* 41: 1967–1972, 1981

50. Tsuruo T, Iida H, Tsukayashi S, Sakurai Y, Increase accumulation of vincristine and Adriamycin in drug-resistant P388 tumor cells following incubation with calcium antagonists and calmodulin inhibitors. *Cancer Res* 42: 4730–4733, 1982

51. Yanovich S, Gervintz D: Involvement of calcium in the enhancement of daunorubicin accummulation in P388 leukemia cells by verapamil and Ca^{++} ionophore A3187. *Proc Am Assoc Cancer Res* 1209, 1984

52. Wilderbing C, Kessel D: Mechanism of circumvention of anthracycline resistance by calcium antagonists. *Proc Am Assoc Cancer Res* 1164, 1984

53. Harker WG, Elisan MH, Bauer DM, Newman RA, Sikic, BI: Effects of verapamil on daunorubicin resistance. Differential sensitization of human tumor cells selected in vitro vs. in vivo. *Proc Am Assoc Clin Oncol* 30: 116, 1984

54. Presant CA, Wiseman C, Gala K, Wynes M: Verapamil plus Adriamycin. A phase I-II clinical study. *Proc Am Soc Clin Oncol* 32: 124, 1984

55. Fine RL, Koizumi S, Curt GA, Chabner BA: Verapamil does not enhance anticancer drug toxicity for human marrow myeloid-macrophage colony forming unit. *Proc Am Soc Clin Oncol* 48: 154, 1984

56. Tsuruo T, Iida H, Nogiri M, Tsukagoshi S, Sahurai Y: Potentiation of chemotherapeutic effect of vincristine in vincristine resistant tumor bearing mice by calmodulin inhibitor chlormipriamine. *J Pharmacobiodyn* 6: 145–147, 1983

57. Panasci L, Ford J, Margolese R: A phase II study of sequential methotrexate and fluorouracil in advanced colorectal cancer. *Cancer Chemother Pharmacol* 15: 164–166, 1985

58. Ellison NM, Bernath AM, Gallagher JG, Porter PA, Rine KT, Lewis GO: Toxicity without benefit for sequential MTX/5FU. *Proc Am Soc Clin Oncol* 4: 26, 1985

59. Danhauser LL, Rustum YM: Chemotherapeutic efficacy of 5-fluorouracil with concurrent thymidine infusion against transplantable colon tumors in rodents. *Cancer Drug Delivery* 1: 269–282, 1984

60. Washtien WL: Thymidylate synthetase levels as a factor in 5-fluorodeoxyuridine and methotrexate cytotoxicity in gastrointestinal tumor cell lines. *Mol Pharmacol* 21: 723–728, 1982

61. Jastreboff MM, Kedzierska B, Rode W: Altered thymidylate synthetase in 5-fluorodeoxyuridine resistant Ehrlich ascites carcinoma cells. *Biochem Pharmacol* 32: 2259–2267, 1983

62. Hutchison DJ: Cross resistance and collateral sensitivity studies in cancer chemotherapy. In: *Advances in Cancer Research*. Haddor A, Weinhouse S (ed). New York: Academic Press, 1963, pp 235–350

63. Schabel, FM Jr, Skipper HE, Trader MW, Laster WR Jr, Griswald DP Jr, Corbett TH: Establishment of cross-resistance profiles in new agents. *Cancer Treat Rep* 67: 905–922, 1983

64. Brockman RW: Mechanisms of resistance. In: *Handbook Experimental Pharmacology* Sartorelli AC, Johns DC (eds). New York, Springer Verlag, 1974, pp 352–410

65. Hall TC: Prediction of response to therapy and mechanisms of resistance. *Sem Oncol* 4: 193–202, 1977

66. Schimke RT: Gene amplification in cultured animal cells. *Cell* 37: 705–713, 1984

67. Flintoff WF, Spindler SM, Siminovitch L: Genetic characterization of methotrexate-resistant CHO cells. *In Vitro* 12: 749–757, 1976

68. Trent JM, Buick RN, Olson S, Horns JC Jr, Schimke RT: Cytologic evidence for gene amplification in methotrexate-resistant cells obtained from a patient with ovarian adenocarcinoma. *J Clin Onc* 2: 8–15, 1984

69. Carman MD, Schornagel JH, Rivest RS, Srimatkandada S, Portlock CS, Duffy T, Bertino JR: Resistance to methotrexate due to gene amplification in a patient with acute leukemia. *J Clin Onc* 2: 16–20, 1984

70. Horns RC Jr, Dower WJ, Schimke RT: Gene amplification in a leukemic patient treated with methotrexate. *J Clin Onc* 2: 2–7, 1984

71. Dedhar S, Hartley D, Goldie JH: Increased dihydrofolate reductase activity in methotrexate-resistant human promyelocytic leukemia (HL-60) cells: lack of correlation between increased activity and overproduction. *Biochem J* 225: 609–617, 1985

72. Dedhar S, Goldie JH: Methotrexate-resistant human promyelocytic leukemia (HL-60) cells express a dihydrofolate reductase with altered properties associated with increased enzyme activity. *Biochem Biophys Res Comm* 129: 536–545, 1985

73. Stewart CS, Burke PJ: Cytidine deaminase and the development of resistance to arabinosyl cytosine. *Nature* (New Biol) 233: 109–110, 1971

74. Cheng YC, Capizzi RL: Enzymology of cytosine arabinoside. *Med Pediatr Oncol* (Supp 1): 27–31, 1982

75. Chou TH, Yost C: Adriamycin resistance in murine leukemia P388 cells and increased DNA repair. *Proc Am Assoc Cancer Res* 26: 217, 1985

76. Fram RJ, Egan EM, Kufe DW: Accumulation of leukemic cell DNA strand breaks with Adriamycin and cytosine arabinoside. *Leuk Res* 7: 243–249, 1983

77. Ward JF, Joner EI, Blakely WF: Effects of inhibitors of DNA strand break repair on HeLa cell radiosensitivity. *Cancer Res* 44: 59–63, 1984

78. Meuth M, Goncalves O, Thom P: A selection system specific for the Thy mutator phenotype. *Somat Cell Genet* 8: 423–432, 1982

79. Trudel M, Van Genechten T, Meuth M: Biochemical characterization of the hamster Thy mutator gene and its revertants. *J Biol Chem* 259, 2355–2359, 1984

80. Weinberg G, Ullman B, Martin DW Jr: Mutator phenotypes in mammalian cell mutants with distinct biochemical defects and abnormal deoxyribonucleoside triphosphate pools. *Proc Nat Acad Sci* 78: 2447–2451, 1981

81. Skipper HE: The cell cycle and chemotherapy of cancer. In: *The Cell Cycle and Cancer*, Baserga, R. (ed). Marcel Dekker Inc, New York, 1971, pp 358–387

82. Tannock IF: Biology of tumor growth. *Hosp Practice* 18: 81–93, 1983

83. Skipper HE, Schabel FM: Tumor stem cell heterogeneity: implications with respect to classification of cancers by chemotherapeutic effect. *Cancer Treat Rep* 68: 43–61, 1984

84. Alexander P: Need for new approaches to the treatment of patients in clinical remission with special reference to acute myeloid leukemia. *Br J Cancer* 46: 151–159, 1982

12. Prognostic value of assays of immune competency

K.P. RYAN and R.O. DILLMAN

A high degree of correlation between assays of immune competence and prognosis has been claimed for patients with various types of malignancy [1–3]. Among the parameters claimed to be correlated with the patients' clinical course are (1) Delayed type cutaneous hypersensitivity reactions to common recall antigens (such as candida, mumps, tuberculin, streptokinase, streptodornase) and to dinitrochlorbenzene (DNCB). (2) Detection of autologous antibodies thought to be directed against specific tumor antigens of tumor products. (3) Absolute lymphocyte count. (4) Detection of immunosuppressive serum blocking factors, usually presumed to be anti-tumor antibody circulating alone, or in complexes with alleged tumor-specific antigen. (5) Blastogenic transformation of autologous lymphocytes by various mitogens such as pokeweed mitogen (PWM), phyto-hemagglutinin (PHA), and conconavalin A (Con A). (6) Reactivity of autologous lymphocytes in mixed culture to heterologous lymphocytes (MCL) or to autologous tumor extract. (7) Levels of circulating polyclonal IgA, IgG, IgM, and IgE.

It is reported that a good prognosis in cancer patients is related to vigorous delayed type hypersensitivity reactions to recall antigens and to DNCB, marked *in vitro* lymphocyte blastogenesis to PHA, and high B-lymphocyte cell levels [4]. A list of *in vivo* and *in vitro* tests which ranged from 'fair' to 'excellent' in terms of their correlation to prognosis was published and both response to therapy and/or subsequent relapse, were claimed to be reliably predicted by such assays. This chapter will critically review the evidence for the prognostic significance of *in vitro* and *in vivo* assays of immunocompetence in cancer patients.

Immunosuppression and cancer

Immunosuppression has been blamed as the cause of second malignancies in patients thought to be cured of a previous primary neoplasm [5–7], and is also widely believed to favour solid tumor proliferation and metastasis [8]. Neoplastic cells are said to trigger host immunosuppression through the generation of suppressive factors or cells that subvert host immunocompetence [9–10]. In spite of such observations, is it justifiable to suggest that immune perturbations seen in an individual cancer patient are solely and directly linked to the clinical behaviour of their neoplasm?

Nutritional impairment can cause immunosuppression with lymphopenia, impaired delayed-type hypersensitivity reactions, and depressed *in vitro* mitogen-induced blastogenesis, all of which have been reported even in patients without cancer [11, 12]. Patients with malignant disease often have severe malnourishment and in malnourished individuals with or without cancer, nutritional restoration is not always correlated with concomitant improvement in previously impaired tests [13]. Increasing age also affects immunity as manifested by a decreasing number of suppressor-cytotoxic T-cells, decrease in intracellular lymphocyte enzyme systems, decreased response in delayed type hypersensitivity reactions, decrease in serum IgM levels, and increasing emergence of auto-antibodies [14, 15].

Radiotherapy, chemotherapy, and major surgery can all affect assays of immunocompetence and may be associated with clinical immunodepression [16, 17]. The total lymphocyte count often falls after only a few days of conventional radiotherapy, with B-cells subsequently recovering more rapidly than T-cells [18]. The suppression of the total T-cell pool may persist for several months or even years [19, 20] whereas humoral immunity tends to be relatively unaffected [20]. Chemotherapy given concomitantly with radiotherapy has been shown to markedly decrease antibody levels [21].

Improvement in skin hypersensitivity reactions has been reported following radiation therapy [22] but this is disputed [23, 24]. Decrease in cell-mediated immunity has been reported following moderate to high dose radiation therapy for up to five years in patients who have obtained a complete remission [26–28], but other studies show no such defect in similarly irradiated individuals [29, 30].

Chemotherapeutic agents have multiple effects on the host immune system, including changes in antigen uptake and recognition, lymphocyte transformation and proliferation, antibody production, and effector cell reactions [29]. Intensive chemotherapy undoubtedly suppresses immune function [30], but even after prolonged continuous chemotherapy, immunity may remain only slightly depressed and eventually becomes normal [31, 32]. The variety of agents used (in terms of their mechanisms of action, the dosage and schedule of administration), and the different national history of each individual tumor make it difficult to predict what immune effects, if any, will occur in any given patient.

Major surgery can have a primary immunosuppressive effect on patients [17, 33] and immunocompetence may be restored after complete tumor removal [34]. Patients undergoing splenectomy are known to have an increased risk of infection by certain organisms, thought by some to be due to the loss of the phagocytosis-stimulating peptide, Tuftsin, which is produced by the spleen [35].

Assessment of immunoreactivity

A number of measures of immunoincompetence in humans have been developed in recent years [36].

Cell-mediated immunity

Tests of cell-mediated immunity (CMI) include *in vivo* skin tests with multiple common antigens to which the patient has almost certainly been previously exposed (such as tuberculin, mumps, and candida) or a direct challenge with the antigen DNCB [37]. Pinsky demonstrated that both DNCB and common recall antigen skin testing weve usually abnormal in advanced cancer, especially in Hodgkin's disease, non-Hodgkin's lymphoma, and head and neck cancer, and that anergy seemed to correlate with a poor prognosis [38]. The converse was not true, and many of the patients studied had multiple medical problems which could have caused their anergic state.

Golub *et al.* tested 52 patients with a variety of solid tumors and attempted to correlate DNCB and common recall antigen skin test reactivity with PHA, PWM, and CON A-induced blastogenesis [39]. No significant correlation was demonstrated, with variable responses being seen across diverse tumor types and stages. This was also reported by Davies *et al.* [40]. Investigators subsequently examined the clinical value of skin testing with autologous human tumor extracts, and while some reported that reactivity correlated with prognosis [41] this observation was refuted by others [42].

In vitro assessment of cell-mediated immunity includes evaluation of lymphocyte transformation responses by T-cell mitogens (such as Con-A and PHA) by measuring uptake of radiolabeled nucleic acids in stimulated lymphocytes. Numerous investigations have shown that lymphocytes from cancer patients often have a diminished response to PHA or Con-A stimulation compared with controls [4, 43]. One study showed that Con-A-stimulated lymphocytes from cancer patients could not mediate chemotaxis of heterologous normal cells as well as did Con-A-stimulated lymphocytes from normal individuals [44].

The so-called mixed lymphocyte reaction (MLR) measures blastogenic response of patients' lymphocytes to antigens on other mononuclear cells and a diminished response in cancer patients may suggest that their immune system is unable to respond to tumor antigens [45]. Unfortunately, such findings have neither been found consistently relevant to prognosis [40], nor functioned effectively as a specific screen for cancer in asymptomatic patients [46].

The most frequently reported alteration in macrophage function in patients with cancer is chemotaxis, which in one study appeared to show high correlation with clinical stage in patients with malignant melanoma [47]. The leukocyte adherence inhibition assay (in which reduced adherence of leukocytes to glass in the presence of serum from cancer patients is measured) has been claimed to show correlation with clinical stage [48]. However, subsequent studies have challenged these observations [49]. Essentially, these assays appear to be non-specific, and present techniques of evaluating macrophage adherence and migration, have little clinical relevance.

Quantitation of total T-cells can readily be performed with monoclonal antibodies, and this has helped to characterize lymphocyte subsets with differing roles in immunosurveillance. Examples include suppressor cells, helper cells, natural killer cells, and natural cytotoxic cells [36].

Several lines of evidence suggest that depressed natural killer (NK) cell activity may facilitate tumor growth and metastases [50]. Tumor cells are reported to activitate T-suppressor cells [51] and also to suppress a number of *in vitro* reactions, including mixed lymphocyte reactivity of spleen cells toward tumor cells (9), macrophage activity [52], natural T-cell activity [53], and even null cells [54]. These observations appear to be much more common in advanced disease than in early disease [55]. Although the growing weight of evidence is in favor of NK cells having an integral role in host resistance, correlation between prognosis and *in vitro* NK cell activity has not yet been reproducibly demonstrated in any series of patients with a given neoplasm.

Control of the immune system is in part governed by the complex interactions of diverse cell types and products they release, known collectively as lymphokines. The interleukin network has illuminated some pathways of T lymphocyte activation and/or proliferation. Interleukin 1 [56] and Interleukin 2 [57] may correct deficient *in vitro* NK cell activity in patients with cancer. Nakayama *et al.* reported defective Interleukin 2 production in peripheral blood leukocytes of patients with metastatic disease, whereas its production in those with loco-regional tumor and in healthy controls was normal [58].

Cameron described a series of patients with head and neck, hematologic or breast cancer in whom the ability of autologous cells to produce macrophage-activating factor was impaired [59]. Furthermore, in some patients, suppressor cells (and/or a soluble suppressor factor) could be identified which had a deleterious effect on the peripheral blood leukocytes of normal controls in *in vitro* assays. As yet, however, there is no clearly defined relationship between assays which measure autologous lymphokine activity and an individual patient's prognosis.

Humoral immunity

Humoral immunity can be evaluated by the following methods: quantitative measurement of individual gamma globulins in patients' sera; assessing antibody production in a patient after antigenic challenge with, for example, tetanus toxoid; detection of surface immunoglobulin in B-cells using anti-immunoglobulin monoclonal antibody; measuring B-lymphocyte transformation *in vitro* after PWM stimulation; various B-cell rosetting techniques.

Whether or not serum immunoglobulin levels have prognostic significance in patients with cancer has been extensively discussed [60]. Immunoglobulin concentrations in serum and secretions have been reported to vary according to stage of the disease and type of therapy but the observations have not established a ratial prognostic significance.

Mononuclear cell infiltration in tumors

Virchow [61] was the first to imply a prognostic significance for mononuclear cell infiltrates in tumor biopsy specimens but this early work was later discredited [62, 63]. Furthermore, the composition of cellular infiltrates varies not only with tumor type but occasionally within different areas of the same tumor. In Hodgkin's disease, however, an indolent natural history, limited stage, and prolonged survival appear to be directly related to the ratio of lymphocytes to abnormal cells found in the biopsy [64, 65].

Eosinophilic infiltration of tumors is infrequent but may indicate a more favorable prognosis, whereas the presence of peripheral eosinophilia is unfavorable [66]. Some investigators evaluating cellular changes in nodes draining breast cancer, claim that lymphocyte predominance in regional nodes is associated with a better prognosis [67]. However, Fisher *et al.* suggest that *in vitro* cytotoxicity of the patient's nodal lymphocytes towards breast cancer target cells is of greater prognostic importance [68].

Circulating immune complexes

Unfortunately, no reproducible and unique human tumor-specific antigens have been described. Furthermore, human tumors are both weakly immunogenic and antigenically heterogeneous, even in the same patient, as shown in specimens from synchronous deposits from carcinoma of the colon [69].

Tumor-associated products, of which CEA is a prototype, have been extensively studied for their diagnostic and prognostic value. Although such antigen levels at the time of diagnosis may provide more precise prognostic information than does clinical staging alone, the information does not lead to more effective management [10]. This view is challenged by Niloff *et al.* who assayed patient sera for the presence of CA-125, a putative ovarian carcinoma antigen, and showed that levels over 35 units/per millimeter were sensitive and specific indicators of intraperitoneal tumor deposits or predictors of future recurrence [71]. The observation was not confirmed in an extensive review of ovarian carcinoma-associated antigens [72]. In another series, sarcoma patients were followed four years postoperatively with a urinary tumor-associated antigen assay, and the reappearance of the antigen seemed to correlate with disease recurrence [73].

Circulating immune complexes can be detected using multiple assays, and levels are reportedly elevated in patients with a broad range of malignancies. Some trials have suggested that their detection at diagnosis or after definitive therapy implies a poor prognosis [74]. However, the clinical relevance of the detection of circulating immune complexes has been extensively reviewed [75], and to date, there is insufficient data to indicate that patients elaborate reproducible, specific or effective antibody responses to autologous tumor. Thus, assays of circulating immune complexes do not yet have proven application to clinical management.

Assays to evaluate *in vitro* autologous antitumor reactivity have been developed. Vanky *et al.* reported that relapse-free survival and median survival was higher in patients with osteogenic sarcoma and soft tissue sarcoma in whom lymphocyte-mediated autologous antitumor reactivity could be demonstrated [76]. In a group of lung cancer patients a similar trend was seen [77] but in neither study were the tests highly specific. The clinical applicability of such assays may be limited in the individual patient because of antigenic tumor cell heterogeneity, and because spontaneous mutation of cell surface antigenic determinants may invalidate the assay when used serially [78].

Immune status in hematologic malignancies

Until recently, it was widely presumed that each hematologic malignancy exhibited a characteristic and unique pattern of immunologic deficiency. Also, that all these malignancies evoked a tumor-specific immune response so that prognosis could be directly related to the degree of immunoincompetency as measured by routine standard assays [79]. In the light of the principles discussed in this chapter, it is difficult to support these conclusions.

Leukemia and Myeloma

Chronic lymphatic leukemia (CLL) is often associated with significant immunosuppression and hypogammaglobulinemia. Fernandez *et al.* compared 18 patients with CLL to 18 normal controls, and reported a marked defect in the primary generation of normal immunoglobulin-secreting B-cells [80]. It was thought that they were overwhelmed by abnormal CLL cells, but no evidence of quantitative or qualitative T-cell abnormalities were noted.

Whelan *et al.* evaluated 27 patients with CLL and found abnormal T-cell ratios and decreased serum immunoglobulin levels to be generally associated with increasing [81] stage. However, exceptions were numerous and no significance in terms of prognosis or clinical management could be demonstrated. Ben-Bassat *et al.* in a study of 70 CLL patients, also showed a tendency for serum IgG and IgA levels to decrease with increasing stage but again, prognosis was not correlated with initial or subsequent serum immunoglobulin levels, leukocyte count, age or sex [82]. In patients with both the chronic and accelerated phases of chronic myelogenous leukemia there is often evidence of defective neutrophil function which may be confounded by chemotherapy [83].

Studies in the early 1970s involving patients with acute leukemia reported that patients with normal and supranormal cell-mediated immunity did better in terms of remission, survival, and relapse-free survival [84]. Also that a sudden decline in immune competency in previously competent patients invariably heralded a relapse [85], while those who had a vigorous blastogenic response to their own leukemic cells manifested a better prognosis [86]. The clinical value of this data is marred by the lack of patient homogeneity in terms of age, morphologic and immunologic type of leukemia, the timing of *in vitro* assays in relation to the patients' clinical course, performance status, and duration and type of chemotherapy. Immunoincompetence in acute leukemia seems to relate more to rigorous chemotherapy [87], with immunologic rebound often noted following termination of therapy [88]. Thus, correlation between immunocompetency and prognosis in acute leukemia is still conjectural, and at present, standard clinical assessment determines management of these patients [88, 89].

Immune incompetence is common in patients with multiple myeloma. In addition to low serum levels of polyclonal immunoglobulins, a depression of total T-cells and T-helper cells (which is intensified by chemotherapy) has been reported in this disease [90]. Fink and Galanos found lower serum anti-lipid A levels in 38 patients with IgG myeloma, 33 patients with IgA myeloma, and 38 patients with Waldenstrom's macroglobulinemia as compared to 34 normals; they showed that the lower the level, the higher the risk of infection [91]. The effect of chemotherapy-induced myelosuppression on serum levels was not examined, and it is clear that both the total tumor burden, and the concomitantly depressed levels of serum immunoglobulins seen in virtually all patients with this disease, remain the major factors which affect prognosis [92].

Hodgkin's Disease

In Hodgkin's disease, cellular immunity is often depressed [98, 94]. When noted on initial presentation, it usually correlates with stage [93–95], and it may also be more common in association with mixed cellularity and lymphocyte-depleted histologies [96]. The exact cause of defects in cell-mediated immunity is not known and they may stem from lymphocyte depletion [97], inherently defective lymphocytes [98], circulating suppressor cells [99] or plasma inhibitors [100]. Response of Hodgkin's disease patients to interleukin 1 has been reported as normal (as has their T-cell proliferative response to exogenous interleukin 2), but in the same study, IL-2 production by patients peripheral mononuclear cells was decreased when compared to age- and sex-matched controls [101].

Kun and Johnson reported that delayed hypersensitivity reactions and serum immunoglobulin levels were normal in 71 consecutive patients treated successfully with radiotherapy five years previously [28]. However, Fuks *et al.* showed a quantitative depression of T-cells and significant impairment of *in vitro* PWM responsivity in the sera of 26 patients in complete remission from 12 to 111 months after curative radiotherapy [19]. MOPP chemotherapy for Hodgkin's disease appears to affect *in vitro* immunocompetence, as shown by a significant reduction in mitogen-induced proliferation and E-rosette formation in lymphocytes from 47 long term survivors previously treated with MOPP. It persisted for up to 11 years [102].

Depression of leukocyte migration inhibition, impaired lymphocyte transformation, and decreased serum immunoglobulins were noted in patients evaluated serially for five years who had previously been treated with chemotherapy and splenectomy [103]. In a similar report by Sutherland *et al.*, multiple immune assays were impaired in a series of 39 patients with Hodgkin's disease treated by splenectomy and radiotherapy; no detrimental effect on prognosis was demonstrated and the majority of such patients were considered cured [104].

In studies of over 500 patients, Kaplan suggested that pre-treatment skin test results have limited prognostic importance [105]. Others, however, have shown that improvement in skin tests [106, 107], or assays of mitogen-induced blastogenesis [108] during therapy, may be associated with a better prognosis. PHA response did not provide a dependable assessment of a patient's immunologic competency or prognosis in a study of 78 patients with Hodgkin's disease [109]. Finally, a study of 35 previously untreated patients with Hodgkin's disease was reported, in which survival was more related to immunocompetency (as defined by responsivity to a broad range of PHA concentrations) than to any other factor including age, sex, clinical stage, lymphocyte count, skin test reactivity, or histologic type [110].

It is not clear that the immunologic deficits reported are secondary to the primary disease or its treatment. The presence of a primary genetic or environmental etiology in Hodgkin's disease is strongly suggested by the demonstration of multiple significant immunologic defects as compared to age- and sex-matched normal controls in 6 healthy twin same-sexed siblings of patients who died from Hodgkin's disease [111]. What is clear is that deficits in multiple assays of cell-mediated immunity are present in patients with Hodgkin's disease who are either untreated, treated, or in prolonged complete remission.

B-cell non-Hodgkin's lymphomas are well known to be associated with defects in humoral immunity, such as production of a non-functioning paraprotein and hypogammaglobulinemia. Disseminated disease is often associated with defects in cell-mediated immunity which are notably exacerbated by chemotherapy [112]. Natural killer cell activity, unimproved by interferon, has been reported [113].

Urasinski *et al.* evaluated a number of immunologic parameters in 51 patients with diverse histologic subtypes of non-Hodgkin's lymphoma and compared them to 25 healthy but unmatched subjects [114]. Depressed levels of IgG, IgA, IgM, antistreptolysins, complement, T- and B-lymphocytes, granulocytes, and impaired skin test reactivity to common recall antigens were demonstrated in all but one patient. This type of report exemplifies the need for longitudinal studies employing thoroughly matched controls, where due consideration is given to the effects of therapy, performance status, and immunohistologic tumor classification. Although there are few data on patients in long term remission with non-Hodgkin's lymphoma, one study implies that prolonged defects are not seen in such patients despite intensive chemotherapy [24].

Immune status in solid cancers

Immune function is generally normal in patients with early stage solid tumors and some studies imply that neutrophil and macrophage function may even be increased in such cases [115, 116]. However, as solid tumors become widely metastatic, there is a trend towards diminution of humoral immunity, and even more, of cellular immunity. It involves delayed-type hypersensitivity to DNCB [20], natural killer-cell activity [117], macrophage function [116], total lymphocyte count, and total T-helper cell count [2]. This decreased immune function seems to be independent of concomitant chemotherapy and/or radiotherapy.

Dillman *et al.* employed 20 assays of immunoreactivity to evaluate immune competency in 72 patients with advanced, previously treated, neoplasms and the results were compared to those of healthy age- and sex-matched controls [45]. As a group, the cancer patients had fewer total lymphocytes, helper cells, a lower helper-suppressor T-cell ratio, and increased suppressor cells. The most frequently abnormal functional assay was the pokeweed mitogen stimulation test. The authors employed three separate statistical methods, all of which showed that a combination of percent lymphocytes, percent I_a^+ cells, percent suppressor cells, number of helper cells, and pokeweed mitogen stimulation was the best predictor of immunoincompetency in a cancer patient. In contrast, total B-cells and quantitative immunoglobulins were found to be normal in cancer patients.

Similar observations were reported by Kaszubowski *et al.* in that previously untreated, solid tumor patients demonstrated a decrease in total lymphocyte count and helper cells with an increase in suppressor cells [118]. Unlike the findings in the study above, I_a^+ cells were decreased in number. The significance of this particular discrepancy may lie not only in the fact that this study evaluated untreated patients, but also that it is not clear if all I_a^+ cells are predominantly helper or suppressor in nature.

Wanebo *et al.* claimed that assays of PHA reactivity could select patients with resectable lung and colon cancer, although this could not be demonstrated in patients with breast or head and neck cancer (2). It was further suggested by Braun *et al.* that serial immune function testing could predict clinical relapse in patients with solid tumors [119]. A rebound overshoot recovery of lymphocyte function after tumor eradication with chemotherapy was observed in a small series and thought to be predictive of response [120, 121].

Immunity may return to normal after eradication of a solid tumor, presumably resulting from improved nutrition and performance status, and removal of the tumor burden and its attendant depressant influence on the patient's general immune condition. However, there are several studies which suggest that *in vitro* defects of immunoreactivity may persist many years after successful treatment [25, 122, 123]. Hersh *et al.* claimed that patients with lung or head and neck cancer were usually more immunoincompetent than patients with other forms of solid tumors (4), but this may result from the high incidence of associated alcoholism, cigarette abuse, malnutrition, and cachexia seen in these patients.

Studies have suggested that squamous cell carcinomas were particularly likely to be associated with a decrease in T-cell number and/or a decreased response to PHA [43, 124]. Olkowski *et al.* reported a large series of patients with squamous cell carcinomas of the head and neck, lung, and cervix who were assessed by a battery of *in vitro* tests carried out prior to radiotherapy, immediately after radiotherapy, and serially [125]. Total T-cells pre-therapy were lower in all patients, whereas B-cells were normal except in patients with lung cancer. Following radiotherapy, a decrease in both levels was seen, with mitogen-induced blastogenesis being decreased in all patients. None of the results were statistically signigicant or related to prognosis in any specific tumor type or individual patient.

Hughes *et al.* studied total lymphocyte count, PHA-induced blastogenesis, and DNCB-induced cutaneous reactivity in a large series, involving 200 patients with breast cancer, 100 with gastric carcinoma, and 100 with colon cancer. He found that other than in advanced and disseminated disease, there was no correlation between these assays levels and clinical stage [126]. Furthermore, pretherapy immunocompetence did not necessarily confer a favorable prognosis.

Lung cancer

Diverse abnormalities in assays of immune reactivity are commonly reported in lung cancer patients. This may, in part, be due to the fact that a large percentage of these patients present with regionally advanced disease, a prolonged history of cigarette smoking, and significant weight loss or poor nutrition. Alsabti compared assays of skin reactivity (using common recall antigens and DNCB) Con-A- and PHA-induced blastogenesis, and mixed lymphocyte culture reactivity, in 48 patients with lung cancer and 94 age-matched healthy controls [127]. Cutaneous reactivity and mitogen stimulation were impaired in patients with squamous carcinoma, whereas the converse was observed in patients with anaplastic histology. No prognostic significance of these findings was shown.

Stage-related impairment of mitogen-induced blastogenesis and cutaneous reactivity to both DNCB and common recall antigens has been reported by others [128]. There was a tendency for assays of lymphocyte function to improve, at least transiently, in patients who appeared to be in remission after surgery or radiation therapy [129].

Breast cancer

Multiple large series examining immunocompetence in breast cancer patients have made conflicting observations. Munzarova *et al:* followed 152 patients for 2 years with a battery of skin tests and found that anergy was more frequent in patients in bad general health, but no prognostic value for skin test reactivity was shown [130]. Papatestas *et al.* retrospectively evaluated total lymphocyte count before and after therapy in 450 patients with breast cancer [131]. The 5 year survival in patients in stage II and III disease was significantly different in those with pre-therapy lymphocyte counts greater than 2000 per mm^3 from those with less than 2000 lymphocytes per mm^3. Abnormal leukocyte adherence inhibition has been reported to reverse several months after mastectomy, with persistent or recurrent adherence abnormalities being associated with an increased risk of recurrent disease [132].

Sophisticated assays of the immunocytologic composition of breast tumor deposits and associated immune effector cells have been used to elicit prognosis information [133, 134]. Lee *et al.* employed monoclonal antibodies to retrospectively analyze 233 specimens of breast carcinoma for the presence of blood group isoantigens [135]. No relationship between any specific antigenic pattern and clinical, epidemiologic, pathologic, or prognostic parameters was seen. Holdsworth *et al.* however, retrospectively analyzed 1001 specimens from patients with invasive carcinoma and claimed that those tumors which exhibited group B and AB isotypes were at highest risk of death or early recurrence [136]. The Eastern Cooperative Oncology Group reviewed 147 specimens from node-positive breast cancer patients and found no correlation between immunohistochemical evidence of CEA tumor cell positivity and the patient's clinical course [63].

Stein *et al.* evaluated assays of cell-mediated immunity in 255 patients with breast cancer at every stage of disease, and also a large number of 5 and 10 year survivors [137]. Early phases of tumor spread were not accompanied by immunoincompetence such as was seen in widely metastatic disease. Furthermore, tumor dissemination preceded immune impairment and thus emerged as a cause rather than a result of immunosuppression. Mandeville *et al.* similarly demonstrated progressive immunoincompetence with advancing stage in a large series of breast cancer patients followed for 5 years using assays of immune reactivity [138].

Gastrointestinal cancer

There are few series which specifically examine immune incompetence in gastrointestinal carcinoma. Kim described 13 patients with stage III gastric carcinoma who underwent radical subtotal gastrectomy followed by a regimen of streptococcal pyogenes extract plus systemic chemotherapy [139]. Survival and immunoreactivity, as measured by DNCB skin tests, T lymphocyte counts, and antibody dependent cell-mediated cytotoxicity, appeared better than in a historical control group treated by surgery alone. Janssen et al. studied serum immunoglobulin levels and C_4 levels in patients with stage I-III gastric carcinoma after undergoing potentially curative resection, and suggested that high post-operative C_4 and C_1 inhibitor levels, as well as low preoperative immunoglobulin levels implied a poor prognosis [140].

Sanz et al. evaluated 88 patients with gastric carcinoma and 63 patients with colon carcinoma, and compared serum IgM, IgG, and IgA levels preoperatively [141]. IgM and IgA were increased in patients with advanced gastric cancer and in all patients with colon cancer. In contrast IgG levels were low in early stage gastric carcinoma patients while a low IgG was seen only in advanced colon carcinoma. Serum immunoglobulin levels did not accurately predict stage, response, or relapse in this study.

Head and neck cancer

Immunocompetence has been frequently measured in patients with head and neck cancer [142, 143]. Sala et al. in a study of 104 patients with squamous cell carcinoma of the larynx, demonstrated that significant immune cellular infiltrates were favorable prognostic signs only in well-differentiated tumors [144]. These observations were partially refuted by Schuller who could not demonstrate any assay of systemic immunity which could identify patients accurately in terms of stage or prognosis [145]. His study further demonstrated that lymphocytes from regional lymph nodes could show significant immunoreactivity that did not correlate with systemic immunity, and did not predict the clinical or biologic behavior of the disease.

Newbill and Johny concluded that there are no assays of immunoreactivity in head and neck cancer patients which can reliably select patients with a good prognosis or those likely to respond to therapy [146]. The conclusion of Wanebo [147] still appears to hold true: (1) Head and neck cancer patients have marked diminution of cell-mediated immunity even early in their course. (2) Defects appear to worsen with stage. (3) Smoking, alcoholism, and malnutrition are major contributors to immunosuppression.

Male genitourinary cancer

Male genitourinary neoplasms are commonly associated with immunoincompetence. Ablin *et al.* examined a broad spectrum of cellular and humoral immune-mediated parameters in prostatic carcinoma patients without prior knowledge of the patient's clinical stage, and found that the so-called 'immune stage' correlated with the patients' clinical stage [148]. Lubaroff *et al.* however, found no difference in the *in vitro* immunity tests between normal males and those with prostatic carcinoma [149]. DNCB reactivity was not impaired in a small series of patients with prostatic carcinoma evaluated by Catalona *et al.* [150] but they later described a positive correlation between DNCB skin test responsivity and PHA-induced blastogenesis in patients with renal cell carcinoma or bladder cancer [151].

Reports of two studies of assays of immunoreactivity in bladder carcinoma patients are typical of the conflicting reports available. Bean *et al.* demonstrated that 75% of the patients with superficiel tumors are DNCB skin test-positive, whereas only 35% of patients with locally advanced or metastatic disease have positive tests [152]. Flamm *et al.* followed 68 patients with biopsy-proven tumors of the urinary bladder for five years from the time of diagnosis [153]. Skin test reactivity to common recall antigens and serum immunoglobulin levels did not differentiate invasiveness or grades of malignance. While highly aggressive tumors were associated with anergy to DNCB, it is not clear that DNCB reactivity selected discriminately for poor prognosis.

More recently, the loss of A, B, and H blood group antigens from the cell surface of transitional carcinoma has been proposed as indicating poorly differentiated tumors with a tendency towards invasive recurrence [154, 155]. However, others have been unable to demonstrate the diagnostic sensitivity of this assay [156, 157].

Gynecologic cancer

In 161 patients with cervical carcinoma, higher serum IgA, C3, and IgM levels, and improved PHA-induced blastogenesis, appeared to correlate with the degree of tumor differentiation [158]. Levin *et al.* used cell-free extracts of autologous tumor for cutaneous testing and showed responsivity in 4 out of 6 patients in complete remission, whereas responses were seen in 0/7 patients in relapse [159]. Piver *et al.* evaluated pretherapy and monthly skin test response to common recall antigens in 51 patients with stage III and IV ovarian carcinoma and found no correlation with response to therapy [160].

Onsrud evaluated serum from 25 patients with ovarian carcinoma for its suppressive effects on normal lymphocytes in an assay of natural-killer cell activity and PHA-induced blastogenesis [161]. Only PHA suppression correlated with the clinical course, with those patients dying within one year of diagnosis showing the most severe suppression, and a possible relationship between the assay and tumor burden. The significance of these observations is limited in that the total number of patients is small, there were no adequate controls, and the effects of performance status and chemotherapy could not be determined.

Malignant melanoma

In a study by Lui *et al.* of 21 patients in various stages of malignant melanoma, it was noted that routine assessments of lymphocyte function or number did not provide clinically relevant data [162]. Byrom *et al.* however, in his study of 85 patients with melanoma showed lower mean levels of total T-lymphocytes and higher mean levels of B-cells than in normal controls [163]. The absolute and percent decrease in T- and B-cells did appear to be related to stage in this study. Balch *et al.* recently reported that diminution of autologous lymphocyte response to interleukin-2 appeared to be stage-related, and also that interleukin-2-induced cytotoxicity of heterologous lymphocytes could be inhibited by a serum-suppressive factor related to tumor growth [164].

Primary cerebral tumors

Depressed cell-mediated immunity with a decrease in T-helper cells and depressed B-cell function has been described in patients with primary brain cancer [165, 166]. In this study, no difference was found in cellular suppressor mechanisms between lymphocytes of normal individuals and those of patients with primary brain malignancies.

Conclusion

Although there is little doubt that quantitative and qualitative immune deficiencies exist in patients with cancer, there are at present no reliable, reproducible, or cost-effective assays which have a clinically meaningful role in the management of patients. Even in Hodgkin's disease, where a clear defect in cell-mediated immunity is present (and is almost certainly a major etiologic factor in the disease) it is still not clear that the studies attaching high prognostic significance to *in vitro* assays are clinically relevant.

Many studies reported to date are poorly controlled, not longitudinal, involve too few patients and are not homogeneous in terms of clinical stage, therapy, or nutritional and performance status. Age effects, poor nutrition and the immune-suppressive effects of chemotherapy, radiation therapy and surgery may all confound attempts at reliable interpretation of assays of immunoreactivity in cancer patients.

References

1. Cochran AJ: *Man Cancer and Immunity.* London, England. Academic Press, Inc. 1978, pp 108–44
2. Wanebo HJ, Pinsky CM, Beattie EJ: Immunocompetence testing in patients with one of the common operable cancer – a review. In: *Immonodiagnosis and Immunotherapy of Malignant Tumors,* Flad HD, Betzler HM (eds). New York: Springer-Verlag, 1979, pp 103–14
3. Hersh EM, Gutterman JU, Mavligit GM *et al.*: Immunocompetence, immunodeficiency and prognosis in cancer. *Ann NY Acad Sci* 276: 386–406, 1976
4. Hersh EM, Mavligit GM, Gutterman JU: Immunodeficiency in cancer and the importance of immune evaluation of the cancer patient. *Med Clin North Am* 60: 623–39, 1976
5. Valagussa P, Santoro A, Kenda R *et al.*: Second malignancies in Hodgkin's disease: a complication of certain forms of treatment. *Br Med J*: 216–19, 1980
6. Pederson-Bjergaard J, Larsen SO: Incidence of acute nonlymphocytic leukaemia, preleukaemia and acute myeloproliferative syndrome up to ten years after treatment of Hodgkin's disease. *N Engl J Med* 307: 965–71, 1982
7. Lerner HJ: Acute myelogenous leukaemia in patients receiving chlorambucil as long-term adjuvant chemotherapy for stage II breast cancer. *Cancer Treat Rep* 62: 1135–38, 1978
8. Eccles SA: Host Immune Mechanisms in the Control of Tumor Metastasis. In: *Tumor Immunity in Prognosis*, Haskill S (ed). New York: Marcel Dekker, Inc. 1982, pp 37–74
9. Ting CC, Hargrove ME: Tumor cell-triggered macrophage-mediated suppression of the T-cell cytotoxic response to tumor-associated antigens. II. Mechanisms for induction of suppression. *JNCI* 69: 873–78, 1982
10. Robbins DS, Fudenberg HH. Human lymphocyte subpopulations in metastatic neoplasia – Six years later. *N Engl J Med* 308: 1595–97, 1983
11. Fauk WP: Nutrition and immunity. *Nature* 250: 283–84, 1974
12. Good RA, Fernandes G. Nutrition, immunity, and cancer – a review. Part I. Influence of protein or protein-calorie malnutrition and zinc deficiency on immunity. *Clin Bull* 9: 3–12, 1979
13. Mullen TJ, Kirckpatrick JR: The effect of nutritional support on immune competency in patients suffering from trauma, sepsis, or malignant disease. *Surgery* 90: 610–5, 1981
14. Dilman VM: Aging, metabolic immunodepression and carcinogenesis. *Mech Ageing Dev* 8: 153–73, 1978
15. Yunis EJ, Fernandes G, Greenberg LJ: Tumor immunology and aging. *J Am Geriatr Soc* 24: 258–263, 1976
16. Campbell AC, Hersey P, Maclennan ICM *et al.*: Immunosuppresive consequences of radiotherapy and chemotherapy in patients with acute lymphoblastic leukemia. *Br Med J* 2: 385–88, 1973
17. Park SK, Brosy JL, Wallace HA *et al.*: Immunosupressive effect of surgery. *Lancet* 1: 53, 1971
18. Petrini B, Wasserman J, Rotstein S *et al.*: Radiotherapy and persistent reduction of peripheral T-cells. *J Clin Lab Immunol* 11: 159–60, 1983
19. Fuks Z, Strober S, Bobrove AM *et al.*: Long-term effects of radiation on T and B lymphocytes in peripheral blood of patients with Hodgkin's disease. *J Clin Invest* 58: 803–814, 1976

186

20. Stratton JA, Byfield PE, Byfield JE *et al.*: A comparison of the acute effects of radiation therapy, including or excluding the thymus, on the lymphocyte subpopulations of cancer patients. *J Clin Invest* 56: 88–97, 1975

21. Weitzman SA, Aisenberg AC, Siber GR *et al.*: Impaired humoral immunity in treated Hodgkin's disease. *N Eng J Med* 297: 245–248, 1977

22. Hancock BW, Bruce L, Ward AM *et al.*: Changes in immune status in patients undergoing splenectomy for the staging of Hodgkin's disease. *Br Med J*: 313–315, 1976

23. Gross L, Mandredi DL, Protos AA: The effect of cobalt-60 irradiation upon cell-mediated immunity. *Radiology* 106: 653–655, 1973

24. Bjorkholm M, Holm G, Mellstedt H: Immunologic profile of patients with cured Hodgkin's disease. *Scand. J Haematol* 18: 361–68, 1977

25. Tarpley JL, Potvin C, Chretian PB: Prolonged depression of cellular immunity in cured laryngopharyngeal cancer patients treated with radiation therapy. *Cancer* 35: 638–644, 1975

26. Hancock BW, Bruce L, Whitham MD *et al.*: The effects of radiotherapy on immunity in patients with cured localised carcinoma of the cervix uteri. *Cancer* 53: 884–887, 1984

27. Kun LE, Johnson RE: Haematological and immunologic status in Hodgkin's disease 5 years after radical radiotherapy. *Cancer* 36: 1912–16, 1975

28. Halili M, Bosworth T, Romney S *et al.*: The long-term effect of radiotherapy on the immune status of patients cured of gynaecological cancer. *Cancer* 37: 2875–78, 1926

29. Bodey GP: Factors predisposing cancer patients to infection. In: *Proceedings of the 13th International Congress of Chemotherapy,* Spitzy KH, Karrer K (eds). 1983, pp 313-318

30. Harris J, Sengar D, Stewart T *et al.*: The effect of immunosuppressive chemotherapy on immune function in patients with malignant disease. *Cancer* 37: 1058–69, 1976

31. Serrou B, Dubois JB, Silva R: Immunological overshoot phenomenon following chemotherapy of solid tumours. *Proc Am Assoc Cancer Res* 15: 125, 1974

32. Borella L, Green AA, Webster RG: Immunologic rebound after cessation of long-term chemotherapy in acute leukaemia. *Blood* 40: 42–51, 1972

33. Smith JA, Hendry HS, Duncan JL *et al.*: Post operative stimulation of cell mediated immunity. *Klin Wochenschr* 63: 1009–18, 1985

34. Anderson WL, Tomasi TB: Immunosuppression in neoplasia. In: *Handbook of Cancer Immunology,* Waters H. (ed). Vol. 7. New York: Garland Publishing, Inc., 1981, pp 27–50

35. Constantopoulos A, Najjar VA, Wish JB *et al.*: Defective phagocytosis due to tuftsin deficiency in splenectomized subjects. *Am J Dis Child* 125: 663–65, 1973

36. Reinherz EL, Rosen FS: New concepts of immunodeficiency. *Am J Med* 71: 511–513, 1981

37. Bolton PM: DNCB sensitivity in cancer patients. A review based on sequential testing in 430 patients. *Clin Oncol* 1: 59–69, 1975

38. Pinsky CM: Skin Tests. In: *Immunodiagnosis of Cancer*, Herberman RB, McIntire KR (eds). Part 2. New York: Marcel Dekker, Inc., 1979, pp 722–737

39. Golub SH, O'Connell TX, Morton DL: Correlation of in vivo and in vitro assays of immunocompetence in cancer patients. *Cancer Res* 34: 1833–7, 1974

40. Davies CJ, Meredith ID, Robins RA *et al.*: Tests of cell mediated immunity in patients with early breast cancer. I. Response to DNCB at time of mastectomy. *Clin Oncol* 4: 227, 1978

41. Oldham RK, Herberman RB: Delayed hypersensitivity skin tests with tumor extracts. In: *Immunodiagnosis of Cancer*, Herberman RB, McIntire KR (eds). Part 2. New York: Marcel Dekker, Inc., 1979, pp 940–963

42. Vanky FT, Stjernsward J: Lymphocyte stimulation by autologous tumor biopsy cells. In: *Immunodiagnosis of Cancer*, Herberman RB, McIntire KR (eds). Part 2. New York: Mark Dekker, Inc., 1979, pp 998–1031

43. Catalona WJ, Sample WF, Chretien PB: Lymphocyte reactivity in cancer patients. Correlation with tumor histology and clinical stage. *Cancer* 31: 65–71, 1973

44. Cole D, Van Epps DE, Williams RC Jr: Defective T-lymphocyte chemotactic factor production in patients with established malignancy. *Clin Immunopathol* 38: 209–21, 1986

45. Dillman RO, Koziol JA, Zavanelli MI *et al.*: Immunoincompetence in cancer patients. *Cancer* 53: 1484–91, 1984

46. Hockings GR, Rolland JM, Nairn Rc *et al.*: Lymphocyte fluorescence polarization after phytohemagglutinin stimulation in the diagnosis of colorectal carcinoma. *J Natl Cancer Inst* 68: 579, 1982

47. Rubin RH, Cosimi AB, Goetz EJ: Defective human mononuclear leukocyte chemotaxis as an index of host resistance to malignant melanoma. *Clin Immunol Immunopathol* 6, 376–88, 1976

38. Halliday WJ, Maluish A, Isbister WH: Detection of anti-tumour cell-mediated immunity and serum blocking factors in cancer patients by the leucocyte adherence inhibition test. *Br J Cancer* 29: 31–35, 1924

49. Burger DR: Leukocyte adherence inhibition. In: *Immunodiagnosis of Cancer,* Herberman RB, McIntire KR (eds). Part 2. New York: Marcel Dekker, Inc., 1979, pp 1124–1146

50. Forbes JT, Greco FA, Oldham RK: Natural cell-mediated cytotoxicity in human tumour patients. In: *Natural Cell-mediated Immunity Against Tumours*, Herberman RB (ed). New York: Academix Press 1980, pp 1031–45

51. Broder S, Mool L, Waldmann TA: Suppressor cells in neoplastic disease. *J Natl Cancer Inst* 61: 5–11, 1978

52. Yamagishi H, Pellis NR, Margalit B *et al.*: Specific and non-specific immunologic mechanisms of tumour growth facilitation. *Cancer* 45: 2929–33, 1980

53. Fujimoto S, Greene MI, Sehon MH: Regulation of the immune response to tumour antigens. II. The nature of immune-suppressor cells in tumour-bearing hosts. *J Immunol* 116: 800–806, 1976

54. Deutsch O, Devens B, Naor D: Immune responses to weakly immunogenic murine leukaemia-virus induced tumours. VIII. Characterization of suppressor cells. *Isr J Med Sci* 16: 538–544, 1980

55. Kadish AS, Doyle AT, Steinhaurer EH *et al.*: Natural cytotoxicity and interferon production in human cancer: Deficient natural killer activity and normal interferon production in patients with advanced disease. *J Immunol* 127: 1817–22, 1981

56. Herman J, Dianrello CA, Kew MC *et al.*: The role of interleukin 1 (IL 1) in tumor-NK cell interactions: correction of defective NK cell activity in cancer patients by treating target cells with IL 1. *J Immunol* 135: 2882–6, 1985

57. Merluzzi VJ, Last-Barney K: Potential use of human interleukin 2 as an adjunct for the therapy of neoplasia. Immunodeficiency and infectious disease. *Int J Immunopharmacol* 7: 31–9, 1985

58. Nakayama E, Asano S, Takuwa N *et al.*: Decreased TCGF activity in the culture medium of PHA stimulated peripheral mononuclear cells from patients with metastatic cancer. *Clin Exper Immunol* 51: 511, 1983

59. Cameron DJ: Impairment of macrophage activating factor (MAF) production in lymphocytes from cancer patients. *Jpn J Exp Med*: 55: 13–19, 1985

60. Ganguly R, Waldman RH: Secretory immunoglobulins and cancer. In: *Handbook of Cancer Immunology*, Waters H (ed). Vol. 4. New York: Garland Publishing, Inc., 1978, pp 313–29

61. Virchow R: *Krankhaften Geschwulste.* Berlin, 1983

62. Woglom WH: Immunity to transplantable tumours. *Cancer Rev* 4: 129–214, 1929

63. Gilchrist KW, Kalish L, Gould VE *et al.*: Immunostaining for carcinoembryonic antigen does not discriminate for early recurrence in breast cancer. The ECOG experience. *Cancer* 56: 351–5, 1985

64. Peters MV, Alison RE, Buch RS: Natural history of Hodgkin's disease as related to staging. *Cancer* 19: 308–346, 1966

65. Johnson RE, Thomas LB, Chretien P: Correlation between clinico-histologic staging and extranodal relapse in Hodgkin's disease. *Cancer* 25: 1071–75, 1970

188

66. Lowe D, Jorizzo J, Hutt MSR: Tumour-associated eosinophilia: A review. *J Clin Pathol* 34: 1343–48, 1981
67. Black MM, Kerpe S, Speer FD: Lymph node structure in patients with cancer of the breast. *Am J Pathol* 29: 505–521, 1953
68. Fisher ER, Kotwal N, Hermann C *et al.*: Types of tumour lymphoid response and sinus histiocytosis: Relationship to five-year, disease-free survival in patients with breast cancer. *Arch Pathol Lab Med* 107: 222–227, 1983
69. Greco RS: The antigenicity of synchronous cancers of the colon and rectum. *J Surg Oncol* 17: 49–56, 1981
70. Fletcher RH: Carcinoembryonic antigen. *Ann Intern Med* 104: 66–73, 1986
71. Niloff JM, Bast RC Jr, Schaetzl EM *et al.*: Predictive value of CA 125 antigen levels in second-look procedures for ovarian cancer. *Am J Obstet Gynecol* 151: 981–6, 1985
72. Smith LH, Oi RH: Detection of malignant ovarian neoplasms: a review of the literature. III. Immunological detection and ovarian cancer-associated antigens. *Obstet Gynecol Surv* 39: 346–60, 1984
73. Huth JF, Gupta RK, Eilber FR *et al.*: A prospective postoperative evaluation of urinary tumor-associated antigens in sarcoma patients. Correlation with disease recurrence. *Cancer* 15: 1306–10, 1984
74. Rossen RD, Morgan AC Jr: Blockade of the Humoral Response: Immune Complexes in Cancer. In: *Handbook of Cancer immunology*, Waters H (ed). Vol. 9. New York: Garland Publishing, Inc., 1981, pp 209–280
75. Salinas FA, Wee KH, Silver HK: Clinical relevance of immune complexes, associated antigen, and antibody in cancer. *Contemp Top Immunobiol* 15: 55–109, 1985
76. Vanky F, Kreicbergs A, Aparisi T *et al.*: Correlations between lymphocyte-mediated auto-tumor reactivities and the clinical course of 46 sarcoma patients. *Cancer Immunol Immunother* 16: 11, 1983
77. Vanky F, Petterffu A, Book K *et al.*: Correlation between lymphocyte-mediated auto-tumor reactivities and the clinical course: II. Retrospective evaluation of 69 patients with lung carcinoma. *Cancer Immunol Immunother* 16: 17, 1983
78. Raffield M, Neckers L, Longo DL *et al.*: Spontaneous alteration of idiotype in a monoclonal B-cell lymphoma. Escape from detection by anti-idiotype. *N Engl J Med* 312: 1653–8, 1985
79. Hersh EV, Gutterman JU, Mavligit GM: Effect of haematological malignancies and their treatment on host defence factors. *Clin Haematol* 5: 425–48, 1976
80. Fernandez A, MacSween JM, Langley GR: Immunoglobulin secretory function of B cells from untreated patients with chronic lymphocytic leukemia and hypogammaglobulinemia: role of T cells. *Blood* 62: 767–74, 1983
81. Whelan CA, Willoughby R, McCann SR: Relationship between immunoglobulin levels, lymphocyte subpopulations and Rai staging in patients with B-CLL. *Acta Haematol* (Basel) 69: 217–223, 1983
82. Ben-Bassat I, Many A, Modan M *et al.*: Serum immunoglobulins in chronic lymphocytic leukemia. *Am J Med Sci* 278: 4–9, 1979
83. Hancock BW, Bruce L, Richmond J: Neutrophil function in lymphoreticular malignancy. *Br J Cancer* 33: 396–500, 1976
84. Hersh EM, Whitecar JP Jr, McCredie KB *et al.*: Chemotherapy, immunocompetence, immunosuppression and prognosis in acute leukemia. *N Engl J Med* 285: 1211–16, 1971
85. Hersh EM, Gutterman JU, Mavligit GM *et al.*: Serial studies of immunocompetence of patients undergoing chemotherapy for acute leukemia. *J Clin Invest* 54: 401–8, 1974
86. Gutterman JU, Hersh EM, McCredie KB: Lymphocyte blastogenesis to human leukemia cells and their relationship to serum factors, immunocompetence, and prognosis. *Cancer Res* 32: 2524–9, 1972

87. Konior GS, Leventhal EG: Immunocompetence and prognosis in acute leukemia. *Semin Oncol* 3: 283–8, 1976

88. Borella L, Casper JT: Immunocompetence in childhood acute lymphocytic leukemia. In: *Handbook of Cancer Immunology*, Waters H (ed). Vol. 4. New York, Garland Publishing, Inc., 1978, pp 103–132

89. Murphy MJ, Haghbin M: Immunological aspects of childhood leukemia. In: *Handbook of Cancer Immunology*, Waters H (ed). Vol. 4. New York, Garland Publishing, Inc., 1978, pp 133–160

90. Bergmann L, Mitrou PS, Weber KC *et al.*: Imbalance of T-cell subsets in monoclonal gammopathies. *Cancer Immunol Immunother* 17: 112–6, 1984

91. Fink PC, Galanos C: Serum anti-lipid A antibodies in multiple myeloma and Waldenstrom's macroglobulinaemia. *Immunobiology* 169: 1–10, 1985

92. MCR Working Party. Prognostic Features in the third MRC myelomatosis trial. *Br J Cancer* 42: 831–840, 1980

93. Hersh EM, Oppenheim JJ: Impaired in vitro lymphocytic transformation in Hodgkin's disease. *N Engl. J Med* 273: 1006–1072, 1965

94. Young RC, Corder MP, Haynes HA *et al.*: Delayed hypersensitivity in Hodgkin's disease. *Am J Med* 52: 63–72, 1972

95. Hancock BW, Bruce L, Sugden P *et al.*: Immune status in untreated patients with lymphoreticular malignancy – A multifactoral study. *Clin Oncol* 3: 57–63, 1977

96. Fisher RI, Young RC: Immunologic aspects of Hodgkin's disease. In: *Handbook of Cancer Immunology,* Waters H (ed). Vol. 4. New York: Garland Publishing, Inc., 1–28, 1978

97. Young RC, Corder MP, Berard CW *et al.*: Immune alterations in Hodgkin's disease. Effect of delayed hypersensitivity and lymphocyte transformation on course on survival. *Arch Int Med* 131: 446–454, 1973

98. Aisenberg AC, Weitzman S, Wilkes B: Lymphocyte receptors for concanavalin A in Hodgkin's disease. *Blood* 51: 439–443, 1978

99. Goodwin JS, Messner RP, Bankhurst AD *et al.*: Postglandin-producing suppressor cells in Hodgkin's disease. *N Engl J Med* 297: 963–968, 1977

100. Sugden PJ, Lilleyman JS: Impairant of lymphocyte transformation by plasma from patients with advanced Hodgkin's disease. *Cancer* 45: 899–905, 1980

101. Ford RJ, Tsao J, Kouttab NM *et al.*: Association of an interleukin abnormality with the T Cell defect in Hodgkin's disease. *Blood* 64: 386–92, 1984

102. Fisher RI, DeVita VT, Bostik F *et al.*: Persistent immunologic abnormalities in long-term survivors of advanced Hodgkin's disease. *Ann Int Med* 92: 595–599, 1980

103. Hancock BW, Bruce L, Whitman MD *et al.*: Immunity in Hodgkin's disease: Status after 5 years remission. *Br J Cancer* 46: 593–600, 1982

104. Sutherland RM, McCredre JD, Inch WR: Effect of splencectomy and radiotherapy on lymphocytes in Hodgkin's disease. *Clin Oncol* 1: 275–284, 1975

105. Kaplan HS: The nature of the immunologic defect. In: *Hodgkin's Disease*, 2nd ed. Cambridge MA: Harvard University Press, 1980, pp 236–279

106. Ciampelli E, Pelu G: Comportamenta della intradermoreazione alla tuberculina nei pazienti affetti da morbo di Hodgkin trattata radiologicamente. *Radiol Med* 49: 683–690, 1963

107. Jackson SM, Garrett JD, Craig AW *et al.*: Lymphocyte transformation changes during the clinical course of Hodgkin's disease. *Cancer* 25: 843–850, 1970

108. De Sousa M, Tan C, Tan R, *et al.*: Immunological parameters of prognosis in childhood Hodgkin's disease. *Proc Am Soc Clin Oncol* 19: 333, 1973

109. Han T, Sokal JE: Lymphocyte response to phytohemagglutinin in Hodgkin's disease. *Am J Med* 48: 728–34, 1970

110. Faguet GB, Davis HC: Survival in Hodgkin's disease: the role of immunocompetence and other major risk factors. *Blood* 59: 938–45, 1982

111. Bjorkholm M, Holm G, De Faire U et al.: Immunological defects in healthy twin siblings to patients with Hodgkin's disease. Scand J Haematol 19: 396–404, 1977

112. Hancock BW, Bruce L, Ward AM et al.: The immediate effects of splenectomy, radiotherapy and cytotoxic chemotherapy on the immune status of patients with malignant lymphoma. Clin Oncol 3: 137–44, 1977

113. Hawylowicz CM, Rees RC, Hancock BW et al.: Depressed natural killer cell activity in patients with malignant lymphoma, and failure of NK cells to respond to interferon treatment. Europ J Cancer 18: 1081–88, 1982

114. Urasinski I, Fiedorowicz-Fabrucy I, Sochacka-Kuzko B: immunological profile in patients with non-Hodgkin's lymphomas. Arch Immunol Ther Exp (Warsz) 31: 467–74, 1983

115. Bruce L, Hancock BW, Richmond J: Neutrophil function in human malignant disease. J Physiol 259: 48–50, 1976

116. Dent RG: The role of the mononuclear phagocyte system in cancer. Hosp Update 6: 469–79, 1980

117. Kadish AS, Doyle AT, Steinhaver EH et al.: Natural cytotoxicity and interferon production in human cancer: Deficient natural killer activity and normal interferon production in patients with advanced disease. J Immunol 127: 1817–22, 1981

118. Kaszubowski PW, Husby G, Tung KSK et al.: T-lymphocyte subpopulations in peripheral blood and tissues of cancer patients. Cancer Res 40: 4648–57, 1980

119. Braun DP, Nisuis SK, and Harris JE: Serial immune function testing to predict clinical disease relapse in solid tumor patients. Cancer Immunol Immunother 15: 155, 1983

120. Harris J, Bagai R, Stewart T: Recovery of Immune function in man following chemotherapy: an index of prognosis and a possible guide for immunotherapy. Blood 38: 805, 1971

121. Harris J, Bagai R, Stewart T: Immunocompetence and response to antitumor treatment. N Engl J Med 286: 494, 1972

122. Stein JA, Adler A, Efraim SB et al.: Immunocompetence, immunosuppression and human breast cancer. Cancer 38: 1171–87, 1876

123. Haim N, Rudik L, Samuelly B et al.: Immune status in patients cured of breast and gynaecological cancer. Clin Oncol 7: 141–47, 1981

124. Twomey PL, Catalona WJ, Chretien PB: Cellular immunity in cured cancer patients. Cancer 33: 435–40, 1974

125. Olkowski ZL, McLaren JR, Skeen MJ: Effects of combined immunotherapy with levamisole and Bacillus Calmette-Guerrin on immunocompetence of patients with squamous cell carcinoma of the cervix, head and neck, and lung undergoing radiation therapy. Cancer Treat Rep 62: 1651–61, 1978

126. Hughes LE, Teasdale C, Forbes JF: Correlation between nonspecific immune competence and clinical outcome of breast, colon, and stomach cancer. In: Immunodiagnosis and Immunotherapy of Malignant Tumors, Plad HD, Betzler HM (eds). Springer-Verlag: New York, 1977, pp 95–102

127. Alsabti EA: In vivo and in vitro assays of immuno-competence in bronchogenic carcinoma. Oncology 36: 151–5, 1979

128. Alberola V, Gonzalez-Moline A, Trenor A et al.: Mechanism of suppression of the depressed lymphocyte response in lung cancer patients. Allergol Immunopathol 13: 213–9, 1985

129. Olkowski ZL, McLaren JR, Mansour KA: Immunocompetence of patients with bronchogenic carcinoma. Ann Thorac Surg 21: 546–51, 1976

130. Munzarova M, Kovaric J, Hlavkova J et al.: DNCB and PPD skin tests and prognosis in 152 patients with breast cancer. A prospective 2-year follow-up. Neoplasma 32: 45–50, 1985

131. Papatestas AE, Lesnick GJ, Genkins G et al.: The prognostic significance of peripheral lymphocyte counts in patients with breast carcinoma. Cancer 37: 164–8, 1976

132. Flores M, Maiti JH, Grosser N, MacFarlance JK et al.: An overvieuw: Anti-tumor immunity in breast cancer assayed by the tube leukocyte adherence inhibition. Cancer 39: 84–505, 1977

133. Baldwin RW: Manipulation of host resistance in cancer therapy. *Springer Seminars in Immuno-pathology* 5: 113, 1982

134. Haybittle JL, Blamey RW, Elston CW *et al.*: A prognostic index in primary breast cancer. *Br J Cancer* 45: 361, 1982

135. Lee AK, DeLillis RA, Rosen PP *et al.*: ABH blood group isoantigen expression in breast carcinoma – an immunohistochemical evaluation using monoclonal antibodies. *Am J Clin Pathol* 83: 208–19, 1985

136. Holdsworth PJ, Thorogood J, Benson EA: Blood groups as a prognostic indicator in breast cancer. *Br Med J* 290: 671–3, 1985

137. Stein JA, Adler A, Efraim SB *et al.*: Immunocompetence, immunosuppression, and human breast cancer . I. An analysis of their relationshio by known parameters of cell-mediated immunity in well-defined clinical stages of disease. *Cancer* 38: 1171–87, 1876

138. Mandeville R, Lamoureux G, Legault-Poisson S etc.: Biological markers and breast cancer. A multiparametric study. II. Depressed immune competence. *Cancer* 50: 1280–8, 1982

139. Kim JP: Immunochemosurgery for gastric cancer. *Semin Surg Oncol* 1: 105–15, 1985

140. Janssen CW Jr, Tender O, Matre R: The prognostic value of postoperative serum immunoglo-bulin and compelement component concentrations following gastric resection for carcinoma. *Acta Chir Scand* 151: 63–7, 1985

141. Sanz ML, Oehling A, Subira ML *et al.*: Immunologic study of carcinoma of the digestive tract. Influence of tumor staging. II. Humoral immunity in the preoperative period. *Allergol Immuno-pathol* (Madr) 10: 95–100, 1982

142. Wanebo HJ, Jun MY, Strong EW: T-cell deficiency in patients with squamous cell cancer of the head and neck. *Am J Surg* 130: 445–51, 1975

143. Scully C. Immunology and oral cancer. *Br J Oral Surg* 21: 136–46, 1983

144. Sala O, Ferlito A: Morphological observations of immunobiology of laryngeal cancer. Eval-uation of the defensive activity of immunocompetent cells present in tumor stroma. *Acta Otolaryng* (Stockh) 81: 353–63, 1976

145. Schuller DE: An Assessment of neck node immunoreactivity in head and neck cancer. *Laryngo-scope* 94: 1–35, 1984

146. Newbill ET, Johns ME: Immunology of head and neck cancers. *CRC Crit Rev Clin Lab Sci* 19: 1–25, 1983

147. Wanebo HJ: Immunobiology of head and neck cancer: basic concepts. *Head Neck Surg* 2: 42–55, 1979

148. Ablin RJ, Guinen PD, Rio ER: Immunologic aspects of malignancy. II. Host immunocompe-tence and relationship to the clinical stage in patients with prostatic cancer. *Allergol Immunopa-thol* (Madr) 4: 247–54, 1976

149. Lubaroff DM, Reynolds CW, Canfield L *et al.*: Immunologic aspects of the prostate. *Prostate* 2: 233–48, 1981

150. Catalona WJ, Smoley JK, Harty JI: Prognostic value of host immunocompetence in urologic cancer patients. *J Urol* 114: 922–6, 1975

151. Catalona WJ, Tarpley JL, Potvin C *et al.*: Host immunocompetence in genitourinary cancer: relation to tumor stage and prognosis. *Natl Cancer Inst Monogr* 49: 105–10, 1978

152. Bean MA, Schellhammer PS, Herr HW *et al.*: Immunocompetence of patients with transitional cell carcinoma as measured by dinitrochlorobenzene skin tests and in vitro lymphocyte function. *Natl Cancer Inst Monogr* 49: 111–14, 1978

153. Flamm J, Sagaster P, Hicksche M: The value of the DNCB test in bladder cancer. Pretreatment evaluation of immune function and 5-year follow-up of patients with urinary bladder cancer. *Urol Int* 39: 257–63, 1984

154. Stephenson TJ, Williams JL, Gelsthorpe K: Monoclonal antibodies to detect A, B and H blood group isoantigens in superficial transitional cell carcinoma of the bladder: a means of predicting invasive recurrences. *Br J Urol* 57: 148–53, 1985

155. Huland H, Kloppel G, Otto U *et al.*: The value of histologic grading and staging, random biopsies, tumor and bladder mucosa blood groups antigens, in predicting progression of superficial bladder cancer. *Eur Urol* 10: 28–31, 1984

156. Gorelick JI, Oyasu R, Golmon ME *et al.*: Correlation of ABH antigenicity and urine cytology results in transitional cell carcinoma of bladder. *Urology* 24: 287–90, 1984

157. Nakatsu H, Kobayashi I, Onishi Y *et al.*: ABO(H) blood group antigens and carcinoembryonic antigens as indicators of malignant potential in patients with transitional cell carcinoma of the bladder. *J Urol* 131: 252–7, 1984

158. Pulay TA, Csomor A: Tumor differentiation and immunocompetence in cervical cancer patients. *Neoplasma* 26: 617–21, 1979

159. Levin L, McHardy JE, Poulton TA *et al.*: Tumour associated immunity and immunocompetence in ovarian cancer. *Br J Obstet Gynecol* 83: 393–9, 1976

160. Piver MS, Blumenson L, Barlow JJ *et al.*: Delayed hypersensitivity reactions vs. chemotherapy and immunotherapy responses in women with ovarian adenosarcoma. *J Surg Oncol* 17: 235–40, 1981

161. Onsrud M: Serum-mediated immunosuppression: a possible tumor marker in patients with ovarian carcinoma. *Gynecol Oncol* 21: 94–100, 1985

162. Lui VK, Karpuchas J, Dent PB *et al.*: Cellular immunocompetence in melanoma: effect of extent of disease and immunotherapy. *Br J Cancer* 32: 323–30, 1975

163. Byrom NA, Campbell MA, Dean AJ *et al.*: Thymosin-inducible lymphocytes in the peripheral blood of patients with malignant melanoma. *Cancer Treat Rep* 62: 1769–74, 1978

164. Balch CM, Itoh K, Tilden AB: Cellular immune defects in patients with melanoma involving interleukin-2-activated lymphocyte cytotoxicity and a serum suppressor factor. *Surgery* 98: 151–7, 1985

165. Cravioto H: Immunology of human brain tumors: a review. In: *The Handbook of Cancer Immunology*, Waters H (ed). Vol. 3. New York: Garland Publishing, Inc., 1978, pp 365–398

166. Rozman TL, Brooks WM, Steele C *et al.*: Pokeweed mitogen-induced immunoglobin secretion by peripheral blood lymphocytes from patients with primary intracranial tumors. Characterization of T helper and B cell function. *J Immunol* 134: 1545–50, 1985

III. Clinical application of prognostic indices

13. Prognostic indices in breast cancer

B.A. STOLL

Three separate components are needed to define the patient's prognosis in breast cancer – the risk and timing of relapse after primary treatment, the sequence of metastases and their sites, and the likely response of such metastases to treatment. Thus, to predict the overall duration of survival in an individual patient, an index needs to include the major variables likely to influence each separate phase. Our prognostic indices in the past have been so unreliable in this respect that breast cancer has despairingly been described as 'a number of entities, masquerading under a single name' [1].

Of the three components, the risk of early relapse is possibly the easiest to predict. It can roughly be assessed from the clinical TNM staging in conjunction with the pathological report on the excised tissue. These are therefore the criteria currently used to identify those patients with resectable tumours who might benefit from the addition of aggressive adjuvant systemic therapy. However, while they help to recognise a group of patients with a high risk of dying within five years because of disseminate micrometastases, they provide little guide to the *biological characteristics* of an individual tumour. It is these which determine the likely sequence, distribution and time pattern of recurrences, and the likelihood of benefit from systemic treatment.

In order to establish an effective prognostic index, we need to:

(a) Distinguish clinical, histopathological, biological and biochemical criteria clearly related to proliferative or metastatic aggressiveness, from those related to the total tumour burden in the body.

(b) Distinguish a prognostic index useful at the time of presentation from one to be applied at relapse.

(c) Assess the relative importance of each predictive factor, (i.e. decide its weighting strength) in determining the duration of relapse-free survival compared to post-relapse survival. With these three distinct aims, predictive criteria will be examined under the following headings:

– Clinical criteria of prognosis at presentation.
– Biological criteria of prognosis at presentation.

– Multivariate analysis of prognostic criteria.
– Prognostic criteria at relapse.

Clinical criteria at presentation (Table 1)

TNM staging of breast cancer aims to identify those tumours offering a possibility of cure by standard therapy. In addition to guiding the choice of therapy, staging also provides an 'educated guess' as to the patient's risk of dying in the first five years, and is therefore used to stratify groups of patients being entered into clinical trials. As a guide either to treatment or to risk of early death, the TNM staging is usually amplified by the pathological report on the excised tissue which confirms the size and local spread of the primary tumour, and the degree and levels of axillary node invasion.

However, in the operable case, clinical stage and pathological node status at presentation bear little or no relation to the progress of the disease once the first recurrence has manifested. Thus, although clinical stage is related to the relapse-free interval, it is not related to the duration of the post-relapse survival [2–5]. Moreover, clinical stage is not related to the proliferative activity of the primary tumour as measured by the labelling index [6, 7].

Clinical stage at presentation is not therefore a measure of the aggressiveness of breast cancer but may be more a measure of its chronological age (see Chapter 3). Stage 2 patients have a greater risk of dying in the first five years after primary treatment than do Stage 1 cases, probably because they have a higher burden of tumour cells in the body. This hypothesis is at present, impossible to prove because current markers of tumour burden and current imaging methods for small metastases are relatively crude, although improvement is expected from techniques using radio-labelled monoclonal antibodies [8]. Future clinical trials aiming to compare survival rates from different primary treatments must there-

Table 1. Clinical and biological criteria of prognosis at the time of breast cancer presentation

Clinical criteria	Biological criteria
Axillary node invasion	Histopathological criteria
Tumour size	Proliferative activity
Internal mammary node invasion	Cytometry
Delay before treatment	Steroid receptor content
Age group and menstrual status	Biochemical tests
Race	Hormone production
Bilaterality	Prostaglandin synthesis
Obesity	Immunological criteria
Reproductive factors	Proto-oncogenes

fore be able to quantify tumour cell burden if we are to stratify subsets of patients in a meaningful manner.

Five year survival rates in breast cancer are dominated by the deaths of patients presenting with more advanced disease and are therefore of little value in assessing the effect of loco-regional treatment upon prognosis. Even longer survival periods are no guide to cure because, of the two-thirds of operated cases who survive 5 years, half will die of their disease between 5 and 25 years following the operation [9–12]. Because of these differences in growth tempo, we need to distinguish from the outset (a) those cases who might benefit from aggressive adjuvant systemic therapy, from (b) those with indolent tumours for which minimal therapy might be compatible with prolonged survival. There is now overwhelming evidence of clonal heterogeneity in breast cancer, and continuous selection will lead to dominance of more malignant phenotypes. As a result, the prognosis in each individual *depends as much on how far biological progression has proceeded by the time of diagnosis, as it does on the presenting stage.*

Thus, two weaknesses – inability to quantify total tumour cell burden in the body and failure to assess growth tempo in the individual tumour – explain why so many clinical trials (even those with long term follow-up) have failed to prove the value of loco-regional or systemic therapy in the cure of operable breast cancer [13]. Patients are currently stratified by dimensional criteria and evidence of local tumour spread, but the biological heterogeneity between tumours in each subgroup is such that benefit from treatment in a particular subset of patients is heavily diluted and easily lost to significance [14]. Not only are clinical trial results inconclusive, but it is also unfortunate for many patients' quality of life that our present state of knowledge does not permit us to recognise relatively indolent tumour.

Axillary node invasion and prognosis

It is widely agreed that invasion of the axillary nodes is the most consistent predictor of early relapse in the patient with breast cancer, but the reason for this is disputed. Devitt [15] suggests that the presence of axillary node invasion indicates that the tumour has overcome the host reactive defences, but this conclusion is not supported by reports that 30–35% of long term survivors had shown histological evidence of axillary metastases at the time of primary surgery [10, 16].

As noted above, the presence of axillary node invasion may indicate a chronologically older tumour rather than a more aggressive tumour, because no difference has been shown between Stages 1 and 2 in the proportion of highly proliferative primary tumours as measured by the thymidine labelling index [6, 7]. Again, no difference has been shown between Stages 1 and 2 in the ratio between locoregional and distant metastases developing ultimately, and this suggests that there is no obvious difference in tumour invasiveness whether or not the axillary nodes are involved by tumour [17, 18].

The involvement of a larger number of axillary nodes (particularly the apical nodes) is associated with a relatively shorter relapse-free interval[19], but the duration of post-relapse survival is almost identical whether the exillary node status at presentation is N_0, N_{1-3} or N_{4+} [20]. There is also no correlation between the proliferative activity of the primary tumour (measured by thymidine labelling) and the number of axillary nodes involved [20]. It is therefore likely that involvement of a larger number of nodes reflects an older tumour, and runs parallel to the extent of disseminated micrometastases and total body tumour burden. It is indeed reported that all patients in a series showing a positive bone scan before mastectomy proved to have evidence of extensive axillary node invasion [21].

It is therefore not surprising that the number of invaded axillary nodes is found to be the most significant prognostic discriminant for relapse-free survival at 10 years in the NSABP report [22]. Also, that in most clinical trials, the least benefit from adjuvant chemotherapy in node-positive premenopausal patients is shown in the subgroups with four or more nodes involved-presumably those with the greatest total tumour burden.

Tumour size and prognosis

While size of the primary tumour and invasion of axillary nodes are the major criteria of TNM clinical staging, the relative strength of each of these factors is not clear. This is because increasing size of the primary tumour is usually correlated with increasing likelihood of node invasion [23], increasing number of nodes involved, and increasing likelihood of apical node involvement [24]. Nevertheless, at 10 year follow-up, multivariate analysis shows that tumour size and nodal status become independent prognostic criteria for survival [22].

It has been reported that smaller tumours are associated not only with a longer relapse-free interval, but also a longer post-relapse survival than are larger tumours [25], which might suggest that tumour size is related to growth aggressiveness. While tumour size is not correlated with histological grading [22], it correlates better with the proliferative activity of the tumour than does lymph node status [26]. Koscielny *et al.* [27] suggest that the size of the tumour at presentation is also related to the probability of metastatic dissemination. Extrapolating back from the observation that the median relapse-free interval is shorter when tumours are larger, they postulate that there is a critical tumour size which dictates when the first metastasis is initiated.

In spite of these overall observations, a large primary tumour does not necessarily carry a poor prognosis for the individual – especially in the case of postmenopausal patients. The mean oestrogen receptor level is found to be higher in T2 and T3 tumours than in T1 tumours in post-menopausal patients [28], and many T3 tumours larger than 6 cms are associated with better overall survival than are smaller tumours [29]. Presumably these represent a subgroup of slowly growing tumours which need to be distinguished from the others by biological criteria. It is the failure to distinguish them which has led to the current confusion as to the optimal treatment for T3 tumours [30].

Internal mammary node invasion and prognosis

Demonstrable invasion of the internal mammary nodes is an important pointer to prognosis, and is found in only 9% of patients with negative axillary nodes compared to 35% of those with involved axillary nodes [31]. In addition, the 10 year survival rate in breast cancer is only 20.5% when both axillary and internal mammary nodes are involved, compared to 45.8% when only the latter are involved [32].

While it may be possible to make an 'educated guess' as to the risk of internal mammary node involvement, based on the size of primary tumour, axillary node status and patient age [32], a more accurate assessment is now possible by scintigraphic imaging of the nodes using radiocolloid [33]. Since internal mammary node invasion is clearly related to prognosis, it has been suggested that future reviews of TNM staging should take their status into account [33].

Delay before treatment and prognosis

The literature shows conflicting conclusions as to the relationship between delay before treatment and duration of survival in breast cancer. Mean delay before treatment is said to be longer in patients with more advanced disease at presentation [9], but long delay before presentation can also be associated with slowly growing disease. In one series, 5 year survival among patients with tumours over 5 cm in diameter, was more common in those with delay for a year or more, than it was for delay of less than 3 months [34].

As a guide to prognosis, attempts have been made to classify tumour growth as either slow or rapid according to duration of symptoms, and to refine the clinical estimate by enquiring for changes observed by the patient after the tumour's first appearance [35, 36]. Such changes include increase in size, change in consistency, development of skin retraction, oedema or ulceration or the appearance of other lumps in the breast, skin, axilla or supracavicular areas (see Chapter 2). It is claimed that clinical estimates of this type can be correlated with 10 year survival rates, especially in node negative cases [36], and that the prognostic information which can be obtained is independent of that obtained from lymph node status, clinical stage or tumour grade.

Feldman *et al.* [37] attempted to correlate the duration of symptoms (other than the lump) with tumour size, invasiveness and nodal status at operation. In 663 patients, they found no clear correlation between the presence of more extensive disease and longer delay in presentation. While a subgroup of slowly growing cancers remained localised even after delay of over 12 months, they concluded that earlier diagnosis must be aimed at if curability was to be increased.

Reports on 30 year follow-up suggest that most patient presenting with 'early' breast cancer have occult metastases by the time of diagnosis. But the outlook may be improved by current techniques of screening for early cancer. Four studies have shown 25–30% reduction in the proportion of Stage 2 cases and also reduction in mortality rates, among women who are regularly screened [38–41]. Since the benefit appears to apply only to women over the age of 50, it has been postulated that younger women may have more aggressive tumours. It has also been suggested that screening may select out only the slowly growing minimal cancers, and that it will provide only short-term reduction in mortality [42]. Against this conclusion is the follow-up report of the New Yok HIP study at 14 years, which continues to claim cumulative reduction in breast cancer deaths in the screened group [38].

Age group, menstrual status and prognosis

Numerous studies have shown inconsistent observations on the relationship between age group, menstrual status and survival rates in breast cancer. Until recently, there was no clear evidence of more aggressive disease in younger women, taking aggressiveness to mean rapid growth. However, increasing ability to measure biological indices of aggressiveness has shown significantly higher tumour proliferative activity in premenopausal than in postmenopausal groups [26, 43]. In each group, the proliferative activity could be correlated both with 6 year relapse-free survival and with overall survival rates [26]. A recent critical review [44] came to the following conclusions on the effect of age on prognosis:

(1) Differences in prognosis between pre- and postmenopausal groups of patients are difficult to detect from 5 year survival rates but are seen better with longer-term follow up. A major cause of conflicting reports is faulty death certification. A recent survey showed that although mortality from breast cancer was recorded as similar in younger as in older patients, in fact 91% of women under 50 died directly from the disease as compared with only 77% of those over 70 [45].

(2) Among premenopausal patients, there is a worse prognosis in the subgroup under the age of 35, but a better mean duration of survival in women going through the menopause shortly after the tumour presents [46]. When *all* preme-

nopausal women are lumped together for analysis, the worse prognosis in one subgroup cancels out the better prognosis in the other.

(3) Tumours in older patients show a lower level of mitotic activity and pleomorphism. In addition, tumours in older patients show higher oestrogen receptor concentrations and lower proliferative activity then do tumours in younger patients.

(4) Prognosis in younger women is more related to the proliferative activity and nuclear ploidy of the tumour. But in older women it is more related to the degree of differentiation and the steroid receptor activity of the tumour.

(5) Older patients are more likely to show their first recurrence loco-regionally, while younger patients are more likely to show their first recurrence at distant sites, and are more likely to show a 'shower' of such metastases. (The observations in (4) and (5) suggest that a higher level of steroid receptor or a higher degree of differentiation is associated with a lesser tendency to distant spread.)

Race and prognosis

In Japanese women, breast cancer is much less common than it is in American women. They also show a higher proportion of early stage and *in situ* cancers, and there is a 74% 5 year survival rate for operable breast cancer in Tokyo compared to 60% in New York [47]. The better prognosis in Japanese women is said to persist even when stage and histological differences are taken into account but a recent study on Japanese women in Hawaii suggests that it disappears in that country when patient groups are matched for stage distribution [48].

The better prognosis noted for the disease in Japan (and also the higher proportion of early stage and *in situ* cancers) may be due either to genetic or environmental factors. An immunological influence is suggested by reports of more lymphoid infiltration within the tumour and sinus hyperplasia in the axillary lymph nodes of Japanese women with breast cancer. An endocrinological influence is suggested by reports of lower serum levels of free oestradiol among Japanese women in general. The latter may also account for their relatively lower incidence of breast cancer after the menopause [49].

Black women in the USA also have a lower incidence of breast cancer, but they have a *lower* survival rate than do Caucasian women in the same country [50]. Investigating the poorer prognosis, Ownby *et al* [51] found no difference in relapse-free periods or total survival between the two groups, when matched for tumour size, stage or grade, and for obesity in the host. They ascribe the higher mortality in blask women to a higher proportion of undifferentiated tumours, more advanced stage at diagnosis, greater frequency of obesity, and more early deaths from other causes.

But breast cancer may also be more aggressive in its growth in black women.

Not only are oestrogen receptor negative (ER −) tumours more frequent in black patients [52], but black postmenopausal patients with Stage 1 ER − tumours show a 67.6% relapse rate at 7 years compared to 29.9% for similar tumours in white women [53]. Thus, ER − tumours appear to be biologically more aggressive in black women, and this, associated with the higher incidence of undifferentiated tumours in black women [34], may be a major factor in their higher mortality rates. As in the case of Japanese women, immunological factors may be implicated.

Bilaterality and prognosis

Only about 1.5% of patients present with synchronous bilateral invasive breast cancer, but an additional 3.5% develop contralateral tumours later [55]. Bilateral breast cancer is more common in younger women (under the age of 50), those with a family history of breast cancer in a first degree relative, and also in association with lobular invasive cancer or proliferative disease in the breast. All these predictive characteristics are said to be relatively weak [56].

Several studies confirm that patients presenting with synchronous bilateral invasive breast cancer have a worse prognosis than those presenting with unilateral disease. For example, Fracchia *et al.* [55] report 84% 10 year relapse-free rates in patients with unilateral Stage 1 breast cancers compared to 71% for those with bilateral Stage 1 disease, and corresponding rates of 62% and 54% respectively for Stage 2 cases. However, in the case of cancer appearing in the second breast at a later date (metachronous bilateral cancer), a recent NSABP study of 1578 cases observed for 10 years suggests that survival is worse only when the contralateral tumour manifests within 2 years of the first tumour [56]. From the presence of *in situ* changes in addition to invasive cancer, the sudy concludes that the vast majority of cancers appearing in the second breast are new primary growths, and that spread across the midline is extremely rare as a cause of contralateral breast cancer.

Since 80% of the second cancers appeared within 5 years of the first tumour, the report also suggests that most metachronous cancers probably originate at the same time as the first tumour, and that their delayed appearance is merely a manifestation of a slower doubling time. Discordance of oestrogen receptor assay between the two sides was found to be more common in metachronous than in synchronous tumours [57], and such a finding would be surprising if most metachronous breast cancers originated by spread across the midline.

Obesity and prognosis

Obesity is claimed not only to increase predisposition to breast cancer but also to worsen prognosis, so that more advanced disease at presentation is found in heavier women [58, 59]. In one series [60], patients weighing under 150 lbs were found to have a 67% cumulative 5 years relapse-free rate compared to 49% for matching stage patients weighing more than 150 lbs, and another group has reported similar observations independently [61]. An adverse effect of obesity of prognosis may be exerted through an associated increase in oestrogen synthesis [62], but there is so far no confirmation of a report that breast cancers in obese women have a lower mean oestrogen receptor level [63].

Obesity may be an independant variable which plays a part in prognostic differences between different racial groups as mentioned above, but multivariate analysis suggests that obesity modifies prognosis only in specific subgroups in breast cancer [64]. Thus, it is found to affect prognosis only in women over the age of 50, while nulliparity appears to be associated with a poor prognosis only among obese women.

Reproductive factors and prognosis

Nulliparous women have a higher incidence of breast cancer than do parous women, especially those whose first pregnancy occurs at an early age. Although earlier reports [65, 66] could find no influence of parity on prognosis, Papatestas *et al.* [63] have reported a poorer 5 year relapse-free survival and a higher proportion of Stage 2 cases among nulliparous than among parous women. They noted also that the association between clinical stage and parity was greater when body weight was taken into account. It has been reported that early age at menarche or a late menopause are both associated with a worse prognosis in breast cancer, in addition to increasing the predisposition to breast cancer [67].

Biological criteria at presentation (Table 1)

Two types of biological marker can provide a pointer either to relapse-free interval or to post-relapse survival; (a) *Biological indices of tumour cell burden in the body*. These permit us to anticipate early clinical relapse and subsequently may provide a measure of overall tumour response to systemic therapy. (b) *Biological indices of tumour aggressiveness – either of invasiveness or proliferative activity*. While invasiveness and early metastasis mainly affect the length of relapse-free interval, the level of proliferative activity also affects the length of post-relapse survival.

It is increasingly being recognises that while higher proliferative activity in a tumour is often associated with evidence of greater invasiveness, they do not necessarily go hand in hand [68]. Thus, histopathological grading is established as a pointer to prognosis, but the importance of distinguishing proliferative activity from invasiveness has been given insufficient attention.

Histopathological criteria and prognosis

It was established 30 years ago that the prognosis in breast cancer patients could be related to histological grading of the primary tumour [69]. More recent investigations have concentrated on nuclear grading, histopathological typing of tumours, the presence of lymphatic or vascular invasion, lymphoid infiltration, necrosis in the tumour or elastosis in the stroma.

The classical histological grading of breast cancer is a composite assessment based on three distinct criteria-degree of tubular formation, nuclear pleomorphism and mitotic frequency in the tumour cells. Early reports suggested that the histological grading of breast cancer could be related to survival rate, and a difference of 30% was shown between survival rates in patients with high and low microscopic grades [69]. However, because of the heterogeneous appearance of different areas of the tumour under the microscope, and the fact that the vast majority of tumours present an unfavourable grade, it has been found difficult in practice to relate the likelihood of early recurrence to histological grade [70].

Nuclear grading is increasingly replacing histological grading in assessing prognosis [71]. It hardly varies throughout the tumour even in the presence of marked variation in tubular formation, and is more clearly correlated with the proliferative aspect of tumour grading in reflecting prognosis [72]. Among the specific nuclear characteristics, mitotic frequency is said to be more accurate than nuclear pleomorphism in predicting relapse [72], but it is more difficult to assess in routine practice.

Some of the less common histopathological types of breast cancer are associated with a significantly better prognosis. Thus, medullary carcinoma is associated with a longer survival than average, in spite of an apparently unfavourable histological and nuclear grading. In addition, tubular carcinoma, classical lobular carcinoma and mucin-producing colloid carcinoma are found more commonly among long survivors [10, 22, 73, 74]. The incidence and number of invaded axillary nodes are usually lower among these rather uncommon types of tumour [74], but lobular carcinoma is said to show a greater tendency to peritoneal and retroperitoneal metastasis [75].

Local invasion of lymphatic vessels is capable of misinterpretation [22] but is seen in approximately one third of cases. Its presence in Stage 1 disease is said to be correlated with systemic (especially visceral) metastases and with a poor prognosis [74, 76–79]. Local invasion of blood vessels also is difficult to interpret because of variations in criteria, but it is less common than lymphatic invasion and its poor prognostic significance is less certain [22, 74, 78]. Absence of a clearly demarcated border to the tumour has an uncertain prognostic significance [78,

80], but is claimed by some to indicate a greater tendency to node involvement and earlier recurrence following mastectomy [72]. Most agree that nipple involvement suggests a poor prognosis [22].

Black and his colleagues [14, 71] have stressed the significance of peripheral and perivenous lymphoid infiltration in the tumour as a good prognostic sign, but others disagree [78]. Fisher *et al.* [81] could not clearly relate it to disease-free interval, but found the presence of lymphoid infiltration to be associated with the presence of tumour necrosis, which itself carries a poor prognosis.

There is considerable disagreement also as to the significance of a lymphoid reaction in non-invaded axillary lymph nodes. Immunological reactions to the presence of breast cancer are common [22, 71, 82] and axillary node lymphocytes respond to mitogenic challenge [70], but the prognostic significance of such reactions is uncertain. While Black *et al.* [14, 17] suggested that sinus histiocytosis was a good prognostic sign. Tsakraklides *et al.* [82] found that lymphocytic predominance was a better indicator of a favourable course. On the other hand, Fisher *et al.* [22] reported that germinal centre predominance (follicular hyperplasia) was associated with a *poor* 10 year disease-free survival rate in node-negative cases.

The presence of elastosis in breast cancer is said to be associated with a longer relapse-free interval [83, 84], a longer survival [74] and a greater likelihood of response to endocrine therapy [85]. On the other hand, the presence of necrosis in the tumour is said to predict early recurrence [80] and shorter survival [22, 74] and is more likely to be associated with aneuploidy and higher proliferative activity [86].

Histopathological criteria may suggest a higher likelihood of *local recurrence* after primary treatment. These include the histopathological type [76, 78], cytological or nuclear grading [76, 78, 87] and lymphatic or blood vessel invasion [76, 78]. Another criterion for local recurrence is the presence of extensive intraductal growth [88], and this is significantly correlated with the presence of multicentric cancer [89].

There is increasing evidence that pre- and postmenopausal tumours differ in their histopathological pattern. While a few have found a similar distribution of high and low grade malignancy in all age groups [34, 77], most recent reports have found more anaplastic tumours among premenopausal patients [70, 90]. It is also reported that the stromal reaction (lymphoid infiltration and elastica formation) is less well marked in premenopausal women [70].

Disagreement between series on histopathological differences between breast cancers in pre- and postmenopausal women may depend on the predominant age group among the premenopausal cases [44]. (A similar observation has been made about differences in proliferative activity between pre- and postmenopausal breast cancers [26].) The biological activity of the tumour can differ markedly in women under the age of 35 from that in women approaching the menopause (see previous discussion on effect of age group on prognosis).

To summarise this section. A report on the nuclear grading of the tumour cells (mitotic frequency and nuclear pleomorphism) provides the best histological reflection of the proliferative activity of the tumour. It is strongly correlated with survival, particularly in the first few years after primary treatment [72, 91]. Evidence is increasing that the proliferative activity of a tumour provides no guide to its invasive or metastatic potential [92, 93]. With regard to metastatic potential, it is claimed that histological evidence of invasion of blood vessels or lymphatics or of dermal infiltration, has an independent prognostic value [79, 84]: also that the degree of tubular formation reflects the cohesiveness of its cellular components [91, 94] which is why highly differentiated tumours are less likely to metastasise. Metastasis genes regulate the cancer cell's ability to express enzymes which facilitate invasion [95].

Proliferative activity and prognosis

Breast cancers show widely divergent doubling times in their primary or metastatic tumours, the median being 120 days. While doubling times are a useful clinical concept, they reflect not only the rate of tumour replication but also the rate at which cells are lost by death or from the surface, or by escaping into the lymphatics or blood vessels. The actual duration of the cell cycle is between 1 and 4 days [96], and the proliferative activity of the tumour can be measured by ^{3}H thymidine labelling of the cells in S phase (DNA synthesis before mitosis).

Three independent groups [6, 7, 97] have shown that a higher thymidine labelling index (TLI) in the tumour is associated with earlier recurrence and shorter mean survival. TLI measurement is reported to be an independent prognostic factor so that the proliferative activity of the tumour is related neither to tumour size nor to axillary node status [6, 7]. On the other hand, a higher TLI is said to be associated histologically with a demarcated tumour border and a well marked lymphoid reaction to the tumour [97]. The mean TLI level is significantly higher in pre- than in postmenopausal patients, and in both groups, the level of TLI is significantly correlated with the risk of subsequent recurrence [26]. The information available from the assay is therefore considerable, but the measurement is laborious.

Cytometry and prognosis

The DNA histogram derived from either single cell methods or flow cytometry, is increasingly being used as a measure of cell kinetics in cancer. The DNA histogram allows discrimination between diploid and aneuploid tumours, provides information on the presence of more than one cell line in the tumour, and can measure the proliferative activity of the individual tumour. It can be carried out on stored paraffin blocks of tissue, so that it can be applied also to retrospective assessment.

Aneuploidy (either more or less chromosomal material than an exact multiple of haploid) is reported in about 70-80% of breast cancers. It is said to be associated with early relapse and a lower survival rate [98, 99] and as a prognostic factor, is claimed by some to be independent of age, menopausal status and clinical stage of the breast cancer at presentation [100, 101]. Although not all agree, aneuploid tumours tend to be histopathologically more highly mitotic and oestrogen receptor poor [102].

Cytometry can also be used to show the proportion of cells in S phase and thus the proliferative activity of the tumour. It correlates well with TLI measurements of proliferative activity [86], and tumours with a high level tend to be more highly mitotic and also oestrogen receptor poor [86, 102, 103]. They are also more likely to show aneuploidy [43, 86, 99]. As in the case of proliferative activity measured by TLI, proliferative activity of the tumour as established by cytometry shows no relationship to the clinical stage at presentation [43, 103]. Again, similar to TLI findings, it is reported that proliferative activity as measured by cytometry is higher in recurrent than in primary tumours, and in premenopausal than in postmenopausal cases of breast cancer [43].

Although the above data suggest that the presence of aneuploidy and high proliferative activity predict a higher likelihood of early relapse in breast cancer, there are some uncertainties; (a) How far is the prognostic information independent of that derived from histopathological criteria? (b) Some reports do not agree that ploidy is inversely correlated with oestrogen receptor level [104–106]. (c) While tumours which are aneuploid or have a high proportion of cells in S phase are associated with earlier relapse, mean survival after relapse is not shorter than in diploid tumours [98, 99]. (d) One report finds that patients with aneuploid tumours are more likely to respond to endocrine therapy and have a longer mean survival than do those with diploid tumours [107].

Serial changes in tumour flow cytometry measurements are being examined in fine needle aspiration biopsies taken from breast cancer under treatment by radiation, endocrine or cytotoxic chemotherapy. Not only may they show changes which will predict response to therapy, but they may also show the appearance of new clones in the tumour cell population associated with resistance to therapy [108].

Steroid receptor content and prognosis

Oestrogen receptor protein (ER) is found in about one half of all breast cancers, and a high level not only predicts the likelihood of response to endocrine manipulation but is also a prognostic variable. Although there is disagreement as to whether ER level is related to the relapse-free interval most studies show that receptor-rich primary breast cancer is associated with a longer overall survival time [109]. This correlation is independent of the size of the primary tumour and the lymph node status [110]. Several of the studies showing lower recurrence rates in ER + than in ER − tumours show that the advantage decreases after 2–3 years and then disappears [110]. Metastasis is presumably *delayed* in ER + cases and not decreased.

Patients with higher levels of progesterone receptor (PgR) in their tumours also show a more prolonged survival time, but again there is conflicting evidence as to whether the relapse-free interval is prolonged. It has been suggested that longer survival in receptor positive cases may be due to (a) delayed relapse; (b) more recurrences in bone or soft tissue − both associated with a better prognosis; (c) greater likelihood of response to endocrine therapy; (d) longer postrelapse survival in patients responding to endocrine manipulation [18].

The level of ER is inversely correlated with proliferative activity in the primary tumour as measures by thymidine labelling [96, 111], but there are conflicting reports on the existence of a correlation between receptor-poor status and histopathological grade in breast cancer. It is reported that as many as 75% of receptor-negative tumours are of grades 1 or 2 (more differentiated tumours) and it is therefore suggested that the two markers may be independent risk factors [112]. They are however, shown to be linked by the observation that receptor status is correlated with *nuclear* grade (especially mitotic frequency in the nucleus) but not with tubule formation [113].

Receptor status of the tumour clearly varies with the patient's age group. All authorities agree that mean ER levels in premenopausal tumours are lower than in postmenopausal tumours, but for anaplastic tumours, the PgR concentration is not lower in premenopausal than in postmenopausal patients [114]. The levels of androgen and corticosteroid receptors also do not appear to be significantly related to menstrual status [115].

Other correlates of steroid receptor status have been reported. Compared to typical ductal tumours, lobular carcinoma shows a higher proportion of ER + and PgR + tumours [75], while medullary carcinoma shows a lower proportion. ER + tumours are correlated with a greater degree of elastosis in the stroma and both are correlated with a longer relapse-free interval [84]. While ER levels in the tumour also show an inverse relationship to the presence of follicular hyperplasia in the axillary nodes [116], ER levels have not been significantly correlated with either lymphatic or blood vessel invasion by the primary tumour [78].

Biochemical tests in relation to prognosis

For breast cancer, we have so far no single biochemical marker in the blood which is directly and consistently related to tumour cell number. If available, such a marker would enable us to stage the tumour, select suitable treatment, detect new spread before it is clinically evident and modify treatment which is failing to control the disease. Nevertheless, various biochemical indices of tumour activity, including enzymes, foetal antigens and secretory products, have been put forward as markers of incipient relapse or as predictors of response to treatment.

The literature shows conflicting results on the value of carcinoembryonic antigen (CEA) assay in monitoring for recurrence after mastectomy. A raised blood level during adjuvant chemotherapy is claimed to predict relapse more reliably than does a raised level of alkaline phosphatase or lactic dehydrogenase [117]. It is also claimed that apparently early breast cancer patients with a raised CEA level either in the tumour or blood show a higher relapse rate [118], but this is not confirmed in a large co-operative trial [119]. A possible reason for inconsistent reports is that while liver metastases are associated with raised CEA levels in the blood in almost all cases, this applies to only about 50% of cases with metastases at other sites [120].

The level of acute phase proteins in the serum is also claimed to predict relapse after primary treatment in breast cancer [121]. An elevated level of these proteins is associated with suppression of cellular immunity, and is common also in benign breast disease. Ceruloplasmin levels are said to be elevated in about 90% of patients with metastatic breast cancer, and the assay has been suggested as a means of monitoring response to therapy or predicting recurrence after mastectomy [122].

Lactic dehydrogenase levels in the serum have been found to correlate with tumour burden in a variety of tumours including breast cancer. Persistently high levels after primary therapy are usually correlated with the presence of persistent tumour and a poor 5 year survival [120], but correlation is not absolute because the enzyme is so widely distributed in normal tissues [123].

A relationship has been claimed between the growth activity of breast cancer and the excretion rate of certain polyamines. Elevated levels are more common with metastatic than with primary breast cancer [124]. While putrescine appears to reflect the proliferative activity of the growth fraction, spermidine is thought to be a marker of cell death. Although increasing levels have preceded disease recurrence in some post-mastectomy cases, the usefulness of polyamines in monitoring breast cancer activity is limited [125].

In a comparison of 21 biochemical markers of disease activity, only three were said to be useful predictors of relapse, and able to provide a lead interval of 3 months or more before the clinical manifestations – carcino-embryonic antigen, alkaline prosphatase and gamma glutamyl transpeptidase [126]. In a similar investigation of biochemical and haematological tests predicting treatment faillure in breast cancer, Lee [120] reported that lower levels of haemoglobin, peripheral lymphocyte count or serum albumin, and raised levels of serum alkaline phosphatase or lactic dehydrogenase were most closely related to the subsequent appearance of recurrence and a low likelihood of 5 year survival. Useful, but less certain, indicators were decrease in serum total protein, and increase in CEA or transaminase (SGOT or SGPT) levels. It was observed that there was less abnormality in the markers in patients with lung and soft tissue metastases than in the case of bone and visceral metastases.

Hormone production and prognosis

The role of prolactin in the growth of human mammary cancer is still not clear. Elevated serum prolactin levels are common, especially during the postmastectomy period both in pre- and postmenopausal patients, but they are attributed to the stress of the diagnosis and treatment. In patients with metastatic breast cancer, raised serum prolactin levels are found in about 60% of postmenopausal patients, yet they are said to be rare in premenopausal cases [127–129].

There are several reports that in advanced breast cancer, mean serum prolactin levels are higher in patients who fail to respond to endocrine therapy [128, 130, 131] but not all agree [132]. There are also reports that an early fall in prolactin level (or TRH − stimulated level) predicts a greater likelihood of response to endocrine therapy [128, 130, 132–4] and that a high initial prolactin level among non responders is associated with a shorter survival [131].

While these findings may appear to suggest that the presence of hyperprolactinaemia may play a role in the failure of endocrine therapy, it has also been proposed that the excess prolactin found among treatment failures reflects the higher tumour burden in the body. Thus, Settatree [132] has noted a correlation between the serum prolactin level and the size of primary breast cancer, and he suggests that local compression of normal breast tissue may stimulate prolactin release from the pituitary gland.

The relationship of adrenocortical secretion to the prognosis of breast cancer is also unclear. An abnormally low urinary androgen metabolite level in relation to corticosteroid metabolites was at one time regarded as a 'discriminant' predicting poor response to endocrine therapy, but is now regarded as evidence of very advanced disease. In early breast cancer, subnormal levels of androgen metabolites are claimed to be associated with a higher recurrence rate [135], yet surprisingly, mean androgen levels are relatively low in Japanese women in spite of their relatively better prognosis [136]. Another report claims that in premenopausal women, *supranormal* levels of testosterone excretion are associated with higher recurrence rates after primary treatment in breast cancer [137]. More investigations of such relationships are required to clarify the inconsistencies.

Prostaglandin synthesis and prognosis

Prostaglandin synthesis by the tumour is thought to be related to its invasive properties, and high levels of prostaglandin production by breast cancer are reported to be associated with increased evidence of local invasion of blood and lymphatic vessels [138, 139]. It has been claimed that in the first 3 years after mastectomy, patients with a higher prostaglandin content of their tumours were more likely to die of metastatic disease [140].

More recent reports confirm the role of prostaglandins in invasion, and in the interaction between platelets and cancer cells which leads to implantation of the metastasis [141]. Thus, a high tumour level of prostaglandin E is said to be a marker of high risk in patients with node-negative breast cancer [142]; it led to a 57.1% rate of blood-borne metastasis and a 28.5% rate of local metastases within a 4 year period. The blood-borne metastases were in bone in 78% of cases in this series.

No clear correlation has been shown between prostaglandin synthesis in breast cancer and its histological grading, but a week correlation has been shown with the oestrogen receptor status of the tumour [143, 144]. It has been suggested that prostaglandin-induced bone resorption may contribute to the establishment and growth of bone metastases [145], and it may be relevant that oestrogen receptor-positive tumours show a relatively higher incidence of bone metastases than do receptor-negative tumours [18].

Immunological criteria and prognosis

The last 30 years have seen numerous reports on the relationship between parameters of immune competence (both *in vivo* and *in vitro* tests) and the prognosis of breast cancer. The evidence is conflicting, but the overall conclusion is that while impaired immunity is common in advanced breast cancer, it provides no specific guide to prognosis. Multivariate analysis has failed to establish a correlation between lymphocyte count and early recurrence [146], but in a small series, a recent report [147] claims that T-lymphocyte reactivity, percentage of EAC-rosettes and ESR level are independently related to relapse-free interval and length of survival.

Proto-oncogenes and prognosis

Recent research suggests that there may be a close correlation between the clinical behaviour of epithelial cancers such as breast cancer, and changes in specific proto-oncogenes in the tumour DNA. Amplification of c-myc or c-erbB-2 has been shown in about 10% of human cancer specimens including breast cancer [148]. The finding is more common in aggressive primary tumours, in metastases than in primary growth and it increases with advancing stage of the disease. Availability of suitable DNA probes, such as radio-labelled monoclonal antibodies against specific oncogenes, may therefore provide vital information on tumour localisation and individual prognosis.

The clinical importance of such observations is that amplification of specific oncogenes is associated with 'progression' of the tumour to a more malignant phase and provides a selective advantage for growth. This effect may be exerted through the gene product, and as an example, that for c-erbB-2 has properties similar to that of epidermal growth factor receptor, a stimulant of epithelial growth. If oncogenes code for growth factors or stimulate their expression, inhibitors of oncogene expression (anti-oncogenes or modulating genes) may enable us either to inhibit tumour cell growth, induce a more differentiated cell type or inhibit metastases genes.

Multivariate analysis of prognostic criteria

Most of the recent attempts to evaluate clinical, histopathological and other biological factors in the prognosis of breast cancer have used multiple regression analysis in order ro recognise the *independent* predictive ability of each factor. Once recognised, major independent prognostic factors can then be combined to make a prognostic index for each patient, using suitable weighting of each variable according to its relative importance. It may then be possible to estimate the likelihood of prolonged survival in an individual from a graph [149].

Various groups have reported multivariate analysis of clinical, microscopic and biological pointers to prognosis at the time of diagnosis [5, 7, 22, 72, 77–79, 86, 91, 146, 147, 149–154] and the variables considered in the analyses include the following:

(1) *Clinical* – extent of primary tumour and nodal status, duration of clinical delay, measures of growth tempo, age and menstrual status of the patient.

(2) *Histopathological* – size and type of primary tumour, number of axillary nodes involved, histological and nuclear grade, presence of elastosis or lymphoid infiltration, evidence of infiltrating margin or vascular or lymphatic invasion.

(3) *Biological* – steroid receptor levels, proliferative activity (rate of DNA synthesis), nuclear DNA content (ploidy).

Practically all the multivariate analyses show that the patient's prognosis (as defined by treatment failure) is most closely related to microscopic axillary lymph node status, and particularly to the number of nodes involved. Of only slightly less importance is the size of the primary tumour. The next most important independent variable is histopathological grading, but in this respect there are conflicting conclusions. While some reports claim it to be even more important than nodal status and tumour size [72, 151], others report that grading does not help in discrimination although lymphatic and blood vessel invasion do so [79]. The NSABP report finds that grading is a prognostic discriminant for disease-free survival at 5 years, but not at 10 years [22] and suggests that 'progression' in malignancy may be responsible.

There is even less agreement about other biological pointers to prognosis. As a result of multivariate analysis, oestrogen receptor assay is claimed by some to provide an independent index [150, 154], while others make a similar claim for measurement of thymidine uptake by the tumour [20]. While Stenkvist *et al.* [91] claim that 2½ years after primary treatment, nuclear ploidy shows more prognostic ability than does histopathological grading, Klintenberg *et al.* [150] claim that ploidy has no independent prognostic ability. Thymidine uptake is claimed by one report to be a major prognostic guide in node-negative cases [26], while another favours steroid receptor assay, which is said to preserve its prognostic ability even after recurrence [5].

In some of the reports, there is a correlation between some of the above criteria in that oestrogen receptor-negative tumours tend to be aneuploid [43, 93]. Also, poorly differentiated tumours tend to be aneuploid, more highly proliferative [93] and more likely to be oestrogen receptor-negative [22].

Prognostic criteria for Stage 1 cases

There is increasing interest in offering adjuvant systemic therapy to younger Stage 1 breast cancer patients with large tumours and biological characteristics reflecting a poor prognosis. A group of histopathologists have expressed doubts as to whether there is sufficient interobserver reproducibility among their reports to provide accurate guidance for individualised therapy of this type [155]. It may result from the fact that only a minute fraction of a heterogeneous tumour is being examined in most such cases. It is uncertain whether receptor assay, thymidine labelling or nuclear ploidy assessment of tumour specimens provide more representative samples of the entire breast cancer.

Looking for a prognostic histological index specifically for Stage 1 cases, the Breast Cancer Study Group [77] has reported that anaplasia and blood vessel invasion independently predict early recurrence, while Nealon *et al.* [152] added an infiltrating tumour border and lymphatic emboli to these criteria. However, Rosen *et al.* [78] were unable to confirm that any combination of these variables could identify a subset of Stage 1 patients with a higher risk of recurrence. Fisher *et al.* [22] report that anaplasia and germinal centre predominance are of worst prognostic significance in Stage 1 cases.

A recent multivariate analysis of 1647 node negative cases shows that large, ER − negative tumours are at the highest risk of recurrence and that age is a much less significant factor [156]. Another recent report shows that measuring ER, PgR, ploidy and S-phase cells provides the best identification of prognosis in node-negative cases [157].

Prognostic criteria for long term survival

Attempts to base a prognostic index on 5 year follow-up studies have a major weakness – the significance of factors which may relate to long-term survival tends to be swamped by the predominant importance of tumour size and nodal status in deciding early deaths. Only after 5 years do these variables become prognostically less important, so that finally the distinction between stages 1 and 2 is lost by 10 years [153] or by 20 years [16]. When histopathological grading is added to clinical staging, its predictive effect is least useful in the first few years after primary treatment when most deaths results from the most widespread tumours [16, 72, 149]. The combination is subsequently more discriminatory than staging alone because grading and staging are independent indices of prognosis [22].

There is little information on a prognostic index specifically for 10 year survival. Boyd *et al.* [36] claim that the degree of delay before treatment is an independent guide to 10 year survival in Stage 1 cases, while Fisher *et al.* [22] make a similar claim for germinal centre predominance in the axillary nodes. While some claim an independent prognostic role for menstrual status [20] others do not agree [150]. It is obvious that further data must be collected about independent prognostic indices particularly in reference to survival for 10 or more years and in Stage 1 cases.

Surprisingly, the NSABP finds histological grade a good discriminant for disease-free survival at 5 years but not at 10 years [22]. (Some have even reported that such grading loses its prognostic ability after 2½ years [91].) A major weakness of histological grading, in contrast to nuclear grading, is that it gives equal weight to all components of the histological assessment (degree of tubule formation, nuclear pleomorphism and mitotic frequency), although each component reflects a different influence on prognosis. While nuclear hyperchromatism and pleomorphism are more related to the proliferative activity of the tumour, the degree of cell differentiation is more related to its potential for invasiveness and metastasis [91, 94].

This last hypothesis is supported by clinical observations that the degree of differentiation and tubule formation in breast cancer are more important than its mitotic frequency in predicting the likelihood of 10 year survival by the patient [22, 153, 154]. Since it is the blood-borne metastases which are the major cause of death in breast cancer, the evidence suggests that certain biological criteria of good prognosis (e.g. differentiation and tubule formation or higher oestrogen receptor level) may be identifying tumours with a tendency to delayed invasion and metastasis. This hypothesis fits in with some of the observed characteristics of breast cancer growth in older patients [44].

Differences in metastatic activity between tumours may be mediated by differences in the local release of specific enzymes or growth factors. Enzymes may be derived either from the tumour cells or from the host cells. There is most experimental evidence for the role of collagenase, plasminogen activator and lysosomal enzymes, and recently a correlation between the ability of tumour cells to produce collagenase and their ability to metastasise has been reported [158]. In addition, plasminogen activator levels in human mammary cancer have been shown to be related to the steroid receptor content of the tumour [159] and may affect the metastatic activity of the tumour.

There may be a role for growth factors in invasion and metastasis. Plasminogen activator levels are increased by epidermal growth factor or by tumour angiogenesis factor, both of which are thought to be involved in the spread of human mammary cancer [160]. It may be relevant that aneuploid tumours are said to show a greater likelihood of node involvement at operation and earlier metastasis, yet survival after relapse is not shorter than in diploid tumours [98]. This observation suggests that ploidy may be related more to the capacity to metastasise before operation than to the rate of growth.

Prognostic criteria at relapse (Table 2)

It is commonly assumed that axillary node involvement at the time of surgery is associated not only with a shorter relapse-free interval but also a shorter post-relapse survival [161], but in fact, the initial staging of breast cancer is of little value as a guide to prognosis once metastases have manifested [3]. Staging is not related to duration of survival following the appearance of either distant metastases [5] or locoregional recurrence [4].

While the relapse-free interval is related to the chronological age of the tumour at the time of diagnosis, its metastatic potential and tumour growth rate, the duration of post-relapse survival is related to the sites and total volume of metastases and to tumour growth rate. But it must be taken into account that tumour progression may have made tumour growth rate more aggressive by the time that the first metastases manifest (see Chapter 7). One cannot therefore assume a long post-relapse survival in patients with a long relapse-free interval [162].

At the time of relapse, assessment of post-relapse survival is currently based on *clinical* factors, particularly the sites of disease involvement, the general health

Table 2. Clinical and biological criteria of prognosis at the time of recurrence or metastasis

Clinical criteria	Biological criteria
Relapse-free survival	Steroid receptor status
Pattern of metastases	Histopathological grading
Response to systemic therapy	Proliferative activity
Age, menstrual status, performance status	Nuclear ploidy

of the patient and the possibility of response to radiation or systemic therapy [161]. Metastases in the liver, brain or mediastinum are usually criteria of poor prognosis, as are also poor performance status or concomitant medical disease. The clinical aggressiveness of the disease is another major factor to be considered in assessing prognosis at time of relapse. It is best assessed from the tempo of growth as measured in overt lesions (see Chapter 1), the order in which vital metastitic sites are involved and the interval between successive metastases. *Biological* criteria which may help in assessing tumour aggressiveness are the histopathological grading, the steroid receptor status and the proliferative activity of the tumour.

Relapse-free interval and survival

It is widely believed that prolonged relapse-free intervals are followed by more prolonged post-relapse survival, but the evidence is conflicting. Finding of such a correlation was reported in several series [2, 87, 163, 164], but other series [165–168] have shown that post-relapse survival is relatively short whatever the relapse-free interval. The dicordant findings may be explained by the observation that relapse-free survival is a guide to survival *only in those cases where the first manifestation of relapse is locoregional* [4, 169, 170]. The overall findings in a series would therefore depend on the proportion in which the first sign of relapse was a locoregional recurrence.

In the case of carcinoma of the cervix similarly there is a correlation between relapse-free interval and post-relapse survival in those cases where recurrence is local, but not it if is extrapelvic (see Chapter 14). It suggests that a locoregional recurrence, which is established at the time of primary treatment, may continue to grow at the same rate after recurrence as it did in its subclinical phase.

Locoregional recurrence in breast cancer may have distinct biological characteristics. Bedwinek *et al.* [169] have noted that patients with a single local recurrences less than 1 cm diameter and with relapse-free intervals greater than 2 years, show much longer delay before the appearance of distant metastases than do other case. It suggests a subset ot tumours where the aggressiveness of both local and metastatic tumour shows little progression after recurrence. Local recurrences in breast cancer are more likely to have high ER levels [18] and this may explain the 26% 5 year survival among patients presenting first with locoregional recurrence, compared to only 5% among those presenting with blood-borne metastases [171].

For distant metastases, the relapse-free interval depends mainly on the timing of surgery in relation to when the metastases were established. As Stage 2 cases are likely to be chronologically older than Stage 1 cases they show a shorter median relapse-free interval than do Stage 1 cases. Nevertheless, even after a prolonged relapse-free interval, there may be a rapid succession of distant metastases due to the tumour having become more aggressive. There is increasing evidence that the cell population of a tumour changes as the disease progresses, and that the overall change is to dedifferentiation (loss of maturation), increased tendency to metastasis and to autonomy [172].

Pattern of metastases and survival

The pattern of metastasis is influenced by the biological characteristics of the tumour cell and this determines its affinity for the stromal tissue at each potential site of metastasis. As a result, the site of first recurrence and the rate of tumour progression are more important determinants of the prognosis than is the choice of therapy [168]. Patient groups are usually stratified by the dominant site of metastasis – soft tissue, osseous or visceral. Visceral involvement is usually associated with the shortest survival, but the organs involved are crucial in assessing the likely prognosis. Metastases in brain or liver are associated with a mean survival of 4-6 months, compared to 10-12 months for lung or pleural invasion and 22-26 months for bone or soft tissue involvement [168]. Visceral metastases are more likely to be ER – while bone and soft tissue metastases tend to have higher ER levels [18].

At each site of involvement, patients with long intervals between first and second relapses have a better prognosis than those with short intervals [168]. The size of metastases also determines prognosis, and the relatively poor prognosis of visceral metastases probably reflects, in part, the larger size of the deposits at the time of their diagnosis. In the case of bone metastases, their presentation with a sclerotic appearance (or the development of such changes subsequently) carries a better prognosis than does a lytic appearance.

Response to systemic therapy and survival

Cytotoxic or hormonal adjuvant therapy after primary surgery may postpone the appearance of relapse. Whether this will lead to a higher proportion of cures is not certain, but improved 9 year survival rates have been shown for CMF-treated cases [173] and improved 6 year survival rates for tamoxifen-treated cases [174]. Patients treated by adjuvant CMF have an increased incidence of brain metastases [175], presumably because the site is sequestered from cytotoxic action.

In the treatment of advanced breast cancer, it is likely that cytotoxic chemotherapy does not prolong mean survival [176, 177], but we can identify characteristics which favour prolongation of survival by systemic therapy in the individual patient. Most studies show that patient with recurrence-free periods shorter than 2 years, respond less frequently to cytotoxic therapy than do patients whose free periods are over 2 years [178]. This pattern is similar to that seen for endocrine therapy [179]. Again, the longer the recurrence-free interval, the longer the mean duration of survival after cytotoxic therapy [180, 181] and patients who respond to prior hormonal manipulation also have a significantly longer survival after chemotherapy [181]. Both observations suggest that the biology of the tumour has a clear-cut influence on length of survival after relapse, and that prolonged survival cannot automatically be ascribed to benefit from systemic therapy.

Response to systemic therapy can occur whatever the localisation of metastasis, and in general, the extent of the disease is more important than the organ site of involvement in predicting an affect on survival [181]. However, sole localisation of metastases in bone is prognostically favourable while visceral localisation is unfavourable [182], and this applies both to endocrine and to cytotoxic therapy.

Considerable evidence shows that response to cytotoxic therapy is not clearly related to oestrogen receptor status of the tumour [178]. However, a cooperative group has reported a 67% response rate for tumours with ER levels higher than 3 fmols/mg cytosol protein, compared to a 58% response rate for those with lower levels, in a group of 324 patients with advanced disease treated by various combinations of CAMFVP [183]. The response rate was higher in older patients, conforming to their higher mean receptor level.

With regard to other biological markers, response to systemic therapy is not clearly related to the initial level of carcinoembryonic antigen (CEA) in the serum, and although there is usually a decline in its level with clinical response to therapy, this is not invariable [123]. It has been reported that higher initial chorionic gonadotrophin levels (HCG) are associated with a poorer response rate to systemic therapy, but it is now suggested that the raised HCG levels observed in breast cancer patients are due to cross reactivity with human luteinising hormone [184]. Successful systemic therapy may be associated with an immediate rise in the level of polyamine excretion followed by a fall, and this applies especially to spermidine levels. Unfortunately not all studies show consistent results [123].

The *degree of regression* will reflect the tumour's content of proliferating cells, the most complete regressions being associated with tumours of a high proliferative cell content. This probably explains why complete regression from combination chemotherapy is said to be more common in patients with relapse-free intervals of less than 5 years than in those where it is over 5 years [185]. Complete tumour regression is said to be associated with a longer survival than is partial regression.

The *rate of regression* following systemic therapy in breast cancer will reflect the doubling time (the rate at which the tumour previously advanced at the site under observation). A slowly growing tumour may take up to 12 months or longer to disappear, while a rapidly growing tumour may regress completely within 2 months. Regression may be delayed for 9–12 months following endocrine therapy [186]. The rate of regression depends also on the tumour volume – larger tumours tend to be relatively avascular in the centre and regression is slower.

Response to endocrine therapy differs from that to cytotoxic therapy mainly in that the former is more closely related to oestrogen receptor-rich tumours, older age of the patient, postmenopausal status and longer relapse-free interval. It is more often delayed in onset, but its mean duration is longer. It is less clearly dependent on small size of tumour and a good performance status of the patient. Endocrine therapy is less effective for metastases in the liver or peritoneal cavity, but is more effective for bone metastases [179].

Age, menstrual status, performance status

The patient's performance status and the number of sites involved by metastases are commonly regarded as measures of the total tumour burden. Pretreatment weight loss, poor performance status, anaemia and hypoproteinaemia have an infavourable effect on survival [180, 181], presumably because they reflect more extensive metastatic disease. While it is widely believed that premenopausal breast cancer is more likely to respond to cytotoxic therapy than is postmenopausal cancer, the report by a cooperative group on 324 patients treated by various combinations of CAMFVP showed a higher response rate in postmenopausal patients [183].

Neither the patient's age nor menstrual status influences survival following chemotherapy [181] but in the case of endocrine therapy, postmenopausal patients tend to survive longer, although this may reflect the slower natural history of the disease in the older patient [44]. The response rate to endocrine therapy is also higher in postmenopausal than in premenopausal women, and within each menstrual group, younger premenopausal and postmenopausal women have a lower reponse rate than do older women [178].

Biological criteria and survival after relapse

At the time when distant metastases first appear, the prognosis for survival is better related to the original histopathological grading, receptor status or proliferative activity of the tumour than it is to the original clinical staging. While some reports find post-relapse survival time most clearly related to grading [5, 187], others favour the proliferative activity of the tumour [7] or the steroid receptor level [3, 188]. Related to the last observation is the report that the longer survival found in patients with steroid receptor-rich tumours is mainly due to prolonged post-relapse survival [188, 189].

Retrospective study of the DNA content (ploidy) of breast cancer tissue in stored paraffin sections has looked for a relationship between ploidy and the response of advanced disease to systemic therapy. One such report shows no significant difference in ploidy between responders and non-responders to cytotoxic therapy [190], but the mean duration of response was greater when aneuploidy was greater. While serum level of carcinoembryonic antigen (CEA) may sometimes help in assessing response to systemic therapy, it is rarely of use late in the disease because 'progression' of the tumour may lead to diminution in this marker level.

There is overwhelming evidence of clonal heterogeneity in most breast cancers leading to the appearance of less differentiated and more malignant phenotypes. Such progression is often associated with activated gene expression for growth factors stimulating tumour activity. Only when we are able to characterise these biological changes in the tumour will we be able to predict the course of breast cancer in the individual patient. Meanwhile, a marker providing an accurate assessment of tumour burden at the time of primary or secondary treatment, would be of more practical value to the clinician than would a prognostic index. It wouls permit rational choice of treatment, the ability to assess the effect of treatment and knowledge of when it is time to stop treatment.

Conclusion

1. Clinical TNM staging of breast cancer at the time of presentation can predict the likelihood of relapse in the first 5 years, but is not clearly related to the proliferative activity of the primary tumour or to the length of post-relapse survival. It is likely to reflect more the chronological age of the tumourand the size of the total tumour burden in the body, rather than the aggressiveness of the tumour.

2. The addition of histopathological criteria may improve the prediction of 5 year survival, especially in earlier stage cases [191], but the relative prognostic importance of the various histopathological criteria need to be distinguished from each other.

3. It is likely that the degree of biological 'progression' of a tumour is the best marker of its aggressiveness, and is therefore best related to post-relapse survival. Measurements of steroid receptor status, nuclear grade and replicating activity are used at present for this purpose, but evidence of chromosomal abnormality and oncogene expression are likely to prove more useful in the future. In our present state of knowledge, it is not clear how far each marker presents independent information, and whether it reflects proliferative or metastatic potential in the tumour.

4. Any initial prognostic index may need revision at the appearance of the first relapse. Changes may have occurred in the biological characteristics of the tumour with time, leading to changes in the tempo of growth and changes in its sensitivity to systemic or radiation therapy.

References

1. Devitt JE: Clinical prediction of growth behaviour. In: *Risk Factors in Breast Cancer*. BA Stoll (ed). Heinemann Medical, London, 1976, p 110
2. Langlands AO, Prescott RJ, Hamilton T: A clinical trial in the management of operable cancer of the breast. *British Journal Surgery* 67: 170–174, 1980
3. Paterson AH, Zuck VP, Szafran O, Lees AW, Hanson J: Influence and significance of certain prognostic factors on survival in breast cancer. *European Journal Cancer* 18: 937–943, 1984
4. Patanaphan V, Salazar OM, Poussin-Rosillo H: Prognosticators in recurrent breast cancer. *Cancer* 54: 228–234, 1984
5. Brunet M, Meeus L, Hacane K: Survival and clinical guiding marks of natural history of breast cancer. *International Journal Breast and Mammary Pathology* 2: 11–14, 1984
6. Gentili C, Sanfilippo O, Silvestrini R: Cell proliferation and its relationship to clinical features. *Cancer* 48: 974–979, 1981
7. Tubiana M, Pejovic MJ, Renaud A, Contesso G, Chavaudra N, Gioanni I and Malaise EP: Kinetic parameters and the course of the disease in breast cancer. *Cancer* 47: 937–943, 1981
8. Redding WH, Coombes RC, Monaghan P, Clink HM, Imrie SF, Dearnaley DP, Ormerod MG, Sloane JP, Gazet JC, Powles TJ, Neville AM: Detection of micrometastatses in patients with primary breast cancer. *Lancet* 2: 1271–1274, 1983
9. Peters MV: The role of local excision and radiation in early cancer. In: *Breast Cancer – Early and Late* MD Anderson (ed), Year Book Medical, Chicago, 1970, p 171
10. Adair F, Berg J, Joubert L and Robbins GF: Long term follow up of breast cancer patients. The 30 year report. *Cancer* 33: 1145–1151, 1974
11. Mueller CB and Jeffries W: Cancer of the breast. Its outcome as measured by the rate of dying and cause of death. *Annals Surgery* 182: 334–341, 1975
12. Haybittle JL: Results of the treatment of female breast cancer in the Cambridge area. *British Journal Cancer* 40, 56–61, 1979
13. Fisher B: Laboratory and clinical research in breast cancer; a personal adventure. *Cancer Research*, 40, 3863–3869, 1980
14. Black MM: Cell mediated response in human mammary cancer. In: *Host Defence in Breast Cancer* BA Stoll (ed). Heinemann Medical, London, 1975, p 48
15. Devitt JE: Lymph node invasion and its significance. In: *Cancer Treatment: End-Point Evaluation* BA Stoll (ed). John Wiley, Chichester, 1980, p 191
16. Fentiman IS, Cuzick J, Millis RR, Hayward JL: Which patients are cured of cancer? *British Medical Journal*, 289, 1108–1111, 1984
17. Levitt SH: Patterns of failure in breast cancer. *Cancer Treatment Symposia* 2: 123–129, 1983
18. Lee Yp TM: Patterns of metastasis and natural course of breast carcinoma. *Cancer and Metastasis Reviews* 4: 153–172, 1985
19. Robbins GF: Long term survivals among primary operable breast cancer patients with metastatic axillary nodes at level III. *Acta UICC* 18, 864–867, 1962
20. Tubiana M: Cell kinetics and radiation oncology. *International Journal Radiation Oncology, Biology, Physics* 8, 1471–1489, 1982
21. Davies CJ, Griffiths PA, Preston BJ *et al.*: Staging breast cancer; role of bone scanning. *British Medical Journal* 2: 603–606, 1977
22. Fisher ER, Sass E, Fisher B and collaborators: Pathological findings from the NSABP Protocol 4: Discriminants for tenth year treatment failure. *Cancer* 53: 712–723, 1984
23. Fisher B and Slack NH: Number of lymph nodes examined and the prognosis of breast cancer. *Surgery, Gynecology, Obstetrics* 131: 79–85, 1970
24. Berg JW, Huvos AG, Axtell LM and Robbins GF: A new sign of favourable prognosis in mammary cancer: Hyperplastic reactive lymph nodes in the apex of the axilla. *Annals Surgery* 177, 8–18, 1973

25. Duncan W and Kerr GR: The curability of breast cancer. *British Medical Journal* 4, 781–786, 1976
26. Silvestrini R, Daidone MG, Gasparini G: Cell kinetics as a prognostic marker in node negative breast cancer. *Cancer* 56, 1982–1987, 1985
27. Koscielny S, Tubiana M, Lee MG, Valleron AJ, Mouriesse H, Contesso G, Sarrazin D: Breast cancer, relationship between the size of the primary tumour and the probability of metastatic dissemination. *British Journal Cancer* 49: 709–715, 1984
28. Kaplan O, Skornick Y, Greif F, Klausner V, Rozin RR: Correlation between oestrogen receptors and tumour size in primary breast cancer. *European Journal Surgical Oncology* 11: 357–360, 1985
29. Gallager HS: Problems in the classification of breast cancer. *Radiological Clinics of North America* 21: 13–26, 1983
30. Koning CS, van der Linden EH, Hart G, Engelsman E: Adjuvant chemo and hormonal therapy in locally advanced breast cancer in a randomised clinical study. *International Journal Radiation Oncology, Biology, Physics* 11: 1751–1767, 1985
31. Handley RS: Observations and thoughts on cancer of the breast. *Proceedings Royal Society Medicine* 65, 437–438, 1972
32. Veronesi U, Cascinelli N, Bufalino R, Morabito A, Greco M, Galluzzo D: Risk of internal mammary node metastases and its relevance to prognosis of breast cancer patients. *Annals Surgery* 198: 681–684, 1983
33. Ege GN and Clark RM: Internal mammary lymphoscintigraphy in the conservative management of breast carcinoma. *Clinical Radiology* 36: 469–472, 1985
34. Bloom HJG: Further studies on prognosis of breast cancer. *British Journal Cancer*: 4, 437–444, 1950
35. Charlson ME, Feinstein AR: The auxiometric dimension. A new method of using rates of growth in prognostic staging of breast cancer. *Journal American Medical Association* 228: 180–185, 1974
36. Boyd NF, Meakin JW, Hayward JL, Brown TC: Clinical estimation of the growth rate of breast cancer. *Cancer* 48: 1037–1042, 1981
37. Feldman JG, Saunders M, Carter AC, Gardner B: The effect of patient delay and symptoms other than a lump on survival in breast cancer. *Cancer* 51: 1226–1229, 1983
38. Strax P: Mass screening for control of breast cancer. *Cancer* 53: 665–670, 1984
39. Verbeek ALM, Hendriks JHCL, Holland R, Mravunac M, Stuurmans F, Day NE: Reduction of breast cancer mortality through mass screening with modern mammography. *Lancet* 1: 1222–1224, 1984
40. Collette HJA, Day NE, Romback JJ, de Waard F: Evaluation of screening for breast cancer by a case control study. *Lancet* 1224–1226, 1984
41. Tabar L, Fagerberg CJG, Gad A and collaborators: Reduction of mortality from breast cancer after mass screening with mammography. *Lancet* 1, 829–832, 1985
42. Feinleib M, Zelen M: Some pitfalls in evaluation of screening programs. *Archives Environmental Health* 19: 412–415, 1969
43. Moran RE, Black MM, Alpert L, Strauss MJ: Correlation of cell cycle kinetics, hormone receptors, histopathology and nodal status in human breast cancer. *Cancer* 54, 1586–1590, 1984
44. Stoll BA: Age group and cancer prognosis. In: *Breast Cancer Treatment and Prognosis* BA Stoll (ed). Blackwell Medical, Oxford, 1986, p 173
45. Melnick Y, Slater PE, Katz L, Davies AM: Breast cancer in Israel: effect of age and origin on survival. *European Journal Cancer* 16: 1017–1023, 1980
46. Host H, Lund E: Age as a prognostic factor in breast cancer. *Cancer* 57, 2217–2221, 1986
47. Morrison AS, Beack MM, Lowe CR, McMahon B, Yuasa S: Some international differences in histology and survival in breast cancer. *International Journal Cancer* 11: 261–267, 1973
48. Stemmerman GN, Catts A, Fukunaga FH, Horie A, Nomura AMT: Breast cancer in women of Japanese and Caucasian ancestry in Hawaii. *Cancer* 56, 206–209, 1985

49. Moore JW, Clark CMG, Takatani O, Wakabayashi Y, Hayward JL, Bulbrook RD: Distribution of 17β estradiol in the serum of normal British and Japanese women. *Journal National Cancer Institue* 71: 749–754, 1983

50. Leffall LD, White JE, Ewing J: Cancer of the breast in Negroes. *Surgery, Gynecology, Obstetrics* 117: 97–103, 1963

51. Owny HE, Russo J, Brooks SJ, Frederick J, Heppner GH, Brennan MJ: Racial differences in breast cancer patients. *Breast Cancer Research and Treatment* 4: 355, Abst. 81, 1984

52. Natarajan N, Nemoto T, Mettlin C, Murphy P: Race-related differences in breast cancer patients. *Cancer* 56, 1704–1709, 1985

53. Gordon NH, Crowe JP, Hubay CE, Pearson OH: Relationship of race and other patient characteristics to early recurrence in Stage 1 breast cancer. *Breast Cancer Research and Treatment* 4: 344, Abst. 39, 1984

54. Mohla S, Sampson CC, Khan T, Enterline JP, Leffall L, White JE: ER and PgR receptors in black Americans. Correlation of receptor data with tumour differentiation. *Cancer* 50: 550–559, 1982

55. Fracchia AA, Robinson D, Legaspi A, Greenall MJ, Kinne DW, Groshen S: Survival in bilateral breast cancer. *Cancer* 55, 1414–1421, 1985

56. Fisher ER, Fisher B, Sass R, Wickerham L and collaborateurs: Pathologic findings from NSABP Protocol 4 – Bilateral breast cancer. *Cancer* 54: 3002–3011, 1984

57. Kiang DT, Kennedy BJ, Snover, DC: Biological and histological characteristics of simultaneous bilateral breast cancer. *Lancet* 2: 1105–1108, 1980

58. Papatestas AE, Mulvihill M, Josi C, Ioannovich J, Lesnick G, Aufses AH: Parity and prognosis in breast cancer. *Cancer* 45, 191–194, 1980

59. Donegan WL, Hartz AJ, Rimmer AA: The association of body weight with recurrent cancer of the breast. *Cancer* 41: 1590–1594, 1978

60. Tartter PI, Papatestas PE, Ioannovich J, Mulvihill MN, Lesnick G, Aufses AH: Cholesterol and obesity as prognostic factors in breast cancer. *Cancer* 47: 2222–2227, 1981

61. Eberlein T, Simon R, Fisher S, Lippman ME: Height, weight and risk of breast cancer relapse. *Breast Cancer Research and Treatment* 5: 81–86, 1985

62. Miller AB: Obesity and cancer of endocrine target organs. *Reviews on Endocrine Related Cancer* 13: 19–24, 1982

63. Papatestas AE, Panvelliwala D, Pertsemlidis D, Mulvihill M, Aufses AH: Association between ER level and weight in women with breast cancer. *Journal Clinical Oncology* 13, 177–180, 1980

64. Papatestas AE, Fagerstrom R, Gotsis W: Prognostic indicators in breast cancer. *British Medical Journal* 290: 1663, 1985

65. McKay EN, Sellars AH: Breast cancer at the Ontario Cancer Clinics, 1938–1956; a statistical review. *Canadian Medical Association Journal* 92: 647–651, 1965

66. Morrison AS, Lowe CR, MacMahon B, Mirra AP, Ravnihae B, Yuasa S: incidence, risk factors and survival in breast cancer. *European Journal Cancer* 13: 209–216, 1977

67. Juret P: Reproductive factors and the natural history of breast cancer. *Reviews on Endocrine Related Cancer* 9: 29–35, 1981

68. Tubiana M and Malaise EP: Growth rate and cell kinetics in human tumours. Some prognostic and therapeutic implications. In: *Scientific Foundations of Oncology* T. Symington and RL Carter (eds). Heinemann Medical, London, 1976, p 126

69. Bloom HJG and Richardson WW: Histological grading and prognosis in breast cancer. A study of 1409 cases of which 359 have been followed for 15 years. *Britisch Journal of Cancer* 11: 359–377, 1957

70. Fisher ER: Pathology of breast cancer. In: *Breast Cancer – Current Approaches to Therapy* WL McGuire (ed). Churchill Livingstone, Edinburgh, 1977, p 43

71. Black MM, Opler SR and Speer FD: Survival in breast cancer cases in relation to structure of

the primary tumour and regional lymph nodes. *Surgery, Gynecology, Obstetrics* 100: 543–549, 1955

72. Baak JPA, Van Dop H, Kurver PHJ, Hermans J: The value of morphometry to classic prognosticators in breast cancer. *Cancer*, 56, 374–382, 1985

73. Dawson PJ, Ferguson DJ, Karrison T: The pathological findings of breast cancer in patients surviving 25 years after radical mastectomy. *Cancer* 50, 2131–2138, 1982

74. Dixon JM, Page DL, Anderson Tj and collaborators: Long term survivors after breast cancer. *British Journal Surgery* 72, 445–448, 1985

75. Howell A, Harris M: Infiltrating lobular carcinoma of the breast. *British Medical Journal* 291: 1371, 1985

76. Fisher ER, Gregorion RM, Fisher B and collaborators: The pathology of invasive breast cancer. NSABP Protocol 4. *Cancer*, 36, 1085–1094, 1975

77. Breast Cancer Study Group: Identification of breast cancer patients with high risk of early recurrence after radical mastectomy. Clinical and pathological correlations. *Cancer* 42: 2809–2826, 1978

78. Rosen PP, Saigo PE, Braun DW, Weathers E, De Palo A: Predictors of recurrence in Stage 1 breast carcinoma. *Annals of Surgery* 193: 15–25, 1981

79. Bettelheim R, Penman HG, Thornton-Jones H, Neville AM: Prognostic significance of peritumoral vascular invasion in breast cancer. *British Journal Cancer* 50: 771–777, 1984

80. Bauer TW, O'Ceallaigh D, Eggleston JC, Moore GW, Baker RR: Prognostic factors in patients with Stage 1, oestrogen receptor negative carcinoma of the breast. *Cancer* 52: 1243–1431, 1983.

81. Fisher ER, Kotwal N, Hermann C, Fisher B: Types of tumor, lymphoid response and sinus histiocytosis. *Archives Pathological and Laboratory Medicine* 107: 222–227, 1983

82. Tsakraklides V, Olson P, Kersey JH, Good RA: Prognostic significance of the regional node histology in cancer of the breast. *Cancer* 34, 1259–1263, 1974

83. Shivas AA and Douglas JG: The prognostic significance of elastosis in breast carcinoma. *Journal Royal College of Surgeons* 17, 315, 1972

84. Weigand RA, Isenberg WM, Brennan MF and study associates: Elastosis as a prognostic indicator in human breast cancers. *Proceedings American Association for Cancer Research* 20: 143, 1979

85. Masters JRW, Millis RR, King RJB, Rubens RD: Elastosis and reponse to endocrine therapy in human breast cancer. *British Journal Cancer* 39, 536-542, 1979

86. McDivitt RW, Stone KR, Craig RB, Palmer JO, Meyer JS, Bauer WC: A proposed classification of breast cancer based on kinetic information. *Cancer* 57: 269–276, 1986

87. Cutler SJ, Black MM, Mark T, Harvey S, Freeman C: Further observations or prognostic factors in cancer of the female breast. *Cancer* 24: 653–667, 1969

88. Sehnitt SJ, Connolly JL, Harris JR, Hellman S, Cohen RB: Pathologic predictors of local recurrence in breast cancer. *Cancer* 53: 1049–1057, 1984

89. Fisher ER, Gregorio R, Redmond C and collaborators: Pathologic findings from NSABP protocol 4. *Cancer* 35: 247–254, 1975

90. Fisher B, Fisher ER, Redmond C *et al.*: The 10 year results from NSABP clinical trials evaluating the use of L-PAM in management of primary breast cancer. *Journal Clinical Oncology* 4: 929–941, 1986

91. Stenkvist B, Bengtsson E, Dahlgvist B, Eklund G, Eriksson D, Jarkrans T, Nordin B: Predicting breast cancer recurrence. *Cancer* 50: 2884–2893, 1982

92. Tickle A, Crawley A, Goodman M: Cell movement and the mechanisms of invasiveness. *Journal Cell Science* 31: 293–297, 1978

93. Holmberg LH, Tabar L, Adami HO, Bergström R: Survival in breast cancer diagnosed between mammographic screening examinations. *Lancet* ii: 27–30, 1986

94. Strauli P, Weiss L: Cell locomotion and tumor penetration. *European Journal Cancer* 13: 1–13, 1977

95. De Vita VT, Lippman M, Hubbard SM, Ihde DC, Rosenberg SA: Effect of combined modality therapy on local control and survival. *International Journal Radiation Oncology, Biology, Physics* 12: 487–501, 1986

96. Meyer JS, Rao BR, Stevens SC, Whilet WL: Low incidence of estrogen receptor in breast carcinoma with rapid rates of cell proliferation. *Cancer* 40: 2290–2298, 1977

97. Meyer JS, Hixton B: Advanced stage and early relapse of breast carcinomas associated with high thymidine labelling indices. *Cancer Research* 39, 4042–4047, 1979

98. Hedley DW, Rugg Ca, Ng ABP, Taylor IW: Influence of cellular DNA content on disease-free survival of Stage 2 breast cancer patients. *Cancer Research* 44: 5395–5398, 1984

99. Coulson PB, Thornthwaite JT, Woolley TE *et al.*: Prognostic indicators including DNA histogram type, receptor content and staging related to human breast cancer survival. *Cancer Research* 44, 4187–4196, 1984

10. Killander D, Borg A, Ewers SB: *Proceedings 3rd EORTC Breast Cancer Working Conference*, Amsterdam, 1983, p 25

101. Auer G, Erikson E, Azaredo E, Caspersson T, Wallgren A: Prognostic significance of nuclear DNA content in mammary adenocarcinomas in humans. *Cancer Research* 44: 394–8, 1984

102. Daver A, Chassevent A, Bertrand G, Larra F: Flow DNA analysis of different cell suspensions in breast carcinoma. Relation of DNA index and cell kinetics to pathological features and steroid receptors. *Journal Steroid Biochemistry* 19: (Supplement) 61S, 1983

103. Raber MN, Barlogie B, Latreille J, Bedrossian C, Fritsche H, Blumenschein G: Ploidy, proliferative activity and estrogen receptor content in human breast cancer. *Cytometry* 3: 36–41, 1982

104. Johannison E, Schaefer P, Scheggia A, Krauer F: Microfluometric assessment of DNA content of breast cancers; relationship with hormone receptors and histological grading. *Senologia* 1: 119–123, 1982

105. Bichel P, Poulsen HS, Andersen J: Estrogen receptor content and ploidy of human mammary carcinoma. *Cancer* 50: 1771–1774, 1982

106. Taylor IW, Musgrove EA, Friedlander ML, Foo MS, Bedley DW: The influence of age on the DNA ploidy levels of breast tumours. *European Journal Cancer and Clinical Oncology* 19, 623–628, 1983

107. Stuart-Harris R, Hedley DW, Taylor IW, Levene AL, Smith IE: Tumour ploidy, response and survival in patients receiving endocrine therapy for advanced breast cancer. *British Journal Cancer* 51: 573–576, 1985

108. Klintenberg C, Bjelkenkrantz K, Mansson JC, Killander D, Nordenskjold B: Cytophotometric analysis of needle aspirates from human tumours during therapy. *Acta Radiologica (Oncology)* 24: 117–122, 1985

109. Editorial: Steroid receptors and prognosis of breast cancer. *Lancet* 1: 887–888, 1984

110. Hähnel R: Oestrogen receptor status, breast cancer growth and prognosis. *Reviews on Endocrine Related Cancer* 5–12, 1981

111. Silvestrini R, Daidone MG and DI Fronzo G: Relationship between proliferative activity and estrogen receptors in breast cancer. *Cancer* 44: 665, 1979

112. Alanko A, Makinen J, Scheinin TM, Tolppanen RM, Vikho R: Correlation of estrogen and progesterone receptors and histological grade in human primary breast cancer. *Acta Pathologica, Microbiologica, Scandinavia*, Section A 92, 311–315, 1984

113. Hähnel R: Progesterone receptor assay in the management of breast and other cancers. *Review on Endocrine Related Cancer* 20: 1–11, 1985

114. Bolla J, Mouriquand J, Chambaz E, Pinet L, Bouchet Y, Sage JC: Prognostic interest of combined study of steroid receptors and cytological grade. *Senologia* 1, 39–42, 1982

115. Allegra JC, Lippman ME, Thompson EB, Simon R, Barlock A, Green G, Huff KK, Do HMT, Aitken SC: Distribution, frequency and quantitative analysis of estrogen, progesterone, androgen and glucocorticoid receptors in human breast cancer. *Cancer Research* 39: 1447–1454, 1979

116. Kosma VM, Syrjanen KJ: Regional lymph node reactions related to hormone receptor status in female breast carcinoma. *Archiv fur Geschwiltsforschung* 55: 123–130, 1985

117. Falkson HC, Falkson G, Portugal MA, van der Watt JJ, Schoeman HS: CEA as a marker in patients with early breast cancer receiving postsurgical adjuvant chemotherapy. *Cancer* 49, 1859–1865, 1982

118. Mansour EG, Hastert M, Park CH, Koehler KA, Petrelli M: Tissue and plasma CEA in early breast cancer. *Cancer* 51: 1243–1248, 1983

119. Gilchrist KW, Kalish L, Gould VE and collaborators: Immunostaining for CEA does not dicriminate for early recurrence in breast cancer. *Cancer* 56: 351–355, 1985

120. Lee Y-TM: Biochemical and hematological tests in patients with breast carcinoma; correlations with extent of disease, sites of relapse and prognosis. *Journal of Surgical Oncology* 29: 242–248, 1985

121. Thompson DK, Haddow JE, Smith DE, Ritchie RF: Elevated serum acute phase protein levels as predictors of disseminated breast cancer. *Cancer* 53: 2100–2104, 1983

122. Schapira DV, Schapira M: Use of ceruloplasmin levels to monitor response to therapy and predict recurrence. *Reviews on Endocrine Related Cancer* (Supplement) 14: 155–157, 1984

123. Bates SE, Longo DL: Tumor markers; value and limitations in the management of cancer patients. *Cancer Treatment Reviews* 12: 163–207, 1985

124. Russell DH, Durie BGM and Salmon SE: Polyamines as predictors of success and failure in cancer chemotherapy. *Lancet*, 2: 797–799, 1975

125. Milano G, Schneider M, Cassuto JP, Viguier E, Pastorini P, Boublil JL, Namer M, Cambon P, Lalanne CM: Polyamines; comments on clinical utility in cancer. *Tumor Diagnostik* 3: 121–125, 1980

126. Coombes RC, Powles TJ, Gazet JC: Screening for metastases in breast cancer; an assessment of biochemical and phydical methods. *Cancer* 48: 310–315, 1981

127. Murray RML, Mozaffarian G, Pearson OH: Prolactin levels with L-DOPA treatment in metastatic breast carcinoma. *Fourth Tenovus Workshop* AR Boyns and K Griffiths (eds). Omega, Alpha Omega, Cardiff, 1972, p 158

128. Willis KJ, London DR, Ward HWC, Butt WR, Lynch SS, Rudd BT: Recurrent breast cancer treated with tamoxifen; correlation between hormonal change and clinical course. *British Medical Journal* 1: 425–428, 1977

129. Rose DP, Pruitt BT: Plasma prolactin levels in patients with breast cancer. *Cancer* 48: 2687–2691, 1981

130. Dowsett M, McGarrick GE, Harris AL, Coombes RC, Smith IE, Jeffcoate SL: Prognostic significance of serum prolactin levels in advanced breast cancer. *British Journal Cancer* 47: 763–769, 1983

131. Ragaz J, Ibrahim E, Leahy M, Spinelli J, Willan AR: Therapy of metastatic breast cancer with aminoglutethimide and tamoxifen; role of systemic oestrogens and pituitary hormones. *Reviews on Endocrine Related Cancer* (Supp.) 14: 259–260, 1982

132. Settatree RS: Prolactin, bromocriptine and tamoxifen in postmenopausal women with breast cancer. *Reviews on Endocrine Related Cancer* (Supplement) 5: 63–70, 1980

133. Szamel I, Hermann I, Borvendeg J, Voncze B, Hindy I, Eckhardt S: Effect of tamoxifen treatment on TRH-induced prolactin release in patients with breast cancer. *Cancer Treatment Reports* 63, 1202 Abstract 296, 1979

134. Pannuti F, Martoni A, Farabegoli G, Piana E, Orsola S: Prolactin levels and hormonal profile in postmenopausal patients with advanced breast cancer during endocrine treatment. *Chemioterapia* 4: 127–134, 1985

135. Thomas BS, Bulbrook RD, Hayward JL, Millis RR: Urinary androgen metabolites and recurrence rates in early breast cancer. *European Journal Cancer* 18: 447–451, 1982

136. Hayward JL, Greenwood FC, Globen G: Endocrine status in British, Japanese and Hawaiian-Japanese women. *European Journal Cancer* 14, 1221–1228, 1978

137. Secreto G, Zumoff B: Supranormal urinary testosterone excretion in premenopausal women with breast cancer. Increased risk of recurrence and higher remission rate after ovariectomy. *Cancer Research* 43: 3408–3411, 1983

138. Bennett A, Charlier EM, McDonald AM, Simpson JS, Stamford IF, Zebro T: Prostaglandins and breast cancer. *Lancet* 11, 124–126, 1977

139. Rolland PH, Martin PM, Jacquemier J, Rolland AM, Toga M: Prostaglandin in human breast cancer; evidence suggesting that an elevated prostaglandin production is a marker of high metastatic potential. *Journal National Cancer Institute* 64: 1061–1065, 1980

140. Bennett A, Berstock DA, Raja B and Stamford IF: Survival time after surgery is inversely related to the amounts of prostaglandins extracted from human breast cancers. *British Journal Pharmacology* 66, 451–458, 1979

141. Donati MB, Rotilio D, Vincenzi E, Poggi A: Incosaenoids and cancer; role of platelet-active prostaglandins in cancer and metastatic growth. *Journal Steroid Biochemistry* 19 (Supplement): 1825–1826, 1983

142. Boublil JL, Namer M, Lelanne CM, Moll JL, Milano G, Krebs BP: Prostaglandins and breast cancer without node involvement. *Journal Steroid Biochemistry* 19 (Supplement): 145, 1983

143. Bishop HM, Haynes J, Evans DF, Elston CW, Johnson J, Blamey RW: Radioimmunoassay of prostaglandin E2 in primary breast cancer and its relationship to histological grade. *Clinical Oncology* 6: 380–381, 1980

144. Fulton A, Roi L, Russo J, Brooks S, Brennan M, Griswold D: Tumor-associated prostaglandins in primary breast cancer. *P.A.A.C.R. Meeting* 140 Abst.: 551, 1982

145. Bennett A: Prostaglandins; relationship to breast cancer and its spread. In: *Endocrine Relationships in Breast Cancer* BA Stoll (ed). Heinemann Medical, London, 1982, p 156

146. Ownby HE, Roi LD, Isenberg RR, Brenna MJ: Peripheral lymphocyte and easinophil counts as indicators of prognosis in primary breast cancer. *Cancer* 52: 126–130, 1983

147. Hacene K, Desplaces A, Brunet M, Lidereau R, Bourguignat A, Oglobine J: Competitive prognostic value of clinicopathologic and bioimmunologic factors in primary breast cancer. *Cancer* 57: 245–250, 1986

148. Yokota P, Yamamoto T, Toyoshima K, Terada M, Sugimura T, Battifira H, Cline MJ: Amplification of c-erbB-2 oncogene in human adenocarcinomas in vivo. *Lancet* 1: 765–767, 1986

149. Blamey RW, Elston CW, Haybittle JL, Griffiths SK: Prognosis in breast cancer: the Nottingham-Tenovus trial. In: *Commentaries on Research in Breast Disease* RD Bulbrook (ed). Alan R Liss, New York, 1983, p 93

150. Klintenberg C, Wallgren A, Bjelkenkrantz K, Carstenssen J, Humla S, Nordenskjold B, Skoog L: DNA Distribution, estrogen receptor and axillary nodes as prognostic predictors in breast carcinoma. *Acta Radiologica Oncologica* 24: 253–258, 1985

151. Freedman LS, Edwards DN, McConnell LA, Downham D: Histological grade and other prognostic factors in relation to survival of patients with breast cancer. *British Journal of Cancer* 40: 44–45, 1979

152. Nealon TF, Nkongho A, Grossi C, Gillooley J: Pathologic identification of poor prognosis Stage 1 cancer of the breast. *Annals of Surgery* 190, 129–132, 1979

153. Wallgren A, Silfverswaard C, Wiklund G: Prognostic factors in mammary carcinoma. *Acta Radiologica* 15: 1–16, 1976

154. Farl FF, Schmidt BP, Dupont WD, Wagner RK: Prognostic significance of ER status in breast cancer in relation to tumor stage, axillary node metastasis and histopathologic grading. *Cancer* 54, 2237–2242, 1984

155. Gilchrist KW, Kalish L, GOuld VE and colleagues: Interobserver reproducibility of histopathological features in Stage 2 breast cancer; an ECOG study. *Breast Cancer Research and Treatment* 5: 3–16, 1985

156. Clark GM, McGuire WL: High risk profile for recurrence and survival in 1647 node-negative breast cancer patients. *Proceedings PASCO Meeting* 22: 61 (Item 253), 1986

157. Dressler LG, Owens M, Seamer L, McGuire WL: Identifying breast cancer patients for adjuvant therapy by DNA flow cytometry and steroid receptors; A 1000 patient study. *Proceedings PASCO Meeting* 22: 61 (Item 238), 1986

158. Liotta LA, Tryggrason K, Garbiss S, Hart I, Foltz CM, Shafie S: Metastatic potential correlates with enzymatic degradation of basement membrane collagen. *Nature* 284, 67–68, 1980

159. Magdalenat M, Mittre H, Martin PM: Plasminogen activator and steroid receptors in human mammary carcinoma. *Journal Steroid Biochemistry* 19 Supplement: 1355, 1983

160. Sainsbury JRC, Farndon JR, Sherbet GV, Harris AL: Epidermal growth factor receptors and oestrogen receptors in human breast cancer. *Lancet* 1: 364–366, 1985

161. Coppin CML, Swenerton KD: Selective treatment in breast cancer. In; *Cancer Treatment – End Point Evaluation* BA Stoll (ed). John Wiley, Chichester, 1983, p 387

162. Stoll BA: Prolonged survival in breast cancer. In: *Prolonged Arrest of Cancer* BA Stoll (ed). John Wiley, Chichester, 1982, p 59

163. Goldenberg IS, Bailar JC, Lowry RH: Survival of women with hormonally treated women. *Surgery, Gynecology, Obstetrics* 119: 785–789, 1964

164. Myers MH, Hankey BF, Mantel N: A logistic-exponential model for use with response time data involving regressor variables. *Biometrics* 29: 257–264, 1973

165. Pawlias KT, Dockerty MB, Ellis FH: Late local recurrent carcinoma of the breast. *Annals Surgery* 148, 192–198, 1958

166. Papaioannou AN, Tang FJ, Vilk H: Fate of patients with recurrent cancer of the breast. *Cancer* 20, 371–376, 1967

167. Stoll BA: Does the malignancy of breast cancer vary with age? *Clinical Oncology* 2: 73–80, 1976

168. Pearlman NW, Jockimsen PR: Recurrent breast cancer. Factors influencing survival including treatment. *Journal Surgical Oncology*, 11, 21–29, 1979

169. Bedwinek JM, Lee J, Fineberg B, Ocwieza M: Prognostic indicators in patients with isolated loco-regional recurrence of breast cancer. *Cancer* 47: 2232–2235, 1981

170. Toonkel LM, Fox I, Jacobson LH, Wallach CB: The significance of local recurrence of carcinoma of the breast. *International Journal Radiation Oncology* 9: 33–39, 1983

171. Karabali-Dalamaga S, Souhami RL, O'Higgins NJ, Soumilas A, Clark CG: Natural history of prognosis of recurrent breast cancer. *British Medical Journal* 2: 730–733, 1978

172. Brawn PN: The dedifferentiation of prostate carcinoma. *Cancer* 52: 246–251, 1983

173. Bonadonna G, Valagussa P: Adjuvant systemic therapy for resectable breast cancer. *Journal Clinical Oncology* 3: 259–275, 1985

174. N.A.T.O. Trial: Controlled trial of tamoxifen as single adjuvant agent in management of early breast cancer. *Lancet* 1: 836–839, 1985

175. Paterson AHG, Agarwal M, Lees A, Hanson J, Szafran O: Brain metastases in breast cancer patients receiving adjuvant chemotherapy. *Cancer* 49: 651–654, 1982

176. Powles TJ, Smith IE, Ford HT, Coombes RC, Jones JM, Gazet JC: Failure of chemotherapy to prolong survival in a group of patients with metastatic breast cancer. *Lancet* 1: 580–582, 1980

177. Paterson AHG, Szafran O, Cornish F, Lees AW, Hanson J: Effect of chemotherapy on survival in metastatic breast cancer. *Breast Cancer Research and Treatment* 1: 357–363, 1981

178. Henderson IC, Canellos GP: Cancer of the breast. *New England Journal of Medicine* 302: 78–90, 1980

179. Stoll BA: Palliation by castration or by hormone administration. In: *Breast Cancer Management – Early and Late* BA Stoll (ed). Heinemann Medical, 1977, p 133

180. Bull JM, Tormey DLC, Li SH, Carbone TP, Falkson G, Blom J, Perlin E, Simon RA: A randomised comparative trial of Adriamycin versus methotrexate in combination drug therapy. *Cancer* 41: 1949–1657, 1978

181. Swenerton KD, Legha SS, Smith T, Hortobagyi GN, Gehan EA, Yap HY, Gutterman JU, Blumenschein GR: Prognostic factors in metastatic breast cancer treated with combination therapy. *Cancer Research* 39: 1552–1562, 1979

182. Brunner KW, Sonntag RW, Martz G: A controlled study on the use of combined drug therapy for metastatic breast cancer. *Cancer* 36, 1208–1219, 1975

183. Corle DK, Sears ME, Olson KB: Relationship of quantitative estrogen receptor level and clinical response to cytotoxic chemotherapy in advanced breast cancer. *Cancer* 54: 1554–1561, 1984

184. Monteiri JC, Ferguson KM, McKinna JA, Greening WP, Neville AM: Ectopic production of human chorionic gonadotrophin like material by breast cancer. *Cancer* 53: 957–959, 1984

185. Decker DA, Ahmann DL, Bisel HF, Edmondson JH, Hahn RG and O'Fallon JR: Complete responders to chemotherapy in metastatic breast cancer. *Journal American Medical Association* 242: 2075–2082, 1979

186. Glick JH, Creech RH and Torri S: Tamoxifen plus sequential CMF chemotherapy versus tamoxifen alone in postmenopausal patients with advanced breast cancer. *Cancer* 45: 735–739, 1980

187. Pater JL, Mores D, Loeb M: Survival after recurrence of breast cancer. *Canadian Medical Association Journal* 124: 1591–1596, 1981

188. Howell A, Holland RNL, Bramwell VHC and colleagues: Steroid hormone receptors and survival after first relapse in breast cancer. *Lancet* 1, 588–591, 1984

189. Alanko A, Heinonen E, Scheinin TM, Tolppanen EM, Vikho R: Oestrogen and progesterone receptors and disease-free interval in primary breast cancer. *British Journal Cancer* 50, 667–672, 1984

190. Mitchel I, Deshande N, Millis R, Rubens RD: DNA content of primary carcinoma and response to endocrine or cytotoxic drug therapies in patients with advanced breast cancer. *European Journal Syrgical Oncology* 11: 251–256, 1985

191. Fuster E, Garcia-Vilanova A, Narbone B, Romero R, Llombart-Bosch A: A statistical approach to an individualized prognostic index for breast cancer survivability. *Cancer* 52–728–736, 1983

14. Prognostic indices in gynecologic cancer

A.J. DEMBO, G.M. THOMAS and M.L. FRIEDLANDER

This discussion will concentrate on the major gynecologic malignancies – endometrial carcinoma, epithelial ovarian carcinoma, and cervical carcinoma. Our understanding of tumor behaviour in these diseases has improved in the last two decades because of surgical staging studies, analyses of relapse patterns after treatment, and the application of multivariate statistical analysis to the evaluation of prognostic factors.

Endometrial cancer

The prognostic factors to be considered in relation to this tumor are anatomic stage, depth of myometrial penetration, histologic differentiation (grade), other histologic parameters (cell type, lymphatic space invasion), patient age, progesterone receptor content, co-morbid factors.

Anatomic Stage

The staging system of the International Federation of Gynecology and Obstretics is widely used (Table I). Approximately 85% of patients have tumors clinically confined to the uterus at the time of presentation [1]. Five-year survival rates by stage are approximately 70-85% for Stage I, 60-70% for Stage II, 20-30% for Stage III and 5% for Stage IV, while overall the 5-year survival rate is 60-70%. The prognostic significance of uterine size in Stage I (i.e., IA *vs* IB) is minor. The greater depth of uterine sounding in Stage IB may be due to factors unrelated to the cancer, such as leiomyomata and multiparity. The slightly worse outcome in Stage IB is probably explained by its association with other unfavorable factors, such as deeper myometrial penetration and higher grade lesions [2].
In practical terms, two subgroups of Stage II exist. The first, 'occult Stage II', is characterized by positive endocervical currettings in the absence of visible or

palpable involvement of the cervix. If the endocervical currettings do not contain endocervical stroma involved by tumor, it is difficult to be certain that the tumor present is not merely free-floating contamination from the endometrial tumor above, and such patients rightly belong in Stage I. The second subgroup, with visible or palpable cervical involvement, is prognostically worse. They are more likely to have deeply invasive tumors and high grade lesions than are patients in Stage I. Their prognosis is similar, or only marginally worse, than that of Stage I patients with tumors of similar grade and depth of myometrial invasion [2].

Stage III also should be divided into two prognostic subgroups. While those with involvement of the parametria, vagina or cul-de-sac have a very high likelihood of dying of their disease, patients whose only extrauterine spread is to the adnexa, probably do not have their prognosis appreciably worsened by this finding [3–5], be it detected preoperatively or in the operative specimen.

Myometrial penetration

For patients with lesions clinically confined to the uterus, the depth to which the tumor invades the myometrium is a strong predictor of outcome. Myometrial penetration is described in a number of ways by pathologists: superficial or deep, the distance from serosa in millimetres, involvement of the inner, middle or outer third, or involvement of the inner half or outer half of the myometrial thickness. The deeper the invasion, the worse is the outcome and penetration through the serosa is almost universally fatal. Deep myometrial invasion (over 50%) is associated with a reduced survival rate [2, 6], a greater risk of pelvic and para-aortic lymph node metastases (see Table 2) [7], a higher clinical stage [2], less tumor differentiation [12] and increasing patient age [6]. Because of these associations, the depth of myometrial penetration is an important determinant of therapy in Stage I.

Table 1. FIGO staging system for endometrial cancer (based on clinical findings and D & C prior to laparotomy/hysterectomy)

Stage I   – confined to body of uterus
    IA – uterine cavity under 8 cm in length
    IB – uterine cavity over 8 cm in length
Stage II – involvement of cervix
Stage III – spread to other pelvic structures
Stage IV – IVA – involvement of bladder or rectal mucosa
    – IVB – spread outside pelvis

Histologic grade

In all grading systems used for describing the degree of histologic differentiation of the tumor, the less differentiated (high grade) lesions predict a worse outcome than the well differentiated (low-grade) ones. The FIGO-system describes grade 1 (well differentiated), grade 2 (moderately differentiated) and grade 3 (poorly differentiated) classes, and worsening tumor grade is associated with:

(a) Lower survival rate and higher relapse rate. In the Mayo Clinic experience in Stage I, 5-year survival rates were 93% for grade 1, 85% for grade 2, and 60% for grade 3 lesions [2].

(b) Higher stage. Malkasian reported that the frequency of grade 3 lesions was inversely related to stage, occurring in 7% of Stage IA, 19% of Stage IB, 37% of Stage II, 30% of Stage III and 57% of Stage IV [2].

(c) Deeper myometrial penetration. Cheon reported deep myometrial penetration in 12% of grade 1, 16% of grade 2, and 46% of grade 3 lesions [8].

(d) Pelvic and para-aortic lymph node metastasis. The Gynecologic Oncology Group (GOG) staging study (protocol 33) results shown in Table 2, correlates tumor grade with risk of nodal involvement [8].

(e) Advancing age [2].

(f) Hematogenous dissemination. Ballon and co-workers reported that while the majority of patients with localized presentations had grade 1 or 2 lesions, 20/33 patients who developed subsequent pulmonary metastases had grade 3 tumors [9].

Other histologic parameters

Adenocarcinoma accounts for 80 to 85% of endometrial cancers but a further

Table 2. Frequency of nodal involvements in stages I and II-occult, according to grade of endometrial cancer and depth of myometrial penetration (GOG Protocol 33) [8]

	Patient No.	Pelvic Nodes (% positive)	Para-aortic Nodes (% positive)
Grade 1	197	4	2
2	216	11	6
3	117	24	12
Myometrial invasion			
none	107	2	1
inner third	211	5	1.4
mid third	89	12	7
outer third	121	29	18

10 to 15% have component of squamous differentiation in addition to the adenocarcinoma component. Terminology in the literature is inconsistent and potentially confusing. Well-differentiated adenocarcinomas sometimes show an element of squamous metaplasia and when the squamous component appears benign, these lesions are usually called adeno-acanthomas and typically behave like grade 1 lesions. However, when the squamous component appears frankly malignant, it is usually referred to as adenosquamous carcinoma [10].

Adenosquamous carcinomas are usually associated with a poor prognosis, because they are often deeply invasive, poorly differentiated and extensive. Their behaviour is usually determined by the grade of the adenocarcinoma component rather than by the squamous component [10]. More recently, it has been suggested that the squamous component of 'adenoacanthoma' does not represent metaplasia, but rather well-differentiated squamous carcinoma. Accordingly, the term adenosquamous carcinoma is now used to describe both adenocanthoma and the original adenosquamous carcinoma, and it is important to specify the degree of differentiation of the lesion.

Approximately 5% of endometrial tumors are morphologically similar to serous carcinomas arising in the fallopian tube or ovary. These 'papillary serous' carcinomas should be distinguished from the commoner adenocarcinomas which may have a papillary configuration. In one series, they comprised 10% of Stage I cases, yet accounted for 50% of the relapses [11]. The pattern of relapse is not infrequently transcoelomic, as with ovarian cancer. Papillary clear cell carcinomas are quite rare, but also tend to have a poor prognosis.

Lymphatic space invasion by tumor in the myometrium is associated with an increased risk of nodal involvement and of tumor relapse.

Patient age

More unfavorable disease presentations call for more aggressive treatment but they often occur in older patients who are less likely to tolerate intensive therapy. Increasing age is associated with worse survival rates (even if corrected for intercurrent deaths), deep myometrial invasion, advancing stage and lower operability rates [6]. Older patients are also more likely to have poorly differentiated tumors [12].

Progesterone receptor content

A high progesterone content in the tumor predicts a better prognosis and a greater likelihood of response to progestagen therapy [13]. However, the usefulness of this assay is limited because of problems in sampling the primary tumor without contamination by normal endometrium, which is usually rich in progesterone receptors. Tumors also show a strong association between progesterone receptor content and degree of differentiation.

Co-morbid factors

The median age of patients with endometrial cancer is about 10 years older than those with cervical or ovarian cancer. In addition the disease has an association with obesity and hypertension. About 20% of patient deaths in the first 5 years after diagnosis are thus due to causes other than endometrial cancer.

There is almost certainly an association between prolonged, unopposed estrogen supplementation after the menopause, and an enhanced risk of developing endometrial cancer [14]. There is an excess of grade 1 lesions in estrogen-associated cancers compared with tumors occurring spontaneously, and there is also a tendency to earlier diagnosis, because estrogen-related withdrawal bleeding provokes diagnostic currettage. For these reasons, endometrial carcinoma associated with estrogen-replacement therapy usually has a favorable prognosis.

Epithelial ovarian carcinoma

The prognostic factors to be considered in relation to this tumor are histologic type and differentiation, anatomic stage, post-resection tumor volume (i.e., residuum), patient age and factors in non-metastatic carcinomas. The first 4 indices are shown in Fig. 1, where a group of patients are classified by each of these factors and the survival curves of each subgroup are shown. Classification of patients by each factor provides prognostically distinct subcategories.

Histologic type and differentiation

Five histologic patterns of ovarian tumors are usually recognized (as shown in Table 3) although admixtures are not infrequent. A sixth, the malignant Brenner tumor, is rare, and probably should be managed no differently from the commoner serous type. Of the methods used to grade the tumors, some are based on mitotic count (e.g., Broders), some on histologic pattern, some on the amount of solid tumor present, and some combine features of nuclear and cytologic grade as well as histologic pattern. Grading systems may be 3- or 4-tier. Most commonly a 3-tier system based predominantly on pattern is favoured, yielding well – (grade 1), moderately – (grade 2) and poorly – (grade 3) differentiated subcategories. Grading is usually based on the worst differentiated areas of the tumor.

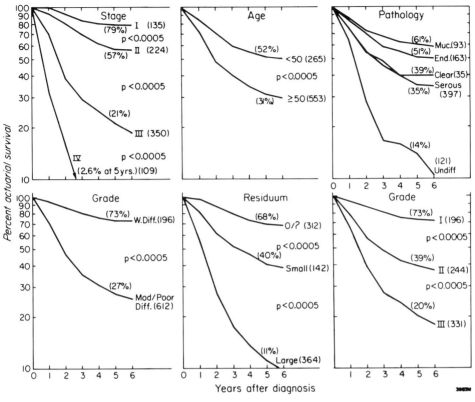

Figure 1. Survival curves of 818 patients with epithelial carcinoma of ovary (PMH, 1971–1978), classified according to stage, residuum, histologic type, grade and age at diagnosis. The percentage in parenthesis above the curve is the 5-year survival rate; the patient number is shown after each survival curve.

In Fig. 1 the survival outcome of patients is shown according to the histologic category and the grade. In general, when clinicians consider the prognostic effect of histologic parameters, there is a tendency to use the tumor grade only, and to disregard the histologic subtype. While this practice simplifies the histologic parameter into 3 subcategories instead of 13 (3 grades for each histologic type

Table 3. Histological types of common epithelial ovarian cancers

Type	Approximate frequency
Serous (Tubal)	50%
Mucinous (Cervical)	10%
Endometroid (Endometrial)	20%
Clear cell	5%
Unclassified and undifferentiated	15%

except the undifferentiated tumors which are always grade 3), it is an oversimplification.

Dembo and co-workers analysed the interactions between histologic type and grade using techniques of multivariate analysis, to adjust for confounding by other factors [15]. They found that grade was highly prognostic (of relapse and death) in the serous tumors, but only minimally prognostic in the mucinous and endometrioid types. Their analysis yielded a 3-tiered classification of histology which took account of the prognostic importance both of histologic type and tumor grade (Table 4). This compound grade-histology classification was a better prognostic discriminant in their experience than grade alone, and this was validated by them on a subsequent cohort of patients [16]. To date, no other investigators have analysed their material in the same way.

Prognostication by histologic parameters is limited by the subjectivity of the pathologist in assigning tumors to a grade or histologic subcategory, as shown by inter- and intra-observer variability [17, 18]. Despite this weakness, the effect of grade is almost always found to be a powerful predictor of survival, relapse and metastatic potential in ovarian cancer [15, 19–21]. The prognostic effect of histology is most clearly seen in patients with early stage disease and successful surgical cytoreduction, because the adverse prognostic effect of large residual tumor volumes tends to dominate the clinical course of those with advanced disease. There is an association between histology and clinical stage in that earlier stages tend to be associated with favorable histologic categories, and vice versa.

A borderline group of epithelial ovarian tumors exists between benign neoplasms (cystadenomas) which do not exhibit either malignant cytologic characteristics or stromal invasion, and malignant tumors (carcinomas) which do. This borderline groups shows absence of destructive stromal invasion even though cytologic features of malignancy are present and metastases can occur [22]. While non-metastatic borderline tumors are almost always cured by operative removal, the metastatic tumors are lethal in about half of the cases, typically running a very protracted course over many years. Histologic criteria cannot identify those borderline tumors which will follow a clinically malignant course, but tumor ploidy studies (see below) may in the future help to distinguish them [23, 24].

Table 4. Compound histologic type-tumor grade classification for epithelial ovarian cancer in use at The Princess Margaret Hospital

% Frequency	Definition	% 5-yr. Survival
22	Grade 1 Serous and Clear-Cell*	82
27	All Mucinous and Endometroid	55
51	Grades 2 + 3 Serous and Clear-cell, and unclassified/undifferentiated	20

* The clear-cell group is very small, and it might be just as satisfactory to place all grades of clear-cell tumor in the worst category.

Anatomic stage

Most commonly used is the FIGO classification (Table 5) which is based on the extent of spread noted at laparotomy. The classification recognizes the principal route of spread of ovarian carcinoma (i.e., transperitoneal) and there is a good correlation between the extent of spread found at operation and the risk of relapse or death from disease. Careful inspection of the peritoneal surfaces in the upper abdomen, routine omental biopsy and sampling of para-aortic lymph nodes, can demonstrate upper abdominal spread in over a quarter of those patients with disease seemingly confined to the pelvis when exploration is limited to the lower abdomen [25].

Removing these 'minimal' Stage III cases from Stages I and II will improve the survival rates for Stages I and II, and its effect likely to exceed the improvement which may have resulted from therapeutic advances [26], although it is often implied that the observed improvement is the result of better treatment alone. Staging provides information predictive of relapse that is independent of histopathology or residuum [15] and is essential for choosing postoperative therapy.

Residuum

The amount of macroscopic tumor remaining after the initial operative attempt

Table 5. Stage classification of ovarian tumors (Simplified from FIGO). Frequency and outcome refer to epithelial tumors. Based on findings at laparotomy.

Stage	% Frequency	% 5 yr. Survival	Description
I	15–20	70–90	Confined to ovaries IA – one ovary IB – both ovaries IC – with ascites or cytologically positive peritoneal washings
II	20–30	40–70	Spread to pelvic peritoneum IIA – direct extension to tubes and/or uterus IIB – pelvic seedings or direct extension IIC – with ascites or positive cytology
III	35–55	5–15	Spread to abdominal peritoneum or retroperitoneal nodes
IV	10–15	0–5	Spread to liver parenchyma, or beyond abdomen
Overall	100	30–35	

at removal is usually defined by the largest diameter of the largest remaining lesion. This indicator shows an inverse relationship to patient survival [27, 28], even though it ignores the number of remaining lesions. The distinction between 'small' versus 'large' residuum used a cut off of 2 or 3 cm in earlier reports, but recently this size has been revised downwards to 1 cm [29]. The older practice grouped patients with no macroscopic residuum (whose prognosis is significantly better than those with small residuum) [15, 16] together with those having lesions under 2 cm in size.

Patients in Stage III who are left with small tumor residua are said to have undergone 'optimal' surgical cytoreduction. A causal association between the resection of large masses to the optimal state and enhanced survival time has been postulated [27, 30] and is indeed, widely accepted in clinical practice. However, since approximately three quarters of such 'optimal' Stage III patients still die of their disease, it remains to be shown which subgroups of patients presenting with large metastases have their cure dependent upon the primary resection of those masses. It is still necessary to disprove the null hypothesis that surgical cytoreduction is merely a means of identifying patients whose disease will follow a more favorable course in response to therapy.

Patient age at diagnosis

The median age at diagnosis of ovarian carcinoma is approximately 53 years. The disease increases in frequency with increasing age and is rare below 20 years of age. Prognosis is worse in older patients, both with respect to relapse and death. Unlike endometrial cancer, most deaths occurring within 5 years of diagnosis of ovarian cancer are due to the primary diagnosis, and cure of relapsed disease is rare. From Fig. 1 it is seen that the survival probability of patients with ovarian cancer is significantly better for those under 50 years of age at diagnosis than those older than 50, and the same applies to the probability of remaining free from relapse.

Multivariate analysis was used to examine the effect of age on the relapse rate, after adjusting for the confounding effect of other variables (stage, residuum, histopathology) [15]. The results showed that the lower risk of relapse in younger patients could be completely explained by the more favorable distribution of variables such as earlier stage, better histology and less residuum. However, the effect of advancing age in reducing the survival time could not be completely explained in this way, suggesting that treatment may be more effective in prolonging survival after relapse in younger patients (possibly because of more vigorous treatment).

Synthesis of stage, residuum and histology

At the Princess Margaret Hospital we have concluded that since outcome is determined by the independent effects exerted by stage, residuum and histopathology, selection of treatment and reporting of results should be based upon all three variables [15, 16]. Similar conclusions have been reached by others [31, 32], but because of differences in staging techniques and histologic classifications between centers, a universal multivariate classification has not been possible.

Prognostic factors in non-metastatic carcinomas

The FIGO classification recognizes several subclasses of Stage I, according to whether tumors are unilateral (IA) or bilateral (IB), whether ascites or positive peritoneal cytology are documented (IC), and whether capsular penetration or cyst-rupture has occurred (ii) or not (i). The distinction between Stages I and II or III based upon invasion into adjacent structures (in the absence of separate metastatic deposits or 'seeding') is somewhat arbitrary, because it is not usually obvious at the time of operation whether the adherence of the tumor to adjacent structures is due to tumor invasion or to some other cause such as endometriosis.

The group at the Mayo Clinic demonstrated that *dense* adherence, no matter the cause, worsened prognosis [33] leading to the common practice of advancing the stage of patients with densely adherent but non-metastatic tumors to Stage II or III, according to whether they are adherent to pelvic (II) or abdominal (III) structures. A more recent analysis from Toronto, which incorporated multivariate statistical analysis, confirmed that dense adherence worsened prognosis independently of the effect of other factors, lending support to the practice of upstaging according to according to adherence [34].

The same analysis showed that tumor grade was the most powerful prognostic factor in Stage I, with a 6-fold relative risk of relapse in grades 2 and 3 compared to grade 1. However in a sample size of over 250 Stage I patients, none of the following factors exerted a significant effect on prognosis: bilaterality, rupture, capsular penetration, ascites, cyst size, or patient age. It is therefore not clear whether any or all of them need consideration for purposes of staging or deciding therapy.

Cervical cancer

Numerous papers have recognized various prognostic factors for carcinoma of the cervix in univariate analyses, but few attempts have been made to show how these factors are interrelated. Moreover, the recognition of these factors has had little impact on the currently accepted FIGO Staging classification for carcinoma of the cervix. End-result reporting of therapy still uses it to classify patients into prognostic groups, ignoring prognostic factors which could subdivide patients of similar FIGO stage into subgroups whose outcome may be widely disparate.

This section will focus on tumor-related prognostic factors including FIGO stage, size and extent of pelvic disease, involvement of the endometrium, nodal involvement, hemoglobin levels and pathology (grade and cell type).

The data used for this discussion will come from the literature and also from a retrospective review of all patients with carcinoma of the cervix treated with radiation therapy at the Princess Margaret Hospital (PMH) between 1976 and 1980.

Stage

The single most significant factor identified in the PMH series and in others in the literature is FIGO stage (see Table 6). In the univariate analysis, stage was highly significant, with the five-year actuarial survival of Stage I patients being 79%, Stage IIA 74%, Stage IIB 64%, Stage III 38%, Stage IVA 9% and Stage–IVB 0% [35]. Overall 60–65% are cured. Although staging investigations may vary between countries and institutes, the compiled FIGO reports show a clear effect on outcome by stage of disease at presentation [36].

The FIGO staging system does not however separate out patient subgroups within each stage who may have better or worse outcomes than the average for the stage. Within each FIGO stage, factors such as bulk of pelvic disease and nodal involvement add prognostic information.

Table 6. Stage classification for cervical carcinoma (Simplified from FIGO; clinical staging)

Stage	Substage	Description
I		Confined to cervix
	IA	Micro-invasive
	IB	Greater than microinvasive (IB – occult: lesion not visible or palpable)
II	IIA	Spread to vagina, upper two-thirds
	IIB	Spread to parametria
III	IIIA	Spread to vagina, lower one-third
	IIIB	Spread to pelvic sidewall
IV	IVA	Mucosa of bladder or rectum
	IVB	Outside of pelvis

Tumor bulk

Bulk or extent of disease within FIGO stage has not been routinely examined in many series, although within Stage I, several observers have correlated the size or volume of cervical tumor with a likelihood of involvement of draining lymph nodes and treatment outcome. Volume of disease appears to be an important prognostic factor even in microinvasive carcinoma (MIC). The pathological entity of MIC describes a subgroup in whom the tumor is associated with absent or minimal ($<1\%$) risk of pelvic nodal involvement. Different criteria have been used to characterize MIC, including the depth of tumor penetration, the absence of confluence and the absence of lymphatic permeation [37]. However, even in these clinically occult tumors, extent may be the most reliable single factor defining MIC, whether measured as the greatest allowable lateral spread (4 mm [38] or 10 mm [39]), two dimensional area (50 mm^2) [38], or tumor volume (500 mm^3) [40].

With Stage IB carcinomas, it has been observed at surgery that lesions $\leqslant 3$ cm in size had an overall incidence of nodal metastases of 21% and survival ranging from 84 to 90% [41], whereas lesions >3 cm had a 35% incidence of nodal metastases and a five-year survival rate of 66% [41]. A similar observation was made for the influence of size of lesion in Stage IIA disease. Thus, Van Nagell *et al.* [42] showed a lower survival rate and nearly a threefold increase in pelvic node positivity when comparing lesions of >2 cm vs <2 cm. Homesley *et al.* reported significantly higher five-year actuarial survival after radiation therapy in those with tumors <4 cm compared to those $\geqslant 4$ cm (95% vs 67%) [43]. Whatever size criteria we used to group patients, it is likely that risk of nodal involvement and death from cancer increases progressively as volume of the lesion increases.

Within FIGO Stage IIB, the extent of disease varies from small lesions with minimal invasion of one medial parametrial region, up to lesions extending out to both lateral parametrial regions. In a series of patients reviewed retrospectively at the Princess Margaret Hospital, we arbitrarily divided tumors according to involvement of the medial half parametrium or the lateral half, and whether it was unilateral or bilateral. Actuarial five-year survivals showed significant differences between those with any lateral parametrial involvement (unilateral or bilateral) vs those with only medial involvement (unilateral or bilateral) [35].

Similarly for FIGO Stage III patients, the division of patients into those with unilateral or bilateral pelvic side wall involvement (which we believe to be an indirect measure of disease volume) defined two distinct prognostic subgroups. Pelvic tumor control rates were significantly better for those with unilateral disease compared to those with bilateral involvement, and those with unilateral had a five-year actuarial survival of 45% compared to 18% for those with bilateral involvement.

Accurate methods of quantitating the volume of pelvic disease need to be developed but even crude indices show that volume of tumor contributes additional prognostic information to that FIGO stage. Some measure of tumor volume should be incorporated into the next modification of the staging system for cervical cancer.

Lymph node spread

Discussion of the prognostic significance of tumor volume showed that volume of disease was predictive of nodal involvement as well as of outcome. It is not known whether bulk and nodal involvement are dependent, or independent, variables with respect to outcome, but it is clear that nodal involvement is another factor predictive of outcome. This is independent of FIGO stage and whether the initial therapy is surgery or irradiation. The general 'rule of thumb' used to estimate the impact of nodal involvement on outcome is that nodal involvement halves the expected survival by stage. This generalization comes from multiple reports in the literature which have shown that within FIGO stage, not only is the presence or absence of nodal involvement critical, but that outcome is dependent on both the number of nodes involved and the anatomic level (from distal to proximal) of the nodes involved.

In a series from the Norwegian Radium Hospital [44], 562 Stage IB patients were treated by preoperative intracavitary radium, radical hysterectomy and pelvic lymphadenectomy, and postoperative external radiation was added if nodal involvement was present. The five-year survival was 92% if no nodes were involved, but 53% for the 21% of patients with positive nodes. The relapse-free rates according to the level of nodal involvement, were 67%, 50% and 0% respectively for bilateral involvement of the obturator, external iliac or common iliac nodes. Collected data from numerous series in the literature demonstrate that for selected patients with para-aortic nodal involvement (identified by extraperitoneal lymph node dissection and treated with extended field irradiation) only 18% will be salvaged on average.

While the likelihood of pelvic and para-aortic nodal involvement increases with increasing FIGO stage of disease, the prognostic significance of nodal involvement is independent of FIGO stage. Although lymphography is not 100% sensitive or specific for the identification of nodal disease in carcinoma of the cervix, it offers significant prognostic information beyond FIGO stage. In the radiation series from the PMH, both the presence of nodal involvement as defined by lymphography, and the level of nodal involvement (be it external iliac vs external plus common iliac vs external plus common plus para-aortic nodes) were significant prognostic factors [35].

Endometrial spread

Involvement of the endometrial cavity has been cited as an adverse prognostic factor [45]. In one series, five year survival rates for FIGO Stage I and II patients with negative D & C findings were 80% and 73% respectively compared to 50% and 45% for those with positive D & C findings. The incidence of distant metastases was also higher in those Stage I and II patients with positive uterine curettings.

There is no report of systematic prospective fractional curettage on all patients, to assess the incidence of endometrial stromal involvement within each FIGO stage, so that the incidence of endometrial involvement by cervical carcinoma is unknown. The above report was based on a subset of patients (302/1300 patients) selected for D & C, but does not specify the selection criteria. It is therefore unknown whether the significance of endometrial involvement is dependent on other factors such as disease volume or nodal involvement. Endometrial involvement may simply represent another measure of increased local extent of disease, without the endometrium *per se* being a specific pelvic site associated with a poorer prognosis.

Hemoglobin level

The prognostic significance of low hemoglobin levels during radiation therapy has been cited by several authors [35, 46, 47]. In the PMH series [35, 46], patients with hemoglobin levels less than 12 gms % had a significantly worse outlook than those with hemoglobin levels > 12 gm %. This finding was independent of FIGO stage. A small randomized study suggested that transfusion during radiation therapy could overcome this effect [46], although other authors [48, 49] found no improvement in the prognosis of anemic patients transfused prior to therapy.

The mechanism by which anemia is related to a deleterious effect on survival is unknown. It has been suggested that anemia may result in an increased proportion of hypoxic, relatively radioresistant, tumor cells which may lead to poorer local control with radiation [46], but this does not explain the poorer outcome in anemic compared to non-anemic patients treated surgically [47]. The unfavourable effect of low hemoglobin levels on survival and local-regional control may result from a nonspecific factor associated with biologically more aggressive disease.

Histology

With respect to histologic cell type, the consensus is that there is a statistically worse survival rate for those patients with adenocarcinoma compared to squamous cell carcinoma [47] and that neuro-ectodermal small cell carcinoma of cervix is associated with a worse prognosis [50, 51]. The evidence for variation for outcome based on the type of squamous cell carcinoma (i.e. large and small cell, keratinizing and non keratinizing) is inconclusive [37]. The prognostic significance of grade within each cell type has also been the subject or controversy. Several authors suggest that dedifferentiated tumors are associated with an increasing incidence of pelvic node involvement and that higher grade lesions are associated with larger tumors and poorer survival [52]. The other microscopic feature of prognostic significance with respect to increasing risk of lymph node metastases and decreasing survival rate, is the presence of lymphatic or blood vessel invasion [37, 53].

In summary: In carcinoma of the cervix, multiple pretreatment factors have been identified to be of prognostic significance, but their interrelationship is not clear because multifactorial analysis of these factors has been rarely carried out. Such analyses on large numbers of patients would enable us to establish prognostic subgroups within FIGO staging.

Tumor ploidy in gynecologic cancer

Aneuploidy has come to be recognised as a common feature of malignant cells and its presence has been associated with an altered biological behaviour in a variety of tumor types [54, 55].

Ovary

Early cytometric studies performed on ovarian tumors suggested an association between clinical stage, tumor grade and ploidy, and indicated that patients with diploid tumors had a favourable prognosis [56, 57]. These studies were however confined to relatively small numbers of patients at a time when there was inadequate staging at diagnosis. Moreover, the importance of the histological features and significance of the 'borderline' group ovarian tumors was not widely appreciated.

Using flow cytometry, Friedlander *et al.* reported that invasive ovarian tumors were commonly aneuploid, and that there was a significant association between stage and ploidy, with early stage tumors tending to be diploid, while advanced tumors were usually aneuploid [58]. In the majority of cases, ploidy was found to be a stable marker, exhibiting consistency within different sites of the primary tumor and metastases and also after subsequent tumor progression [59]. Diploid tumors were shown to have a significantly lower S phase fraction than aneuploid tumors but there are problems with accurately estimating S phase in tumor specimens, and it is possible that the values of S phase in diploid cells may in some instances have been falsely lowered by admixture with normal noncycling diploid cells.

In a flow cytometric study of paraffin-embedded tumor blocks from patients with advanced (FIGO Stages III and IV) ovarian cancer, 69% of tumors were shown to be aneuploid and 31% diploid. Patients with diploid tumors (mean survival of 123 weeks) had a significantly longer survival than those patients with aneuploid or multiploid tumors (median survival 52 and 63 weeks respectively), and multivariate analysis showed that tumor ploidy was the most powerful determinant of survival [60]. Further analysis indicated that the relatively good prognosis associated with diploid tumors was limited to those patients with Stage III disease while patients with Stage IV disease had a poor prognosis irrespective of ploidy [61].

In a similar study performed on paraffin-embedded tumor blocks from patients with early stage (FIGO Stages I and II) disease, a significant association between ploidy and tumor grade was evident, with well differentiated tumors being more commonly diploid while poorly differentiated tumors tended to be aneuploid. There was a significant effect of both grade and ploidy on survival, but because of the relativity small numbers, multivariate analysis was not performed to assess the relative importance of stage, histological grade, subtype and ploidy [61, 62].

Recently two other groups have reported similar findings. In a prospective flow cytometric study of ploidy in patients with Stage III and IV ovarian cancer, Volm *et al.* found that patients with aneuploid tumors had significantly shorter survival than those with diploid tumors [63]. Similar findings were reported using Feulgen cytophotometry to analyse DNA content in patients with FIGO Stage I and II ovarian cancer [64].

Borderline ovarian tumors account for 15% of ovarian tumors and as a group are characterised by an indolent course even when spread beyond the ovaries occurs [65]. The diagnosis can be difficult even for the experienced pathologist and there is evidence that cellular DNA content may be a useful adjunct to the histopathological diagnosis of borderline malignancy. In a study of 44 borderline ovarian tumors analysed for ploidy, Friedlander *et al.* demonstrated that 95% of tumors were diploid and associated with a good prognosis while two patients (5%) with aneuploid 'borderline' tumors died with progressive disease within a relatively short period of time [23]. Hall and Fu found a 31% incidence of aneuploidy among 16 borderline malignant serous tumors and demonstrated a close association of ploidy with FIGO stage and survival [66]. Two of 11 diploid borderline tumors recurred, in contrast to 4 of the 5 aneuploid tumors.

Similar results attesting to the potential value of ploidy in the assessment of borderline ovarian tumors have been reported in two other studies [64, 67]. It should however be emphasized that as a diploid DNA content can occur in frankly invasive ovarian tumors, the DNA content alone cannot be used as the sole means of differentiating borderline from invasive tumors. Nevertheless, the finding of an aneuploid population in a borderline ovarian tumor should be useful in predicting which 'borderline' tumors are more likely to have a more aggressive biological behaviour.

Uterine cervix

A number of studies have correlated tumor ploidy with survival among patients with cervical carcinomas. Using static cytometry Atkin reported that patients with near diploid tumors had a worse prognosis than those with high ploidy squamous cell carcinomas of the cervix [56, 58], but in the case of adenocarcinomas, the survival rate of patients with low ploidy was 45% in contrast to 18% in the high ploidy group [56]. In a similar study on patients with adenocarcinomas of the cervix Fu *et al.* reported 80% five-year survival for patients with low ploidy tumors, and 22% five-year survival for the high ploidy group [69].

Of the more recent reports on the use of flow cytometry in carcinomas of the uterine cervix, Jakobsen has reported a study involving 171 patients with squamous cell carcinoma of the cervix in which patients with low ploidy tumors had a significantly better prognosis than those with high ploidy tumors [70]. These findings are quite different to those reported by Atkin using static cytometry, and it is unlikely that the difference can be accounted for by the different techniques as there is a good correlation between ploidy as determined by both static and flow cytometry [71]. The differences may be due to different follow-up times or treatment techniques. Jakobsen has also reported a significant correlation between the DNA index and the incidence of pelvic lymph node metastases in patients with Stage IB and IIA tumors, with high ploidy tumors having a higher likelihood of metastases [72]. This finding could have important implications for the choice of treatment.

There may be a place for determining ploidy in intraepithelial cervical neoplasms. Fu *et al.* using Feulgen cytophotometry, investigated biopsy speciement from 100 women with cervical dysplasia and carcinoma *in situ* who were followed for more than a year without therapy [73]. There was a strong association between ploidy and outcome in that the vast majority of persisting lesions were aneuploid, as were all the cases in which there was progression to invasive cancer. Among women whose lesions regressed, the DNA content was usually diploid or polyploid.

Jakobsen has also investigated patients with cervical dysplasia and reported that lesions characterised by mild or moderate dysplasia were almost always diploid, while 80% of cases of severe dysplasia or carcinoma *in situ* were aneuploid [74]. These findings are in accordance with cytogenetic investigations which showed that only 29% of cases of carcinoma *in situ* had a chromosome number in the diploid range [75]. Analysis of ploidy may be of value in indicating which intraepithelial neoplasms have a high propensity to progress to invasive cancer, and this merits further study.

Endometrial cancer

There have been few studies to date on cellular DNA content in endometrial carcinoma. Atkin found that near-diploid tumors were more likely to be well differentiated and to be associated with a better prognosis than were high ploidy tumors [56].

Moberger *et al.* confirmed these findings and suggested that ploidy correlated better with outcome than did either clinical stage or grade; the eight year survival rates were 79% for patients with diploid tumors and 18% for patients with aneuploid tumors [76]. Naus *et al.* have demonstrated the ability to determine ploidy on paraffin-embedded endometrial tumors using flow cytometry [77]. Their initial report confirms the results of the static cytophotometric studies and this should encourage retrospective flow cytometric studies on stored specimens of endometrial tumors from patients whose outcome is known.

References

1. Morrow CP, DiSaia PJ, Townsend D: Current management of endometrial cancer. *Obstet Gynecol* 42: 399–406, 1973
2. Malkasian GD: Carcinoma of the endometrium: Effect of stage and grade on survival. *Cancer* 41: 966–1001, 1978
3. Mackillop WJ, Pringle JF: Stage III endometrial carcinoma. A review of 90 cases. *Cancer* 56: 2519–2523, 1985
4. Bruckman JE, Bloomer WD, Marck A, Ehrmann RL, Knapp RC: Stage III adenocarcinoma of the endometrium: Two prognostic groups. *Gynecol Oncol* 9: 12–17, 1980
5. Potish RA, Twiggs LB, Adcock LL, Prem A: Role of whole abdominal radiation therapy in the management of endometrial cancer: Prognostic importance of factors indicating peritoneal metastases. *Gynecol Oncol* 21: 80–86, 1985
6. Nilsen PA, Koller O: Carcinoma of the endometrium in Norway 1957–1960 with special reference to treatment results. *Am J Obstet Gynecol* 105: 1099–1109, 1969
7. Morrow CP, Creasman WT, Homesly H, Yordan E, Park R, Bundy B: Recurrence in Endometrial Cancer as a Function of Extended Surgical Staging Data. In: *Gynecological Oncology*, Morrow CP, Smart GE (eds). Springer-Verlag, 1986
8. Cheon HD: Prognosis of endometrial cancer. *Obstet Gynecol* 34: 680–684, 1969
9. Ballon SC, Berman ML, Donaldson RC, Growdon WA, Lagasse LD: Pulmonary metastases of endometrial cancer. *Gynecol Oncol* 7: 56–65, 1979
10. Ng ABP, Regan JW, Storaasli JP, Wentz WB: Mixed adenosquamous carcinoma of the endometrium. *Am J Clin Pathol* 59: 765–781, 1973
11. Hendrickson M, Ross J, Eifel PJ, Cox RS, Martinez A, Kempson R: Adenocarcinoma of the endometrium: Analysis of 256 cases with carcinoma limited to the uterine corpus. *Gynecol Oncol* 13: 373–392, 1982
12. Malkasian GD, Annegers JF, Fountain KS: Carcinoma of the endometrium Stage I. *Am J Obstet Gynecol* 136: 872–883, 1980
13. Creasman WT, McCarty KS, Sr., Barton TK, McCarty KS, Jr.: Clinical correlates of estrogen- and progesterone-binding proteins in human endometrial adenocarcinoma. *Obstet Gynecol* 55: 363–370, 1980

248

14. Antunes CMF, Stolley PD, Rosenstein NB, Dacies JL, Tonascia JA, Brown C, Burnett L, Rutledge A, Pokempner M, Garcia E: Endometrial cancer and estrogen use – report of a large case-controlled study. *N Eng J Med* 300: 9–13, 1979
15. Dembo AJ: The role of radiotherapy in ovarian cancer. *Bull Cancer* (Paris) 69, 3: 275–283, 1982
16. Dembo AJ: Abdominopelvic radiotherapy in ovarian cancer: A 10-year experience. *Cancer* 55: 2290–2295, 1985
17. Hernandez E, Bhangavan BS, Parmley TH, Rosenshein NB: Interobserver variability in the interpretation of eptihelial ovarian cancer. *Gynecol Oncol* 17: 117–123, 1984
18. Baak JPA, Lindeman J, Overdiep SH, Langley FA: Disagreement of histopathological diagnoses of different pathologists in ovarian tumors – with some theoretical considerations. *Europ J Obstet Gynec Reprod Biol* 13: 51–55, 1982
19. Santesson L, Kottmeier HL: General classification of ovarian tumours. In: *Ovarian Cancer*, Gentil F and Junguerira AC (eds). U.I.C.C. Monograph Series. New York: Springer-Verlag, 1968, Vol. 11, p 1
20. Malkasian GD, Decker DG, Webb MJ: Histology of epithelial tumours of the ovary: Clinical usefullness and prognostic significance of histologic classification and grading. *Semin Oncol*, 2: 191–201, 1975
21. Sorbe B, Frankendal B and Veress B: Importance of histologic grading in the prognosis of epithelial ovarian carcinoma. *Obstet Gynecol* 59: 576–582, 1982
22. Colgan TJ, Norris HJ: Ovarian epithelial tumors of low potential malignancy: A review. *Int J Gynecol Oncol* 1: 367–382, 1983
23. Friedlander ML, Russell P, Taylor IW, Hedley DWE, Tattersall MHN: Flow cytometric analysis of cellular DNA content as an adjunct to the diagnosis of ovarian tumors of borderline malignancy. *Pathology* 16: 301–306, 1984
24. Baak JPA, Agrafojo B, Kurver PHI *et al*: Quantitative analysis of borderline and malignant mucinous tumours. *Histopathology* 5: 553–560, 1981
25. Piver MS, Barlow JJ, Lele SB: Incidence of subclinical metastasis in Stage I and II ovarian carcinoma. *Obstet Gynecol* 52: 100–104, 1978
26. Bush RS: Ovarian cancer: Contribution of radiation therapy to patient management. *Radiology* 153: 17–24, 1984
27. Griffiths CT: Surgical resection of tumor bulk in the primary treatment of ovarian carcinoma. *Natl Cancer Inst Monogr* 42: 101–104, 1975
28. Smith JP, Day TG: Review of ovarian cancer at the University of Texas Systems Cancer Center, M.D. Anderson Hospital and Tumor Institute. *Am J Obstet Gynecol* 135: 984–993, 1979
29. Pater J, Shelley W, Willan A, Kirk ME, Carmichael J, Krepart G, Levitt M, Roy M: The effect of histologic subtype, grade and residual tumour diameter on survival and negative second look rates in patients with Stage III and IV carcinoma of the ovary. *Proc Am Soc Clin Oncol* 3: 166 (Abstract C-646), 1984
30. Wharton J, Herson J: Surgery for common epithelial tumors of the ovary. *Cancer* 48: 582-589, 1981
31. Swenerton KD, Hislop TG, Spinelli J, LeRiche JC, Yang N, Boyes DA: Ovarian carcinoma: A multivariate analysis of prognostic factors. *Obstet Gynecol* 65: 264–269, 1985
32. Schray M, Martinez A, Cox R, Ballon A: Radiotherapy in epithelial ovarian cancer: Analysis of prognostic factors based on long term experience. *Obstet Gynecol* 62: 373–382, 1983
33. Webb MJ, Decker DG, Mussey E *et al*.: Factors influencing survival in Stage I ovarian cancer. *Am J Obstet Gynecol* 116: 222–228, 1973
34. Dembo AJ, Prefontaine M, Miceli P, Bush RS: Prognostic factors in Stage I epithelial ovarian carcinoma. *Proc Am Soc Clin Oncol* 5: 124 (Abstract 483) 1986
35. Thomas G: Princess Margaret Hospital (unpublished data)
36. International Federation of Gynecology and Obstretics. Annual report on the results of treatment in gynecological cancer. 18th vol. 1973–1975

37. Clement PB, Scully RE: Carcinoma of the cervix: Histologic types. *Seminars in Oncology*, Vol. 9, No. 3 (Sept), 1982
38. Burghardt E: *Early Histological Diagnosis of Cervical Cancer*. Philadelphia, Saunders, 1973
39. Lohe KJ: Early squamous cell carcinoma of the uterine cervix. *Gynecol Oncol* 6: 10–30, 1978
40. Burghardt E, Holzer E: Diagnosis and treatment of microinvasive carcinoma of the cervix uteri. *Obstet Gynecol Survey* 34: 836–838, 1979
41. Piver SM, Chung WS: Prognostic significance of cervical lesion size and pelvic node metastases in cervical carcinoma. *Obstet Gynecol*, Vol. 46, No. 5, Nov. 1975
42. Van Nagell JR, Donaldson ES, Parker JC *et al.*: The prognostic significance of cell type and lesion size in patients with servical cancer treated by radical surgery. *Gynecol Oncol* 5: 142, 1977
43. Homesley HD, Raben M, Blake DD *et al.*: Relationship of lesion size to survival in patients with Stage IB squamous cell carcinoma of the cervix uteri treated by radiation therapy. *Surgery, Gynecology & Obstetrics* 150, 1980
44. Martimbeau PW, Kjorstad KE, Iversen T *et al.*: Stage IB carcinoma of the cervix, The Norwegian Radium Hospital, 1986–1972: Study of results when pelvic nodes are involved. *Abstract. Society of Gynecologic Oncologists*. Eleventh Annual Meeting, 1980
45. Perez CA, Zivnuska F, Askin F *et al.*: Prognostic significance of endometrial extension from primary carcinoma of the uterine cervix. *Cancer* 35: 1493–1504, 1975
46. Bush RS, Jenkin RDT, Allt WEC *et al.*: Definitive evidence for hypoxic cells influencing cure in cancer therapy. *Br J Cancer* 37 (Suppl III): 302–306, 1978
47. Kapp DS, Fisher D, Gutierrez E *et al.*: Pretreatment prognostic factors in carcinoma of the uterine cavity: a multivariate analysis of the effect of age, stage, histology and blood counts on survival. *Int J Radiat Oncol Biol Phys* 9: No. 4, 1983
48. Vigario G, Kurshara SS, George SW: Association of hemoglobin levels before and during radiotherapy with prognosis in uterine cervix cancer. *Radiol* 106: 649–652, 1973
49. Evans JC, Bergsjo P: Influence of anemia on the results of radiotherapy in carcinoma of cervix. *Radiol* 84: 709–716, 1965
50. Finck FM, Denk M: Cervical carcinoma: Relationships between histology and survival following radiation therapy. *Obstet Gynecol* 35: 339–343, 1970
51. Wentz WB, Lewis CG: Correlation of histologic morphology and survival in cervical cancer following radiation therapy. *Obstet Gynecol* 26: 228–232, 1965
52. Chung CK, Stryker JA, Ward SP *et al.*: Histologic grade and prognosis of carcinoma of the cervix. *Obstet Gynecol* 57, No. 5, 636–642, 1981
53. Van Nagell JR, Donaldson ES, Wood EG *et al.*: The significance of vascular and lymphocytic infiltration in invasive cervical cancer. *Cancer* 41: 228–234, 1978
54. Friedlander ML, Hedley DW, Taylor IW: Clinical and biological significance of aneuploidy in human tumours. *J Clin Pathol* 37: 961–974, 1984
55. Barlogie B, Raber MN, Schumann J *et al.*: Flow cytometry in clinical cancer research. *Cancer Res* 43: 3982–3997, 1983
56. Atkin NB: Prognostic significance of ploidy level in human tumours. 1. Carcinoma of the uterus. *J Natl Cancer Inst* 56: 909–910, 1976
57. Bader S, Taylor HC, Engle ET: Deoxyribonucleide acid (DNA) content of human ovarian tumours in relation to histological grading. *Lab Invest* 9: 443–459, 1960
58. Friedlander ML, Taylor IW, Russell P, Musgrove EA, Hedley DW, Tattersall MHN: Ploidy as a prognostic factor in ovarian cancer. *Int J Gynecol Pathol* 2: 55–63, 1983
59. Friedlander ML, Taylor IW, Russell P, Tattersall MHN: Cellular DNA content – a stable marker in epithelial ovarian cancer. *Br J Cancer* 49: 173–179, 1984
60. Friedlander ML, Hedley DW, Taylor IW, Russel P, Coates AS, Tattersall MHN: Influence of cellular DNA content on survival in advanced ovarian cancer. *Cancer Res.* 44: 397–400, 1984

61. Hedley DW, Friedlander ML, Taylor IW: Application of DNA flow cytometry to paraffin-embedded archival material for the study of aneuploidy and its clinical significance. *Cytometry* 6: 327–333, 1985
62. Friedlander ML, Taylor IW, Hedley DW, Tattersall MHN: The biological significancer of cellular DNA content in ovarian cancer. *Proc Am Assoc Cancer Res* 25: 34, 1984
63. Volm M *et al.*: Prognostic relevance of ploidy and proliferation in ovarian carcinoma. *Cancer Res* 45: 5180–5185, 1985
64. Erhardt K, Auer G, Bjorkholm E *etal.*: Prognostic significance of DNA content in serous ovarian tumours. *Cancer Res* 44: 2198–2202, 1984
65. Hart WR: Ovarian epithelial tumours of borderline malignancy (carcinoma of low malignant potential). *Hum Pathol* 8: 541–549, 1977
66. Hall TL, Fu YS: Applications of quantitative microscopy in tumour pathology. *Lab Invest* 53: 5–21, 1985
67. Weiss R, Richart R, Okagaki T: DNA content of mucinous tumours of the ovary. *Am J Obstet Gynecol* 103: 409–424, 1969
68. Ng ABP, Atkin NB: Histological cell type and DNA value in the prognosis of squamous cell cancer of uterine cervix. *Br J Cancer* 28: 322–331, 1973
69. Fu YS, Reagan JW, FU AS, Janiga KE: Adenocarcinoma and mixed carcinoma of the uterine cervix. II. Prognostic value of DNA analysis. *Cancer* 49: 25712577, 1982
70. Jakobsen A: Prognostic impact of ploidy level in carcinoma of the cervix. *Am J Clin Oncol* 7: 475–480, 1984
71. Strong P, Lindgren A, Stendahl U: Comparison between flow cytometry and single cell cytophotometry for DNA content analysis of the uterine cervix. *Acta Radiologica Oncology* 24 (Phase 4): 337–341, 1985
72. Jakobsen A: Ploidy level and short time prognosis of early cervix cancer. *Radiather Oncol* 1: 271–275, 1984
73. Fu YS, Reagan JW, Richardt RM: Definition of precursors. *Gynecol Oncol* 12: 220–231, 1980
74. Jakobsen A, Kristensen PB, Poulsen HK: Flow cytometric classification of biopsy specimencts from cervical intraepithelial neoplasia. *Cytometry* 4: 166–170, 1983
75. Spriggs AI, Bowey CE, Cordell RH: Chromosomes of precancerous lesions oif the cervix uteri: New data and a review. *Cancer* 27: 1239–1254, 1971
76. Moberger B, Auer G, Forsslund G, Moberger G: The prognistic sifnificance of DNA measurements in endometrial carcinoma. *Cytometry* 5: 430–436, 1983
77. Naus GJ, De Vere White R, Richart RM, Deitch AD: Predictive value of flow cytometric DNA content analysis of paraffin-embedded tissue in endometrial carcinoma. *Lab Investig* 52: 48A (Abstract) 1985

15. Prognostic indices in prostatic cancer

G. WILLIAMS

Prostatic cancer is the third leading cause of male death from cancer [1] but its course is so unpredictable that many unsuspected tumours are discovered post-mortem, and patients with untreated small, well-differentiated tumours may never show metastases [2, 3]. On the other hand, rapidly growing or metastatic tumours may be associated with a more anaplastic pathological category [4]. Median survival after diagnosis of metastatic disease is short (12–18 months), though approximately 20% of patients with metastatic disease survive for five years or more [5].

The behaviour of a tumour is a function of tumour-host interaction. While host factors such as age, race, or serum hormone concentrations may influence the prognosis, such information is of little help in determining the prognosis of the individual patient. Tumour factors influencing individual prognosis are better defined and this chapter considers those which significantly affect the outcome and also the likelihood of response to current therapy. However, at the outset, it must be recognised that within any tumour there is considerable clonal heterogeneity, so that sub-populations of morphologically identical cells may have different malignant potential [6].

Age, race and prognosis

Deaths from carcinoma of the prostate are seldom seen in those under 50 years, but increase markedly with increasing age [7]. The patients age at diagnosis is not significantly related to crude survival [8] but in patients older than 70, increasing tumour volume is associated with a significantly increased number of poorly differentiated tumours [9]. This predominance is more striking in the elderly black population, than in the older white population.

A feature of prostatic cancer in the United States is a 50% higher incidence for the black population in areas where blacks make up the majority of the non-white population [10]. Furthermore, the mortality rate for blacks is 54% compared to

64% for whites [11] while mortality rates for Chinese and Mexican Americans, and for American Indians are lower than those for the black or white populations. In 1974/5, the age-corrected mortality rate ranged from 1–2 per hundred thousand in Asian countries, to a peak of 22 per hundred thousand in Sweden [12].

Stage at presentation

The volume of a prostatic tumour is directly related to the prognosis. In their early phase, tumours of the prostate have a slow growth rate, and metastases are unusual before a tumour volume of 1 ml is reached [13] In a study of 138 malignant prostates removed either at radical prostatectomy or necropsy, only tumours with a volume of greater than 4 ml were associated with metastases, a volume achiebed in only 13 of the necropsy tumours [9]. Thus, precise determination of tumour volume and the presence of capsule invasion should help in the estimation of prognosis in the individual.

The two commonly-used clinical staging classifications are that of the American Urological Association, originally described by Whitmore [14], and the TNM classification [15]. The two systems are compared in Table I. The TNM classifi-

Table 1. Comparison of staging systems

	AUA staging system		TNM staging system
A1	Microscopic focus of well differentiated adeno-carcinoma in up to three foci of transurethral specimen or enucleation; clinically not apparent on rectal examination	T0	No tumour palpable
A2	Tumour not well differentiated or present in more than three areas		
B1	Asymptomatic palpable nodule <1.5 cm; normal surrounding prostate; no capsular extension; normal acid phosphatase	T1	Tumour intracapsular (normal gland surrounds tumour)
B2	Diffuse involvement of gland; no capsular extension; normal acid phosphatase	T2	Tumour confined to gland smooth nodule deforming contour
C	Extensive local tumour with penetration through the capsule, contiguous spread; may involve seminal vesicles, bladder neck, lateral side wall of pelvis; acid phosphatase may be elevated; normal bone scan	T3 T4	Tumour beyond capsule Tumour fixed to other pelvic organs
D1	Metastases to pelvic lymph nodes below aortic bifurcation; acid phosphatase may be elevated	N1-2	Regional lymph node metastases
D2	Bone or lymph node metastases above aortic bifurcation of other soft tissue metastases	M1	Distant metastases

cation has considerable advantages in separating the assessment of the primary tumour from that of nodal or other metastases. However, the T0 category is unsatisfactory in lumping together foci of well differentiated adenocarcinoma and diffuse anaplastic carcinoma in spite of their different prognostic significance.

For the higher T categories, digital rectal examination is a poor guide to tumour volume and CT scanning or a rectal ultrasound probe are not generally available for routine monitoring. Our present measurement of tumour volume is therefore inadequate for the majority of patients, although it is the basis of the clinical staging system widely used for predicting clinical behaviour and determining therapy.

Patients with A1 disease appear to have a normal life expectancy, but those with A2 disease have a similar clinical course to those with C or D disease. Patients with stage B1 disease treated by radical prostatectomy have a five year survival of 85% [16], whereas 50% of those with stage C are dead by five years, and 50% of those with stage D by three years [17].

A number of studies have assessed the prognostic value of lymph node involvement, based on either clinical or surgical assessment. In view of the high incidence of false-negative and false-positive reports by non-invasive techniques in assessing node involvement, only those studies [18] which include a staging or radical lymphadenectomy are reviewed. Whitemore *et al.* [19] found that 40% of patients with positive nodes treated by lymphadenectomy and ^{125}I implantation to the prostate 'failed' within two years, and 75% had evidence of distant metastases within five years. In another series, 50% of patients with positive nodes developed distant metastases within two years [20]. In patients treated by ^{125}I implantation and lymphadenectomy, survival rates were much lower in those with positive nodes [21].

Although survival rate is related to the number of nodes involved [22] the risk of developing distant metastases appears to be unrelated to this variable. Lymphadenectomy can be considered as a useful prognostic indicator rather than of any therapeutic value. Adjuvant treatment with external radiation does not appear to improve survival rates when nodes are positive [20] while in the absence of adjuvant treatment, survival rate is not influenced by tumour volume or by seminal vesicle involvement [22].

Patients with skeletal metastases at the time of diagnosis have a clearly worse prognosis compared to those without such metastases [8]. In the diagnosis of skeletal metastases the use of radio-isotope bone scans has considerable advantages over conventional X-rays and some suggest that the bone scan is more reliable than the serum acid phosphatase level, and often provides evidence of progression of metastases before any other index [23, 24].

In judging prognosis, performance status may be as useful as staging. In 211 patients, a strong correlation with prolonged survival was found in patients who had good appetites, were fully active and did not need strong analgesics [25].

Histopathological criteria

A numer of studies have shown a strong correlation between histopathological category and prognosis [26, 27, 28]. In one series, five year survival rates in patients with histological grades of 1–4 were 59.5, 34.1, 16.2 and 5.6% respectively, independantly of staging [28]. Not only do poorly differentiated tumours have a poor prognosis, but they are also less likely to respond to hormone therapy compared to well differentiated tumours. Esposti has reported a 10% five year survival rate in patients with poorly differentiated tumours compared to 65% survival in high category tumours [29] but the prognosis of those with moderately differentiated tumours cannot be predicted with any degree of confidence.

However, even among patients with poorly differentiated tumours, there are some long-term survivors. Because of clonal heterogeneity in prostatic carcinoma, the reported grading of a tumour does not always reflect the prognosis for the individual patient. This may apply especially when the diagnosis is made by prostatic aspiration or needle biopsy, as only small, possibly unrepresentative, areas of tumour are obtained. Even when tissues are obtained by radical prostatectomy or transurethral resection, multiple sections are required to give an overall picture.

Gleason's method of grading, allowing extremes of glandular differentiation to be scored separately for each section, has tried to overcome the problems of tissue heterogeneity [30]. However, reports vary as to the value of the Gleason score in prognosis, some series showing no correlation between the Gleason score and response to treatment [31, 32, 33]. Metastatic disease is associated with a poor prognosis and in a study of 138 prostatic cancers, only those with a Gleason score of 4 or 5 had developed metastases [9].

It may be possible to improve our predictive ability by the use of lectins or monoclonal antibodies to identify the surface characteristics of morphologically identical cells with different invasive or metastatic potential. One technique claimed to assess metastatic potential is a computerised method to assess nuclear roundness [34] which is said to have distinguished patients with tumours confined to the prostate who subsequently showed spread, from those who did not. Blood vessel invasion shown in histological sections is considered to indicate a poor prognosis [35]. The presence of lymphocytic infiltration and the character of tumour cell borders may also be useful prognostic indicators [36].

Cell DNA content

The cell nuclei in malignant tumours may have an increased DNA content [37, 38] and the aggressiveness of some tumours may be related to the DNA content [39, 40, 41]. Using a rapid scanning microspectrophotometer, Zetterberg and Esposti [42] showed that the majority of cells in moderately differentiated prostatic cancers had a DNA content in the normal diploid range, though some had a grossly abnormal DNA content (heteroploid or aneuploid cells.) They subsequently showed correlation between abnormal DNA content and poor survival, and also between DNA content in the diploid and tetraploid range and a high response rate to endocrine therapy [43].

Using flow cytometry for analysing DNA content, Bichel et al. drew similar conclusions [44]. Studying serial biopsies of the tumour (after initiation of endocrine therapy, they also showed that a significant reduction in DNA content was correlated with good clinical response to therapy [44, 45, 46]. Techniques which depend upon the scanning of single cells are time-consuming and the development of new apparatus which combines the speed of flow cytometry and the accuracy of single cell scanning may advance the determination of prognosis and management in patients with prostatic cancer.

Endocrinological criteria

Hormonal levels

Mean plasma concentrations of testosterone, 17β-oestradiol, FSH, LH and prolactin in patients with carcinoma of the prostate are said to be identical to those of age-matched controls, but levels of growth hormone are said to be significantly higher in those with metastatic disease [47]. The finding of a low serum testosterone level at diagnosis predicts a poor prognosis and such patients do not respond as well to endocrine treatment aimed at androgen reduction [48].

Hormone receptors

Androgens are necessary for the continued growth of prostatic cancer, and their effects are mediated by intracellular receptor protein in both cytoplasm and nucleus. The most active androgen within the prostate is dihydrotestosterone, and high concentrations of receptors for this androgen are found in the epithelial cells [40]. Because androgen exerts its effect in the cell nucleus, measurement of the nuclear androgen receptor content may better distinguish androgen-sensitive tumours from those which are not.

Results to date on androgen receptor measurements in prostatic tumours are conflicting, and the numbers studied are small. Measuring cytosolic androgen receptor content, two studies have reported no correlation with hormonal response [50, 51], while two have reported that patients with the lowest receptor content failed to respond to hormone therapy [57, 53]. Three studies have reported on the nuclear androgen receptor level and all have found high levels to be associated with a significantly prolonged response to endocrine therapy, compared to those patients with a low nuclear androgen receptor concentration [54, 55, 56]. (None of these studies have included more than 26 patients.) A more specific assay which could measure *functional* nuclear receptors would be more reliable in predicting hormone dependence. Prolactin [44], oestrogen [57], and progesterone [55] receptors have also been identified in the prostate but their role as prognostic indicators are still undetermined.

Tumours which contain high levels of dihydrotestosterone have been shown to respond uniformly well to anti-androgen therapy [58]. Using a combication of nuclear androgen receptor levels together with multiple biochemical assays, a better prognostic index can be achieved. In a study of 16 patients treated by endocrine therapy, seven patients had a mean response of 7.7 months and nine a mean response of 18.6 months. The mean nuclear androgen receptor content differed between the two groups, but with considerable overlap of individual levels. By combining an index of multiple biochemical assays with the nuclear androgen receptor content, the two groups could be almost completely separated [59].

Tumour markers as prognostic criteria

Tumour markers of a high degree of sensitivity and specificity would contribute considerably to rational management of patients with prostatic cancer and provide an accurate guide to prognosis. Until recently, serum acid phosphatase was the only tumour marker routinely available. It is of doubtful value as a marker of response to treatment, although in some patients it is useful as a prognostic guide [60, 61]. This section examines currently available biochemical tumour markers and evaluates their role as prognostic criteria.

Acid phosphatase

Acid phosphatase is a phospho-hydrolase, present in large quantities in the exocrine secretion of the normal prostate. Iso-enzymes of acid phosphatase are present in every tissue in the body, and as a result, there are many possibilities for false positive reports [62]. The observation that L-tartrate may specifically inhibit other acid phosphatase iso-enzymes has given rise to assays measuring the prostatic fraction of this enzyme [63], despite the finding of the tartrate-labile fraction in a number of phosphatases of extra-prostatic origin [64].

Early studies to evaluate prostatic acid phosphatase (PAP) as a tumour marker showed that up to 85% of patients with metastatic disease had elevated levels [65, 66] compared with only 11% of patients with localised disease. Among 570 controls, only 3% had elevated PAP levels. Huggins and Hodges noted a decrease of serum acid phosphatase levels in response to oestrogen therapy or orchidectomy and a rise following androgen administration [67]. When patients without evidence of metastases were divided into those with normal and those with elevated acid phosphatase levels, twice as many patients with an increased value were dead of prostatic cancer within three years [68].

A poor prognosis is attached to the findings of an elevated acid phosphatase level [69] and patients with a negative bone scan but an elevated acid phosphatase level have a 60% chance of lymph node involvement, in contrast to only 25% of patients with a normal acid phosphatase level [10]. In a series of 343 patients, acid phosphatase levels were measured prior to lymph node sampling [60]. Of the total, 318 were found to have normal acid phosphatase levels and of these 70 had positive nodes. Of the 25 patients with increased acid phosphatase levels, 15 had positive nodes and the rest were negative, but nevertheless, the vast majority of *both* groups showed bone metastases within two years.

False-positive and false-negative results have been reported. Griffiths [71] noted a 14% false-negative rate when extensive metastatic disease was present, but almost all the false-negative group had anaplastic tumours, leading to the conclusion that poorly differentiated tumours are less likely to secrete acid phosphatase. The role of serial measurements during the course of treatment has been reported [72]. If an elevated level is decreased to normal with therapy, survival is likely to be prolonged; decrease by 50% but not to normal is a weaker, but still optimistic sign whereas a stable or rising acid phosphatase level is suggestive of disease progression.

Nevertheless, such statements may have little relevance to individual patient management. An elevation of acid phosphatase from the normal level preceded the development of a positive bone scan in only 19% of patients in one series [73]. A National Prostatic Cancer Project study utilising total acid phosphatase assay concluded that the test was not sensitive enough to monitor response to treatment [74], and a similar conclusion has been drawn by the EORTC study group.

With the purification, characterisation and production of its antibodies, a number of immunoassays measuring serum and bone marrow prostatic acid phosphatase are now available. At the present time, the sensitivity and specificity of these techniques are uncertain [75] and they offer no added advantage in assessing prognosis or response to treatment.

Measurement of bone marrow acid phosphatase level has been used to detect early bone metastasis in patients with apparently localised disease. Using enzymatic techniques a large number of false-positive results were reported [76] but the immuno-chemical assay of bone marrow acid phosphatase has been shown useful in predicting the future appearance of distant metastases [77], In one study, only three of 86 patients with negative serum and bone marrow acid phosphatase assays showed progression, whereas four of eleven with a normal serum, but increased bone marrow acid phosphatase, progressed [78].

Alkaline phosphatase

Alkaline phosphatase is considered a non-specific tumour marker, being neither organ – nor tumour – specific. However, it has been suggested that alkaline phosphatase conforms more closely to the ideal marker, with the highest specificity and sensitivity in carcinoma of the prostate [79]. Up to 91% of patients with bone metastases have an elevated alkaline phosphatase level and its presence before treatment is associated with a poor prognosis [80, 81]. High pre-treatment levels of bone and total alkaline phosphatase may reflect a high tumour burden.

A consistently elevated liver alkaline phosphatase level (greater than three times the upper limit of normal) may indicate the presence of liver metastases and a poor prognosis [81]. Merrick *et al.* [73] in a series of 220 patients found that, though the survival of patients with a raised acid phosphatase level at presentation was significantly shorter than those with normal values, the differences were even greater when considered in conjunction with alkaline phosphatase level level. Multivariate analysis showed that the level of alkaline phosphatase alone could be related to the differences in survival [73]. Alkaline phosphatase is also used as a marker of response to therapy, and Bishop *et al.* showed that serial alkaline phosphatase estimations are essential in the follow-up of treatment for bone metastases and probably render serial bone imaging studies superfluous [82].

Prostate specific antigen (PSA)

A prostatic-tissue specific antigen has been identified and characterised [83] but is expressed by both normal and neoplastic prostatic cells. Nevertheless, elevated pre-treatment levels of PSA in patients with metastatic prostatic cancer have been shown to correlate with a poor prognosis [84]. It has also been found useful in follow-up so that in patients undergoing radical prostatectomy for presumed localised disease, there was a clear relationship between elevated PSA and the subsequent appearance of metastases [85].

Tissue polypeptide antigen (TPA)

TPA is a cytoskeleton protein synthesised during cell division and released from cells undergoing rapid growth [86]. It is not tumour-specific, but has predictive ability in that prostatic cancer patients with normal serum TPA levels fare better than those in whom the TPA level is elevated [81], Costello and Kumar [88] studied the 24 hour urine excretion of this polypeptide and found good correlation with both the stage of prostatic cancer and survival. Using a combination of tumour stage, initial performance status and 24 hour TPA concentration, a score could be achieved for each patient, and worsening of prognosis occurred with an increasing score.

In a series of 40 patients with prostatic cancer, it was shown that serum levels of TPA and prostatic acid phosphatase, tumour stage and ESR were all useful prognostic markers but in both single test and multivariate life table analysis, TPA was the most reliable prognostic indicator [88]. Eight of eleven patients with elevated TPA levels, but only seven of twenty-nine with normal TPA levels, died from widespread prostatic cancer [8].

Carcino-embryonic antigen (CEA)

Increased serum levels of carcino-embryonic antigen have been found in between 25% and 59% of patients with carcinoma of the prostate [89, 90, 91] and this variable incidence makes CEA assay too non-specific to be a useful prognostic indicator. However, with the advent of hybridoma technology, a more precise and specific detection of this antigen in prostatic tissue can now be performed. In a preliminary retrospective study, 25 of 30 randomly-chosen specimens of benign prostatic hypertrophy were found to be negative for CEA and five had focally weak staining, whereas 31 of 36 carcinomas had diffuse positive staining. A good correlation between moderate and strong staining and increase in tumour grade and presence of metastatic disease has also been reported [92]. Further studies are necessary to confirm the above results.

Non-specific markers

Many non-specific markers have been identified in the serum and urine of patients with prostatic and other cancers. Some of these markers correlate well with tumour burden, response to treatment and progression of disease, and can be considered as monitors of progress.

Polyamines. In a series of 20 patients, erythrocyte polyamine levels reflected tumour load and correlated well with tumour response or progression [93]. Serum and urinary spermidine levels may also be of some value as a monitor of response [94, 95].

Lactic dehydrogenase. Consistent elevations of fractions IV and V of this enzyme were found in patients with metastatic prostatic cancer which showed complete regression after therapy [96].

Creatine kinase. The iso-enzyme B/B is found almost exclusively in the genito-urinary tract, and elevated levels often accompany neoplasia. Elevated levels most frequently occur with poorly differentiated tumours [91] and in patients with advanced disease [98]. Because of its low specificity and sensitivity, its main role is as a monitor of the course of the disease in individual patients.

Hydroxyproline excretion. This has been shown to be a useful marker of collagen breakdown in bone metastases from prostatic carcinoma, and as such, a monitor of progress [99].

Effect of treatment on prognosis

The likelihood that a patient with advanced prostatic cancer will respond to endocrine therapy remains unchanged at around 70–80‰. Duration of response to therapy averages about 18 months, while relapse and progression to death occurs usually in two to three years. Only 25% of treated patients survive five years, with no more than 10% surviving 10 years [100, 101] and there is no convincing evidence that any form of endocrine therapy prolongs survival. There is little difference in response rates between treatments by oestrogens, orchidectomy or LHRH analogues and the main differences relate to adverse effects and patient acceptance.

Bishop *et al.* [33] examined serial prostatic histology in a group of 146 patients treated with one of two different forms of endocrine therapy. He found that it bore no relationship either to progression of metastatic disease or to survival, and was an unreliable measure of response of advanced local disease to hormone therapy. We await confirmation by others of the superior results claimed by Labrie and his colleagues [102, 103] from the use of total androgen ablation, in improving both the response rate and prognosis for patients with prostatic cancer.

Conclusion

Clinical factors such as performance status, appetite and analgesic requirements may be as useful in judging prognosis as are the sophisticated procedures involved in tumour staging. Nevertheless, there is no doubt that patients with locally advanced disease and those with lymph node or bone metastases have a worse prognosis than those with disease confined to the prostate. Again, well differentiated tumours are more likely to respond to endocrine therapy than those which are poorly differentiated. On the whole, tumour grading systems which take into account the overall cell pattern have not been universally accepted as a better indicator of prognosis.

Of the various biochemical tumour markers such as PSA, TPA and CEA, alkaline and acid phosphatases, only the last two have reached wide acceptance as useful markers. Patients with pre-treatment elevation of acid and alkaline phosphatase levels show a worse prognosis, but there are still patients who show a prolonged survival despite these adverse prognostic features.

To assess the prognosis for the individual, we need to establish the malignant potential of individual cells within a tumour. Measurement of tumour cell DNA content, nuclear androgen receptor concentrations, and intra-cellular enzyme levels have been studied in only small numbers of patients but these early results appear to provide better prognostic indicators than the traditional measurement of tumour grade, stage and serum acid phosphatase level.

References

1. Mortality statistics cause, England and Wales 1978. DH 2, No 5, H.M.S.O., London, 1983
2. Stamey TA: Cancer of the prostate, an analysis of some important contributions and dilemmas. *Monogr Urol* 3: 67–94, 1982
3. Franks LM: Latent carcinoma of the prostate. *J Pathol Bacteriol* 68: 603–616, 1954
4. Gleason DF: Histologic grading and clinical staging of prostatic carcinoma. In: *Urologic Pathology: The Prostate*. Tannenbaum M. (ed): Philadelphia, Lea & Febiger, pp 171–194, 1977
5. Bayard S, Greenberg R, Showalter D, Byar D: Comparison of treatments for prostatic cancer using an exponential type life model relating survival to concomitant information. *Cancer Chemotherapy Rep* 58: 845–859, 1974
6. Fidler IJ: Tumour heterogeneity and the biology of cancer invasion and metastases. *Cancer Res* 38: 2651–2660, 1978
7. Franks LM: Etiology, epidemiology and pathology of prostatic cancer. *Cancer* 32: 1092–1095, 1973
8. Lewenhaupt A, Ekman P, Eneroth P, Nilsson B, Nordstrom L: Tissue Polypeptide Antigen (TPA) as a prognostic aid in human prostatic carcinoma. *Prostate* 6: 285–291, 1985
9. McNeal JE, Kindrachuck RA, Freiha FS, Bostwick DG, Redwine EA, Stamey TA: Patterns of progression in prostate cancer. *Lancet* i, 60–63, 1986
10. Blair A, Fraumen JF: Geographic patterns of prostatic cancer in the United States. *J Natl Cancer Inst* 61: 1379–1384, 1978
11. Ries LG, Pollack ES, Young JL: Cancer patient survival: surveillance, epidemiology and end results programme 1973-79. *J Natl Cancer Inst* 70: 693–707, 1983
12. Silverberg E: Cancer statistics, 1980. *CA* 30: 23–38, 1980
13. McNeal JE: Origin and development of carcinoma in the prostate. *Cancer* 23: 24–34, 1969
14. Whitmore WFJnr: Hormone therapy in prostatic cancer. *Am J Med* 21: 697–713, 1956
15. U.I.C.C., Union Internationale Contre le Cancer. TNM classification of malignant tumours, 3rd edition, International Union against Cancer, Geneva, 1978
16. Jewett HJ: Radical perineal prostatectomy for palpable clinically localised non obstructive cancer. Experience at The John Hopkins Hospital, 1909–1943. *J Urol* 124: 492–497, 1980
17. Hanash KA, Utz DC, Cook EN, Taylor WF, Titus JL: Carcinoma of the prostate. A 15 year follow-up. *J Urol* 107: 450–453, 1972
18. Hoekstra WJ, Schroeder FH: The role of lymphangiography in the staging of prostate cancer. *Prostate* 2: 433–440, 1981
19. Whitmore WF Jnr, Batata MA, Hilaris BS: Prostatic irradiation by Iodine 125 implantation, p 195–205. In: *Cancer of the Genito-urinary Tract* Johnson DE, Samuels ML (eds). Raven Press New York, 1979
20. Kramer SA, Cline WA Jnr, Fernham R, Carson CC, Cox EB, Hinshaw W, Paulson DF: Prognosis of patients with stage D1 prostatic adenocarcinoma. *J Urol* 125: 817–819, 1981

262

21. Whitmore WF Jnr: Interstitial radiation therapy for carcinoma of the prostate. *Prostate* 1: 157–160, 1980

22. Utz DC: Radical excision of adenocarcinoma of the prostate with pelvic lymph node involvement: surgical gesture or curative treatment. *Urology Suppl* 24: 4–11, 1984

23. Fitzpatrick JM, Constable AR, Sherwood T, Stephenson TJ, Chisholm GD, O'Donohue EPN. Serial bone scanning: the assessment of treatment response in carcinoma of the prostate. *Br J Urol* 50: 555–561, 1978

24. Stone AR, Merrick MV, Chisholm GD: The bone scan as a monitor of prostatic disease. *Clinical Oncology* 6: 349–360, 1980

25. Williams G. (In preparation)

26. Murphy GP, Whitmore WF: A report of the workshops on the current status of the histological grading of prostatic cancer. *Cancer,* 44: 1490–1494, 1979

27. Ansell ID: Histopathology of prostatic tumours. In: *Endocrinology of Prostate Tumours* Ghanadian R (ed). 15–33, MTP Lancaster, 1982

28. Pool TL Thompson GJ: Conservative treatment of carcinoma of the prostate. *J Am Med Assoc* 160: 833–837, 1956

29. Esposti PL: Cytologic malignancy grading of prostatic carcinoma by transrectal aspiration biopsy. *Scand J Urol Nephrol* 5: 199–209, 1971

30. Gleason DF: Classification of prostatic carcinoma. *Cancer Chemotherapy Reports* 50: 125–128, 1966

31. Kramer AS, Spahr J, Brendler CB, Glenn JF and Paulson DF: Experience with Gleason's histolpathologic grading in prostatic cancer. *J Urol* 124: 223–225, 1980

32. Catalona WJ, Stein A, Fair WR: Grading errors in prostatic needle biopsies: relation the accuracy of tumour grade in predicting pelvic lymph node mestatases. *J Urol,* 127: 919–922, 1982

33. Bishop MC, Ansell ID, Taylor MC, Thomas AL: Serial prostatic histology. A valid marker of resonse to hormone treatment. *Br J Urol* 57: 453–457, 1985

34. Diamond DA, Berry SJ, Jewett HJ, Eggleston SC, Coffey DS: A new method to assess metastatic potential of human prostatic cancer: Relative nuclear roundness. *J Urol,* 128: 729–734, 1982

35. Kwart AM, Sims JE: Blood vascular invasion. A poor prognostic factor in adenocarcinoma of the prostate. *J Urol* 119: 138–140, 1978

36. Epstein NA, Fatti LP: Prostatic carcinoma. Some morphological features affecting prognosis. *Cancer* 37: 2455–2465, 1976

37. Leuchtenberger C, Leuchtenberger R, Davis AM: A microspectrophotometric study of deoxyribose nucleic acid, (DNA) content in cells of normal and malignant human tissues. *Am J Pathol* 30: 65–68, 1954

38. Barlogie B, Prewincko B, Schumann J, Gohde W, Dosik G, Latreille J, Johnston DA, Freireich EJ: Cellular DNA as a marker of neoplasia in man. *Am J Med* 69: 195–203, 1980

39. Lamb D: Correlation of chromosome counts with histological appearances and prognosis in transitional cell carcinoma of the bladder. *B M J,* 1: 273–277, 1967

40. Atkin NB, Richards BM: Clinical significance of ploidy in carcinoma of cervix. Its relation to prognosis. *B M J* 2: 1445–1446, 1962

41. Atkin NB: Modal deoxyribose nucleic acid value and survival in carcinoma of the breast. *B M J* 1: 271–272, 1972

42. Zetterberg A, Esposti PL: Cytophotometric DNA analysis of aspirated cells from prostatic carcinoma. *Acta Cytol* (Baltimore) 20: 46–57, 1976

43. Zetterberg A, Esposti PL: Prognostic significance of nuclear DNA levels in prostatic carcinoma. *Scand J Urol Nephrol* (Suppl) 55: 53–58, 1980

44. Bichel P, Fredriksen P, Kjaer T, Thommesen P, Vindelu LL: Flow microfluorometry and transrectal fine needle biopsy in the classification of human prostatic carcinoma. *Cancer* 40: 1206–1211, 1977

45. Leistenschneider W, Nagel R: Estrocyt therapy of advanced prostatic cancer with special reference to control of therapy with cytology and DNA cytophotometry. *Eur Urol* 6: 111–115, 1980

46. Leistenschneider W, Nagel R: Control of response to estromustine phosphate therapy through cytology and DNA analysis of cell nuclei in a prospective syudy. *Urology* 23 Suppl.: 81–88, 1984

47. British Prostate Study Group. Evaluation of plasma hormone concentrations in relation to clinical staging in patients with prostatic cancer. *Br J Urol* 51: 382–389, 1979

48. Allen JM, O'Shea JP, Mashiter K, Williams G, Bloom SR: Advanced carcinoma of the prostate. Treatment with a gonadotrophin releasing hormone agonist. *Brit Med J* 286: 1607–1609, 1983

49. Keenan EJ, Kemp ED, Ramsey EE, Garrison LB, Pearse HD, Hodges CV: Specific binding of prolactin by the prostate gland of the rat and man. *J Urol* 122: 43–46, 1979

50. Wagner RK: Critical evaluation of receptor assays in relation to tumours. In: *Research on Steroids* Vermeulen A, Klopper A, Sciarra F, Jungblut P, Lerner L (eds). North Holland Publishing Co, Amsterdam, Vol 7, 205–224, 1979

51. de Voogt HJ, Dingjam P: Steroid receptors in human prostate cancer: a preliminary evaluation. *Urol Res* 6: 151–158, 1978

52. Ekman P, Snochowski M, Zetterberg A, Hogberg B, Gustafsson JA: Steroid receptor content in human prostatic carcinoma and response to endocrine therapy. *Cancer* 44: 1173–1181, 1979

53. Mobbs BG, Johnson IE, Connolly JG: The effect of therapy on the concentration and occupancy of androgen receptors in human prostatic cytosol. *Prostate* 1: 37–51, 1980

54. Trachtenberg J, Walsh PC: Correlation of prostatic nuclear androgen receptor content with duration of response and survival following hormonal therapy in advanced prostatic cancer. *J Urol* 127: 466–471, 1982

55. Concolino G, Marocchi A, Margiotto G, Conti C, Di Silverio F, Tenaglia R, Ferraro F, Bracci U: Steroid receptors and hormone responsiveness of human prostate carcinoma. *Prostate* 3: 475–482, 1982

56. Ghandian R, Auf G, Williams G, Davis A, Richards B: Predicting the reponse of prostatic carcinoma to endocrine therapy. *Lancet* ii: 1418, 1981

57. Hawkins RF: Steroid receptors in the human prostate 1. Estradiol 17-Beta, binding in benign prostatic hypertrophy. *Steroids* 26: 458–469, 1975

58. Geller J, Albert J, de la Vega P, Loza D, Stoeltzing W: Dihydrotestosterone concentration in prostate cancer tissue as a predictor of tumour differentiation and hormone dependency. *Cancer Res* 38: 4349–4352, 1979

59. Brendler CB, Issacs JT, Follansbee AL, Walsh PC: The use of multiple variables to predict response to endocrine therapy in carcinoma of the prostate: a preliminary report. *J Urol* 131: 694–700, 1984

60. Ganem EJ: The orognostic significance of an elevated serum acid phosphatase level in advanced prostatic carcinoma. *J Urol* 76: 179–182, 1956

61. Whitesel JA, Donohue RE, Mani JH, Mohr S, Scanavino DJ, Augspurger RR, Biber RJ, Fauver HE, Wettlaufer JN, Pfister RR: Acid phosphtase. Its influence on the management of carcinoma of the prostate. *J Urol* 131: 70–72, 1984

62. Ozar MB, Isaac CA, Valk WL: Methods fot eh elimination of errors in serum acid phosphatase determinations. *J Urol* 74: 150–157, 1955

63. King EJ, Jegatheesan KA: A method for the determination of tartrate labile prostatic acid phosphatase in serum. *J Clin Path* 12: 85–89, 1959

64. Yam LT: Clinical significance of the human acid phosphatases: a review. *Am J Med* 56: 604–616, 1974

65. Gutman AB, Gutman EB: An 'acid' phosphatase occuring in the serum of patients with metastasizing carcinoma of the prostate gland. *J Clin Invest* 17: 473–478, 1938

66. Sullivan TJ, Gutman EB, Gutman AB: Theory and application of the serum 'acid' phosphatase

determination in metastasizing prostatic carcinoma; early effects of castration. *J Urol* 48: 426–458, 1942

67. Huggins C, Hodges CV. The effect of castration of oestrogen and of androgen injection on serum phosphatases in metastatic carcinoma of the prostate. *Cancer Res* 1: 293–297, 1941

68. Nesbit RM, Baum WB: Serum phosphatase determination in diagnosis of prostatic cancer. A review of 1150 cases *J.A.M.A.* 145: 1321–1324, 1951

69. McNeil BJ, Polak JF: An up-date on the rationale for the use of bone scans in selected metastatic and primary bone tumours. In: *Bone Scintigraphy* Pauwels EK, Schutte HE, Taconis WK (eds). Pp 186–207, 1981, Leiden University Press

70. Paulson DF and the Uro/Oncology Research Group. The impact of current staging procedure in assessing disease extent of prostatic adenocarcinoma. *J Urol* 121: 300–302, 1979

71. Griffiths JC: Prostate specific acid phosphatase reevaluation of radio-immune assay in diagnosing prostate disease. *Clin Chem* 26: 433–436, 1980

72. Scardino P: Serum acid phosphatase assays and other tumour markers of prostatic cancer. In: *Prostate Cancer: Video Conference Guide Book.* American Urological Association Offices of Education, pp 109–113, 1982

73. Merrick MV, Ding CL, Chisholm GD, Elton RA: Prognostic significance of alkaline and acid phosphatase with skeletal scientiography in carcinoma of the prostate. *Br J Urol* 57: 715–720, 1985

74. Johnson DE, Prout GR, Scott WW, Schmidt JD, Gibbons RP, Murphy GP: Clinical significance of serum acid phosphatase levels in advanced prostatic carcinoma. *Urology* 8: 123–126, 1976

75. Pontes JE: Biological markers in prostate cancer. *J Urol* 130: 1037–1047, 1983

76. Khan R, Turner B, Edson M, Dolan M: Bone marrow acid phosphatase: another look. *J Urol* 117: 79–80, 1977

77. Schellhammer PF, Warden SS, Wright GL, Sieg SM: Bone marrow acid phosphatase by counterimmune electrophoresis: pre-treatment and post-treatment correlations. *J Urol* 127: 66–68, 1982

78. Belville WD, Mahan DE, Sepulveda RA, Bruce AW, Miller CF: Bone marow acid phosphatase by radio-immuno assay. Three years of experience. *J Urol* 125: 809–811, 1981

79. Urwin GH, Percival RC, Yates AJP, Watson ME, Couch M, McDonald B, Forrest ARW, Williams JL, Kanis JA: Biochemical markers and skeletal metabolism in carcinoma of the prostate. *Br J Urol* 57: 711–714, 1985

80. Wajsman Z, Chu Tm, Bross D, Saroff J, Murphy Gp, Johnson DE, Scott WW, Gibbons RP, Prout GR, Schmidt JD: Clinical significance of seum alkaline phosphatase iso enzyme levels in advanced prostatic carcinoma. *J Urol* 119: 244–246, 1978

81. Killian CS, Vargas FP, Pontes EJ, Beckley S, Slack NH, Murphy GP, Chu TM: The use of serum iso enzymes of alkaline and acid phosphatase as a possible quantitive tumour markers of tumour loas in prostatic cancer. *Prostate* 2: 187–206, 1981

87. Bishop MC, Hardy JG, Taylor MC, Wastie ML, Lemberger RJ: Bone imaging and serum phosphatases in prostatic carcinoma. *Br J Urol* 57: 317–324, 1985

83. Wang MC, Valenzuda LA, Murphy GP, Chu TM: Purification of a human prostate specific antigen. *Invest Urol* 17: 159–163, 1979

84. Kuriyama M, Wang MC, Lee CI, Papsidero LD, Killian Cs, Inaji H, Slack NH, Nishiura T, Murphy GP, Chu TM: Use of human prostate specific antigen in monitoring prostate cancer. *Cancer Res* 41: 3874–3876, 1981

85. Pontes JE, Chu TM, Slack K, Karr J, Murphy GP: Serum prostatic antigen measurement in localised prostatic cancer: correlation with clinical course. *J Urol* 128: 1216–1218, 1982

86. Luning B, Nilsson U: Sequence homology between TPA and intermediate filament proteins. *Acta Chem Scand* (B) 37: 731–753, 1983

87. Mross K, Mross B, Wolfrum DI: Der Wert der TPA Brstimmurg bei Malignom patienten. *Lab Medizin* 7: 231–236, 1983

88. Costello CB, Kumar S: Prognostic value of tissue polypeptide antigen in urological neoplasia. *J Roy Soc Med* 78: 207–210, 1985

89. Guinan P, Ablin RJ, Barakat H, John T, Sadoughi N, Bush IM: Carcinomo-embryonic antigen in patients with urologic cancers. *Urol Res* 1: 101–105, 1973

90. Neufeld L, Dublin A, Guiman P, Nabon GR, Ablin RJ, Bush IM: Carcino-embryonic antigens in the diagnosis of prostate carcinoma. *Oncology*, 29: 376–381, 1974

91. Fleisher M, Grabstald H, Whitmore WF Jnr, Pinsky CM, Oettgen HF, Schwartz MK: The clinical utility of plasma and urinary carcino-embryonic antigen in patients with genito-urinary disease. *J Urol* 117: 635–637, 1977

92. Ghazizadeh M, Kagawa S, Izumi K, Maebayashi K, Takigawa H, Salkit Kawano A, Kurokawa K: Immunohistochemical detection of carcino-embryonic antigen in benign hyperplasia and adeno-carcinoma of the prostate with monoclonal antibody. *J Urol* 131: 501–505, 1984

93. Killian CS, Vargas FP, Beckley S, Wajsman Z, Murphy GP, Chu TN: Analysis of serial erythrocyte polyamines by automated reverse phase liquid chromatography (HPLC). *Clin Chem Abstract* 122: 26: 983, 1980

94. Chaisiri P, Harper M, Blamey R, Peeling WB, Griffiths K: Plasma spermidine concentrations in patients with tumours of the breast or prostate or testis. *Clin Chem Acta* 104: 367–375, 1980

95. Hradec CE, Jiranek J, Macek K: Urinary spermidine levels in cases of carcinoma of the prostate–preliminary report. *Scand J Urol Nephrol* (Suppl) 55: 71–73, 1980

96. Prout GR Jnr, Macalalag EV Jnr, Denis LH, Preston LW Jnr: Alterations in serum lactate dehydrogenase and its fourth and fifth iso enzymes in patients with prostatic cancer. *J Urol* 94: 451–461, 1965

97. Silverman L, Chapman J, Jones M, Dermer GB, Pullano T, Tokes ZA: Creatine Kinase BB and other markers of prostatic carcinoma. *Prostate* 2: 109–119, 1981

98. Fair W, Heston W, Kadmon D, Crane D, Catalona W, Ladenson J, McDonald JM, Noll B, Harvey G: Prostatic cancer acid phosphatase, creatine kinase – BB and race, a prospective study. *J Urol* 128: 735–738, 1982

99. Mooppan MMU, Kim H, Wang JC, Tobin MS, Wax SH: Use of urinary hydroxyproline excretion as a tumour marker in diagnosis and follow-up of prostatic carcinoma. *Prostate* 4: 397–405, 1983

100. Robinson MRG, Shearer RJ, Ferguson JD: Adrenal secression in the treatment of carcinoma of the prostate. *Brit J Urol*, 555–559, 1974

101. Reiner WG, Scott WW, Eggleston JC, Walsh PC: Long term survival after hormone therapy for stage D prostatic cancer. *J Urol* 122: 183–184, 1979

102. Labrie F, DuPont A, Belanger A: Complete androgen blockade for the treatment of prostate cancer. In: *Important Advances in Oncology*, VT De Vita Jnr, Hellman S, Rosenberg SA, (eds), JB Lippincott Co. Philadelphia, 1985, p 193–217

103. Complete androgen blockade at start of treatment causes a dramatic improvement of survival in advanced prostatic cancer. In: *Proceedings of the International Symposium on LHRH and its Analogues: Basic and Clinical Aspects*, Labrie F, Belanger A, Dupont A (eds) Exceprta Medica, 1984: p 1–12

16. Prognostic indices in lung cancer

M.H. ROSEN and A.P. CHAHINIAN

In the case of lung cancer, advances in therapy have had minimal impact on survival. In the past 25 years, the relative 5 year survival has risen from 8 to only 13% for white Americans [1], and it is clear that certain prognostic factors have far greater impact on survival than many of the currently available treatments. It is therefore essential when assessing the benefits of therapy, to clarify the influence of these factors both on survival and on response to therapy.

General prognostic factors

Performance status

Karnofsky [2] quantified clinical response to therapy by measuring the patient's degree of independence. This scheme is presented in Table 1 with the corresponding Zubrod score. Tabulated in the right-hand column is the median survival in weeks for patients with inoperable lung cancer as reported by Stanley [3] for the Veterans Administration Lung Study Group (VALSG).

Zelen [4] emphasized the paramount predictive value of performance status (PS) in patients with inoperable bronchogenic carcinoma. In reviewing the results of prospective randomized trials of chemotherapy, he described the linear relationship between the logarithm of the median survival and the PS score. This relationship was particularly strong in patients with extensive disease, where PS scores as low as 20 were represented in significant numbers. Patients with inoperable but limited disease were clustered at higher performance scores where the data are far less convincing. For a specific histologic type, variations dependent on PS were far more significant than differences based on histology, and the relative importance of PS in multivariate analyses is later presented separately for small cell lung cancer (SCLC) and non small cell lung cancer (NSCLC).

Table 1. Performance status (PS) and survival in lung cancer (Adapted from [2] and [3])

Definition	Zubrod score	PS %	Criteria	# of Pts	Median survival (weeks)
Able to carry on normal activity and to work. No special care is needed.	0	100	Normal; no complaints; no evidence of disease.	88	34.1
		90	Able to carry on normal activity; minor signs or symptoms of disease.	635	27.1
Unable to work. Able to live at home, care for most personal needs. A varying amount of assistance is needed.		80	Normal activity with effort; some signs or symptoms of disease.	948	24.0
	1	70	Cares for self. Unable to carry on normal activity or to do active work.	1117	20.9
	2	60	Requires occasional assistance, but is able to care for most of his needs.	892	13.8
		50	Requires considerable assistance and frequent medical care.	626	9.1
Unable to care for self. Requires equivalent of institutional or hospital care. Disease may be progressing rapidly.	3	40	Disabled, requires special care and assistance.	479	6.7
		30	Severely disabled; hospitalization is indicated although death not imminent.	202	4.6
	4	20	Very sick; hospitalization necessary; active supportive treatment necessary.	35	3.2
		10	Moribund; fatal processes progressing rapidly.		
	5	0	Dead		

Gender, age and race

Ederer and Mersheimer [5] reported a significant survival advantage for women with lung cancer in data for 7547 white men and 1260 white women collected from 99 hospitals by the End Results Evaluation Program of the National Cancer Institute. Women with localized disease (confined to the site of origin) had a 5 year survival of 41% as compared to 21% in their male counterparts. Women with localized disease who underwent resection had a 68% survival at 5 years, versus 35% in men. These data were reviewed by Connelly *et al.* [6] who confirmed the female advantage in cases with resected local disease. (They shifted many of the patients from local disease to regional disease categories, thereby abolishing the advantage in the latter group.) Among patients with localized disease, women had a higher rate of lobectomy than men and a better 5 year survival rate (68% versus 26%) but survival following pneumonectomy did not differ significantly between men and women.

Advancing age has a modest negative impact on survival in resectable cases, as shown in a large series [7–9] of patients. For instance, in resected Stage I patients, Williams [8] noted that patients over age 70 had a 5 year survival of 62% compared to 72% for the younger group. In inoperable patients the difference in survival in the older age group was minimal [10] or nonexistent.

Axtell and Meyers [11], collected data from 3 central tumor registries and 6 individual hospital registries and showed a trend (statistically insignificant) for higher survival among white patients. Page and Kuntz [12], could detect no difference in survival between 15,262 whites and 1980 blacks treated at Veterans Administration (VA) Hospitals in the United States. The noted that in VA facilities the same of level of care is administered, free of charge, to eligible veterans, regardless of race or economic attainment, whereas elsewhere, differences in treatment meted out to black patients of relatively low socioeconomic status might skew survival data.

Table 2. Effect of weight loss on median survival in lung cancer

Median survival (weeks)

Tumor type	Weight loss				Reference
	0	0–5%	5–10%	>10%	
NSCLC	20	17	13	11	[13]
SCLC	34	26	26	17	[14]

Weight loss

Weight loss is common in lung cancer and adversely affects survival and 59% of patients with inoperable disease entered into prospective clinical trials [13] reported some degree of weight loss. There is evidence of both increased caloric demand and decreased nutritional intake in cancer and with increasing levels of weight loss, there is a progressive decrease in median survival in lung cancer (Table 2). Weight loss and poor performance status often coexist in patients with advanced disease and the prognostic importance of weight loss is primarily noted in patients of good performance status (Table 3). Thus, the presence of weight loss in fully ambulatory patients (PS 0–1) is associated with a 10 week survival disadvantage, while in debilitated patients (PS 2–4), little difference is noted. Again, the presence of weight loss is far more significant in patients with limited disease [10].

Clinical symptoms

The majority of patients with lung cancer present with symptoms related either to the local or metastatic disease and the nature of their symptoms should therefore yield information relevant to the prognosis. Feinstein devised the following staging scheme for symptoms [15]: (i) Asymptomatic; (ii) Primary symptoms present for more than 6 months – cough, hemoptysis, or symptoms of an associated pneumonia; (iii) Primary symptoms present for less than 6 months; (iv) Systemic symptoms remote from the local process, but not from spread beyond the primary site. These include malaise, anorexia and weight loss; (v) Metastatic symptoms caused by extension beyond the primary site, either directly or distantly. Symptoms caused by local extension include hoarseness due to a paralyzed vocal cord or dysphagia, while bone pain and neurologic disturbances are defined as metastatic symptoms.

In 956 patients with lung cancer treated at the Yale Medical Center between

Table 3. Relationship between weight loss, performance status (PS) and median survival (Adopted from [3])

Median survival (weeks)

Tumor type	PS 0–1(Zubrod)			PS 2–4		
	No weight loss	Weight loss	P value	No weight loss	Weight loss	P value
SCLC	39	29	<.01	19	25	NS*
NSCLC	28	18	.18	14	10	<0.05

* NS: Not significant

1953 and 1958, 5 year survival correlated with this symptom staging (Table 4). Stage II patients had a marginally better 5 year survival rate than Stage III patients, presumably because Stage II patients have symptoms which are slowly progressive, thus indicating a less aggressive tumor. This concept is supported by the correlation of symptom-stage with tumor doubling time [16] so that rapidly growing tumors with short doubling times are associated with higher symptom stage. However, Huhti [17], prospectively followed 446 patients staged by this method and demonstrated consistently better survival at Stage III than at Stage II. Symptom staging may be most useful in patients found to have negative nodes at resection. In this group of patients, Senior and Adamson [18] confirmed that patients with longer histories of local symptoms survived longer after diagnosis.

Tumour doubling time

Collins *et al.* [19] established the model of exponential growth of tumors in man through roentgenographic study of 24 cases of pulmonary metastases. By plotting tumor diameter on semilogarithmic coordinates, they demonstrated that the tumour doubling time (TDT) remained constant throughout the clinical course of the disease. The constant quality was confirmed by Chahinian and Israel [20] in 86% of the tumors in a series of 150 cases of primary and metastatic lung tumors. Since approximately 40 tumor doublings are necessary for death of the host in most cases of lung cancer [21], theoretically two serial tumor measurements should yield an approximate survival estimate. Since a tumor of 1 cm in diameter has already undergone 30 doublings and should lead to death in 10 more doubling times, a typical TDT of 100 days [16] would predict survival of 3 years.

For 56 patients retrospectively reviewed by Mizuno *et al.* [22], the overall survival correlated well with predicted survival time based on TDT. Resected patients survived longer than predicted by TDT showing the survival benefit of surgery. TDT has been found to correlate with Feinstein's symptom staging [16]

Table 4. Relationship of survival to symptomatic staging in lung cancer (Adapted from [15])

Symptom stage	5 Year survival (%)	
	all patients	resected patients
I	32 (11/34)	37 (28/75)
II	18 (17/93)	
III	10 (9/88)	24 (26/108)
VI	8 (18/212)	
V	0.6 (1/169)	— (1/10)

and is a simple but powerful prognostic indicator in lung cancer (see [23] for review).

Pulmonary function

The adequacy of pulmonary function at presentation is a major criterion of resectability. The M.D. Anderson Group [24] studied pulmonary function in 251 patients with all stages of lung cancer. Patient were resected if they met anatomical criteria for resectability, and had adequate pulmonary function. The latter was defined as a forced expiratory volume in 1 sec ($FEV_{1.0}$) calculated for the postoperative state which exceeded one third of the predicted normal value. The postoperative $FEV_{1.0}$ was determined by Xenon-133 perfusion and ventilation studies which yielded appropriate regional values.

Preoperative pulmonary function did not differ significantly according to stage. An $FEV_{1.0}$ less than 40% of normal was associated with a higher short-term mortality rate, but did not significantly affect long-term survival. Survival after resection for lung cancer is more dependent on anatomical staging, assuming that lung function is adequate to allow surgery to be undertaken safely.

Immune competence

Reactivity to delayed cutaneous hypersensitivity tests, including the tuberculin skin test, is a marker both of previous infection and immunologic competence. In populations with a high incidence of PPD positivity, lower frequencies of reactivity among cancer patients serve as a marker of decreased immune competence. In patients with lung cancer, survival correlated with tuberculin reactivity in both resected [25] and unresected [26] patients.

Consistently shorter median survival is noted in patients who are preoperatively PPD negative, and recovery of tuberculin reactivity postoperatively portended better survival. The association between reactivity and longer survival prompted a large randomized sudy of the utility of adjuvant intrathoracic BCG therapy in lung cancer [9] but no benefit was seen. Nevertheless, the findings show the value of skin testing as a marker of host well-being, comparable to performance status. Active or quiescent tuberculosis confers no survival advantage in lung cancer patients.

Tobacco smoking is a major etiologic factor in lung cancer [27] but intensity of exposure has not been found to influence prognosis when lung cancer has developed. Cessation of smoking at diagnosis (at least, in small cell lung cancer) has a positive impact on survival and response to chemotherapy [28]. The advantage however, is small and reaches statistical significance only for the group that stopped smoking prior to the diagnosis of SCLC.

272

Biological markers

Various HLA types have been reported to be positively correlated with the frequency of lung cancer and with the duration of survival. HLA B_{12} has been reported to be more frequent in small cell [29] and non-small cell cancer [30] than in the general population. HLA B_5 was more prevalent in small cell lung cancer [31]. Similarly, HLA-AW$_{19}$, HLA-B$_5$ [32, 33] and HLA-BW$_{22}$ [31] were associated with longer survival while HLA-A$_1$ was a predictor of poor survival [29]. Svejgaard *et al.* [34] have pointed out that when a battery of antigens is screened for association, chance alone may dictate success in the absence of true significance. For example, if the required P value is 0.04, the probability is better than 50% that such an association will be demonstrated when 17 antigens are examined. They recommended multiplying the P value by the number of antigens studied and by this criterion, no association between HLA type and lung cancer can be demonstrated.

DNA patterns characteristic of the various stages of the cell cycle may be recognized by flow cytometry. Application of this method to lung cancer specimens suggests that tumors with a high proportion of cells in the synthetic proliferative stages (S, G2/M) are correlated with a poor prognosis. Abe *et al.* [35] demonstrated that small cell tumors with a high degree of aneuploidy are associated with short survival. This difference was larger in the limited disease group, where those patients with aneuploid tumors had a median survival of 44 weeks compared to 75 weeks for those with diploid tumors. For non-small cell tumors, Volm *et al.* [36] found that diploidy conferred a marked survival advantage independent of stage.

Non-small cell lung cancer (NSCLC)

Histology

The World Health Organization has adopted a classification for primary epithelial tumors of the lung [37]. The most common histologic types are squamous cell carcinoma, adenocarcinoma, small cell carcinoma and large cell carcinoma, representing 46.2%, 24.2%, 17.1% and 9.0% respectively [38]. In Mountain's series [38], the 2 year survival for these histologic types was 26%, 19%, 4% and 23% respectively.

In a group of 449 patients evaluated at Yale by Feinstein [39], patients with squamous cell carcinoma were least likely to present with symptoms of distant metastases and were most likely to be resectable. In resected patients with TNM Stage I disease, the Lung Cancer Study Group [9] reported lower recurrence and death rates in squamous cell carcinoma (Table 5). However, in the Mayo Clinic study, in 495 patients with resected Stage I lung cancer, survival did not vary with histologic type [8, 40].

Campobasso *et al*. [41] concluded that resected patients with advanced regional squamous cell carcinoma fared better than patients with other histologic types. The data in Table 6 is for patients with tumors greater than 4 cm spreading to contiguous structures, of tumors of any size with nodal involvement. Patients with distant metastases are excluded. In summary, although the differences are modest, patients with squamous cell carcinoma are more frequently resectable and achieve higher cure rates.

Staging

Staging provides a coded anatomical designation of the tumor at presentation, but to be useful in predicting the outcome, each stage should contain patients with similar prognoses and response to treatment. The TNM code is based on tumor size, nodal involvement and presence or absence of metastases. Mountain [42] reviewed 2155 histologically proven cases of bronchogenic carcinoma, and the primary tumor size and extent were classified as follows:

T_o: Primary tumor cannot be demonstrated.

T_x: Tumor demonstrated only on cytology, but not visualized.

T_{1s}: Carcinoma *in situ*.

T_1: Tumor that is 3 cm or less, without involvement of visceral pleura or invasion proximal to a lobar bronchus.

T_2: Tumor greater than 3 cm or any tumor extending to the hilar region or invading the visceral pleura. Secondary atelectasis or pneumonia cannot involve an entire lung.

T_3: Any tumor involving an adjacent structure or extending to within 2 cm of the carina; and any tumor causing atelectasis or pneumonia of an entire lung or pleural effusion.

The 5 year survival rate for T_1 lesions was 39% [42]. Patients with adenocarcinoma or squamous cell carcinoma had significantly better survival rates than those with large cell carcinoma. In the T_2 category only 21% survived 5 years and

Table 5. Recurrence and death rates in resected stage I lung cancer (Adapted from [9])

Type	Number	Recurrence rate per person year	Death rate per person year
Squamous	171	0.101	0.083 $p < 0.001$
Adenocarcinoma	184	0.181	0.114
Large cell	11	0.505	0.239
Mixed	18	0.219	0.279

again, those with squamous histology had the highest survival (28%). In this category, adenocarcinoma and large cell have similarly poor 5 year survivals (11 and 16%, respectively). Only 7% of the patients with T_3 tumors survived 5 years yet this category includes the prognostically favorable subset of superior sulcus tumors which often respond to local therapy [42–43].

Regional lymph nodes in this system are designated as follows: N_0: No nodal involvement; N_1: Ipsilateral hilar nodal involvement; N_2: Mediastinal lymph node involvement. For both N_0 and N_1 categories, 5 year survival was highest in patients with squamous histology. For the N_2 group, survival at 5 years was 3.5% and did not vary significantly with histologic type. In 440 patients surviving complete resection for more than 1 month, Naruke et al. [44], reported 18.1% survival after 5 years in the N_2 group, but he identified a prognostically favorable group with negative subcarinal nodes. The degree of nodal involvement has prognostic value so that patients with intranodal disease had a 5 year survival of 43% compared to 4.3% when disease extended outside the nodal capsule [45].

Distant metastases in NSCLC virtually exclude the possibility of long-term survival. The M designation includes M_0: No metastatic spread; M_1: Distant metastases present. In the absence of metastatic disease, 25% of all patients survived 5 years. When extrathoracic disease is present, survival rates at 5 years approach zero [42]. Analysis of 428 patients at M.D. Anderson Hospital [10] examined the effects of different metastatic sites on survival. Patients with extensive disease had an overall median survival of 14 weeks, but patients with metastases to liver, bone or contralateral thorax had median survivals of 8, 9 and 10 weeks, respectively. Patients with brain metastases had a median survival of 13 weeks – not significantly different from the overall survival.

The various permutations of TNM factors were grouped in prognostically similar categories [38] as shown in Table 7. Survival within stages was similar for the different TNM groups, with one notable exception. $T_3N_0M_0$ (216 patients), was remarkable for a 12 month survival rate of 38% and an 18 month survival rate of 24%. These values are significantly higher than those of other TNM groups within Stage III. This group contained superior sulcus tumors which generally present with pain earlier in the course of the disease. In 170 patients with superior sulcus tumors, Martini [43] reported an overall 5 year survival of 14%.

Table 6. Post-operative survival in regional disease (Adapted from [41])

Histologic type	Number	Survival rate (%)		
		2 years	3 years	5 years
SCC	128	39	34	24
Adenocarcinoma	42	36	17	14
Large cell	87	12	7	6

Biological markers

The most useful antigenic marker in non-small cell lung cancer is carcinoembryonic antigen (CEA). The level is often elevated whatever the histologic type of bronchogenic carcinoma, but most commonly and to the highest levels, in adenocarcinoma [46]. Concanon *et al.* [47], reporting preoperative CEA levels in 149 patients, noted that a level of 6 ng/ml represented a critical cut-off point. Patients with a CEA level greater than 6 were all dead within 3 years while all long-term survivors (>3 years) had initial levels less than 6. The predictive value of the CEA level was noted only in TNM Stages I and II. For patients with a CEA level less than 6, 5 year survival rate was about 50% for a group of 38 patients, as compared to no survivors at 3 years among 8 patients with CEA levels greater than 6. In Vincent's series [46], CEA elevation was predictive of relapse, with a level >6 preceding recurrence by 3 months in 50% of the relapse patients and a level >8 preceding death by months in 50% of the cases.

Lung cancer is the most common cause of Cushing's syndrome secondary to ectopic ACTH production and numerous investigators have identified the glycopeptide precursor, proACTH, in carcinoma tissue as well as in the serum of lung cancer patients. Its poor specificity and sensitivity for lung cancer, particularly among patients with chronic pulmonary disease [48], rules out its usefulness in screening for lung cancer among high risk populations. When found to be elevated, it is not a useful prognostic indicator.

Neuron-specific enolase (NSE) is a glycolytic enzyme which is widely distributed in mammalian neuroendocrine cells [49]. In a group of 54 patients with NSCLC, Ariyoshi detected elevated levels of NSE in only 6, all of whom demonstrated large-cell elements. In these patients, elevations in NSE heralded relapse, but initial levels dit not correlate with prognosis.

Relation to surgical treatment

Early reports [7, 50] reviewed the impact of prognostic factors on survival after

Table 7. TNM stage and survival

Stage	Number of TNM groups	Patients	(%)	Survival (%)			
				12 months	18 months	2years	5 years
I	$T_1N_0M_0$, $T_2N_0M_0$ $T_1N_1M_0$	543	34	66	56	46	40
II	$T_2N_1M_0$	111	7	49	35	29	17
III	Any T_3, N_2 or M_1	961	60	20	11	10	9

surgery for NSCLC but their data was limited by the lack of a uniform staging system. They noted the positive effect on survival of female gender, absence of nodal invasion and lesser degrees of resection but the effects of age, histology and weight loss were not consistent. With the advent of uniform staging [42], the confounding effect of disease extent can be controlled, thus clarifying the role of other prognostic parameters.

Stage I

Two large series of resected Stage I NSCLC patients are available for review. One study from the Mayo Clinic [8] reported survival data on 495 patients enrolled prospectively, but staged retrospectively. The second paper contributed by the Lung Cancer Study Group (LCSG) [9] followed 392 prospectively staged patients, and reported recurrence rates as well as survival data. These patients were randomized to receive placebo or intrapleural BCG immunization and isoniazid. No difference was seen between these treatment arms and all statistics were pooled. The two studies reported similar survival rates – 78.6% at 2 years [9] and 56% at 5 years [8].

Advancing age adversely affected survival in both series. The advantage of squamous histology was marked in the LCSG, particularly in patients with positive hilar nodes (T_1N_1). While women did better in both series, statistical significance was not achieved in the Mayo Clinic study. The only initial laboratory parameter that predicted recurrence was an elevated CEA level. History of heart disease and liver tenderness shortened survival as correlates of significant right-sided heart disease.

When all the indices were followed serially, changes in two factors were highly associated ($p < 0.001$) with recurrence and death [9]: (a) A fall in performance status from high ($\geqslant 90\%$) to low ($\leqslant 80\%$); (b) An elevation in leukocyte count $> 9100/mm^3$. Based on the LCSG data, Gail et al. suggested division of Stage I patients into 3 risk groups. The highest risk group is characterized by non-squamous histology, T_1N_1 or T_2N_0 and poor performance status (PS less than or equal to 80%). The highest risk group had a 3 year survival rate of less than 50%, while survival rates in the better risk categories ranged from 73–85%.

Stage II

Patients with Stage II (T_2N_1) NSCLC represented only 6% of staged patients in Mountain's series of 1824 adequately-assessed patients [38]. Five year survival after surgical resection may range as high as 38–50% [44, 51]. In Martini's series [44] of 75 T_1N_1 and T_2N_1 patients, survival rates did not differ significantly between the two groups. Long term survival of this order has encouraged adjuvant use of radiation and chemotherapy but so far, there is no conclusive benefit proved for such therapy, and its indiscriminate use outside of clinical trials cannot be encouraged.

The LCSG has reported encouraging data on adjuvant chemotherapy in resected Stage II and III lung cancer [52]. One hundred and forty-one patients with Stages II-III adenocarcinoma and large cell carcinoma were randomized to receive combination chemotherapy (cyclophosphamide, doxorubicin and cisplatin), or immunotherapy with intrapleural BCG and levamisole. After a mean observation period of 1.7 years, a significant prolongation of disease-free survival was noted for the chemotherapy arm. Overall survival rates did not differ significantly, however, and further investigation is clearly needed.

Stage III

Tumours that are classified as Stage III, by virtue of tumor invasion of contiguous structures (T_3) or the presence of distant metastasis, are not generally amenable to complete resection. Two types of tumor are however, occasionally cured by surgery with or without the addition of other modalities:

(1) Superior sulcus tumors which invade contiguous structures ($T_3N_1M_0$ and $T_3N_1M_0$). Five year survival rates range from 15% for patients undergoing palliative surgery and radiotherapy, to >50% in the small subset of patients undergoing curative surgery following radiotherapy [43]. Surgical therapy clearly has a role in carefully selected patients.

(2) N_2 tumors (mediastinal nodes positive). The poor survival data reported by Mountain [38] for this group of patients has discouraged many surgeons from attempting resection. However, most patients in that series were not staged by mediastinoscopy or computerized tomography, and the results of thoracotomy were not used at all for staging. Martini [53] reported 48% 3 year survival rate in those N2 patients thought to have Stage I disease preoperatively. Patients with small tumors (T_1) had a 3 year survival rate of 74%%. Routine mediastinoscopy and computerized tomography were not performed.

Bergh [45] confirmed curative potential in patients with subclinical nodal metastases, noting that patients with intranodal disease had 43% (15/35) survival at 5 years. However, when perinodal disease was shown, the 5 year survival rate was a dismal 4% (2/47). The level of mediastinal lymph node involvement is significant prognostically. Naruke [44] obtained a 5 year survival rate of 29% (9/31) when subcarinal nodes were negative, as compared to 9% (3/31) when these nodes were involved. Favorable predictive factors for curative resection are: (1) failure of routine evaluation to detect mediastinal nodal involvement; (2) absence of perinodal involvement at surgery; (3) absence of subcarinal nodal involvement.

Relation to chemotherapy

Early trials of single agent chemotherapy by the Veterans Administration Lung Group (VALSG) demonstrated a range of median survivals, from a low of 13.6 weeks for hexamethylamelamine to a high of 18.9 weeks for cyclophosphamide [4]. This difference was dwarfed by the impact of prognostic factors such as performance status and weight loss. In a randomized study of combination chemotherapy (methotrexate, doxorubicin, cyclophosphamide and carmustine versus placebo), Cormier [54] reported a 35% response rate and improved survival in the treated group. Generally, Phase II trials of combination chemotherapy have reported response rates as high as 40%.

Statistical analyses of such trials have shown significantly longer survival among the responders as compared to non-responders but as pointed out by Aisner and Hansen [55], this sleight-of-hand merely selects a group of patients with biologically favorable disease. When the trials are advanced into Phase III testing, as in a recent collaborative group study [56], the response rates range from 20–30% but with no significant impact on median survival. This randomized study also proved that toxicity tends to be severe in patients with a performance status of less than 80%. Chemotherapy in NSCLC should best be administered as part of a controlled randomized trial in patients with a performance status of 80% or better.

Relation to radiotherapy

Patients with regional disease are suitable for curative radiotherapy if resection is ruled out by disease extent, advanced age, or associated medical problems [57, 58]. The necessary dose seems to be in the range of 50–60 Gy administered at a rate of 2 Gy per day [57–59]. Long-term survival rates (>5 years) range from 6% [58] to 10% [57]. As in the case of chemotherapy, there are few reported studies randomizing patients to radiotherapy versus placebo, and to assess the effect on survival, we have to compare responders and non-responders. One such study [59] randomized 481 patients with Stage III NSCLC to 4 different regimens. Patients who experienced a complete regression of disease had a median survival of 75 weeks compared to 29 weeks for non-responders. Clinical characteristics predictive of prolonged survival are ranked in Table 8. Tumor size is not significant as a predictive factor if allowance is made for performance status, histology and weight loss.

Multivariate analyses

Stanley [61] reviewed data for 2 large cooperative studies of inoperable NSCLC. The Veterans Administration Lung Study Group (VALSG) randomized 2671 patients among various single agent and combination regimens. Data on 78 prognostic factors were collected, and 49 were significant with a P value <0.05. As noted earlier, the P value is inordinately influenced by the large number of patients studied and to circumvent this problem, he introduced the (psi)-statistic [13] which was designed to escape the influence of sample size, scale, and the number of levels of a factor.

Using this method, *initial performance status, extent of disease, prior weight loss* and *reduced appetite* were found to be the most important factors. Using a Cox model, 95% of the prognostic information was retained with the Zubrod scale (0–5). Condensing the coding to ambulatory versus non-ambulatory patients lost most of the prognostic value. The only significant laboratory parameter was the initial lymphocyte count. Patients with a lymphocyte count under $1000/mm^3$ had a median survival of only 7 weeks compared to 18 weeks for those with counts above $3000 \; mm^3$.

The Eastern Cooperative Oncology Group (ECOG) entered 1391 patients into protocol 2375 which screened new agents and combinations. Application of the (psi)-statistics yielded the same 4 factors as noted above. In this study, histology was more significant, ranking 10th using the (psi)-statistic and 3rd on stepwise analysis of the Cox model.

Small cell lung cancer (SCLC)

Histology

Recognition of the prognostic value of histopathology in small cell lung cancer (SCLC) has been hampered by nosology. Table 9 presents the current system adopted in 1977 together with the frequency of each subtype. The subset of patients with tumors combining elements of both small and large cell carcinomas has a poorer response rate to chemotherapy (58% vs. 91%), a poorer complete response rate (16% vs. 46%) and a shorter median survival (6 vs. 10.5 months.) [62]. In the group studied by Radice et al these patients represented 12% of all small cell cases, and this finding was confirmed by Hirsch *et al.* [63]. Other workers [64–65f] have failed to demonstrate any histologic impact on survival when this subtype was not analyzed separately.

Table 8. Prognostic indices in lung cancer patients treated with radiotherapy (Adapted from [60])

Prognostic factors	Median survival (weeks)		P value
	with characteristic	without characteristic	
Karnofsky performance factor $\geqslant 80$	44	34	0.0006
Squamous histology	56	33	0.0007
Weight loss $<5\%$	42	32	0.01
Tumor <6 cm in diameter	51	29	0.05

Staging

In his review of data accrued prior to the development of effective chemotherapy, Mountain [42] concluded that patients with SCLC should be assigned to Stage III because the survival experience was universally disastrous. Patients are most commonly categorized according to the VALSG criteria [3], as having either limited disease (LD: confined to one hemithorax) or extensive disease (ED).

Median survival in LD ranges from 8 to 12 months, compared to a range of 4 to 10 months for ED [14, 66–69]. Patients with LD have a higher complete remission (CR) rate with combination chemotherapy than is seen in ED. CR rates in LD between 9% and 64% have been reported compared to a range between 10% and 36% in ED [14, 67]. Similarly, Vogelsang [69] reported 2 year survival rates of 21% in LD compared to 3.8% in ED. Long-term survival (>5 years) is much poorer, but conforms to this pattern (12% in LD vs. 1.3% in ED) [70].

Visceral sites of metastatic disease, including brain, liver and bone marrow, are associated with short survival and poor response to treatment [27, 71–72]. In his review of reported cases of metastasis to these sites, Meyer [71] could identify only one survivor for each site at 30 months. Bone marrow involvement severe enough to cause thrombocytopenia was associated with a median survival of 68 days, compared to 231 days in the marrow-negative group [72]. When 3 or more sites of metastasis were identified, median survival was months less than in the LD group [67]. Conversely, patients with solitary bone lesions, bilateral supraclavicular lymphadenopathy, or ipsilateral pleural effusions [67–68, 71] are prognostically similar to patients with limited disease.

Biological markers

SCLC has many biochemical similarities to APUD (Amine Precursor Uptake and Decarboxylation) neuroendocrine cells, including abundant NSE. Carney *et al.* [73] reported high NSE levels (greater than or equal to 12 ng/ml) in 69% of 94 patients with SCLC. Among patients with limited disease (LD), 15 of 38 (39%)

Table 9. Frequency of histologic subtypes in small cell lung cancer (Adapted from [62] and [63])

	Frequency % [63]
WHO Type 21: oat cell	38–74
22: intermediate, including	
polygonal	23–30
fusiform	15–29
combined small cell/large cell	12–14
23: combined oat cell-tumors containing elements of	
adenocarcinoma or squamous cell carcinoma	rare

had elevated NSE levels, as compared to 49 of 56 (87%) patients with extensive disease (ED). Although NSE levels correlated with disease activity for individual patients, response rates to chemotherapy did not vary with initial NSE levels. Therefore, NSE levels may be useful in monitoring individual patients as an index of disease activity, but not as a predictor of response or of survival at the time of presentation.

CEA is an excellent monitoring adjunct in SCLC and is readily available. In a group of 85 patients studied at the Dana Farber Institute [74], elevated CEA levels (>2.5 ng/ml) were seen in 88% of patients with extensive disease, but in only 55% of patients with limited disease. Of 34 patients with CEA levels >5.0, 22 responded clinically, and all showed a fall in CEA values. All of the 12 non-responders had progressive increases in CEA levels. Of 55 patients demonstrating progressive disease, 44 (80%) had a rise in CEA level. There were no false-positive elevations in CEA. Although survival and response rates did not correlate with CEA at presentation, CEA measurements during treatment were useful in quantifying disease activity and response to treatment.

Various ectopic hormones are present in a minority of patients with SCLC. ProACTH, calcitonin and vasopressin [75] may contribute to the development of Cushing's syndrome, hypercalcemia and the syndrome of inappropriate anti-diuretic hormone (SIADH) secretion, respectively. There is no evidence for the prognostic utility of these markers, although serial determinations in any given patient may prove useful once clinical correlation is established. Bombesin, a tetradecapeptide first isolated in amphibians, promotes gastric and pancreatic secretion in experimental animals, and is occasionally found in the serum of SCLC patients. It acts as an autocrine growth factor *in vitro* [76]. Clinical correlates are being studied.

Table 10. Multivariate analysis showing significance of prognostic factors in small cell lung cancer

Prognostic factors	Veterans administration lung study group (VALSG) [61]	Eastern cooperative oncology group (ECOG) [14]	Cancer and acute leukemia group B (CALGB) [68]
Performance status	2	1	2
Disease extent	3	3	1
Weight loss	1	4	NE
Female sex	NE*	2	NS

NE: Not evaluated.
NS: Not significant.
*:   All patients were men.

Oncogenes

Oncogenes are ubiquitous and amplification of these genes is often detected in tumors. High levels of amplification have been correlated with advanced stages of neuroblastoma. Gazdar [77] has identified morphologically variant cell lines (SCLC-MV) which show marked oncogene amplification. Nine variant lines and a median of 26 c-myc copies per cell compared to a median of 1 copy for 23 typical lines (SCLC-C). This finding is particularly interesting because the SCLC-MV line is derived from patients with rapidly growing small cell lung cancers and short survival. Preliminary data from the same group [78] suggested an association between poor prognosis and amplification of c-myc and n-myc oncogenes. Such findings await confirmation.

Relation to treatment

The mainstay of treatment in SCLC is combination chemotherapy [79], and regimens containing at least 3 agents produce response rates exceeding 80%, and significant prolongation of survival when compared to untreated controls. As sole modalities of treatment, surgery [80] and radiotherapy [60] have no effect on survival. While Meyer [75] achieved an 80% survival rate at 30 months in a small group of patients with TNM Stages I-II from a combination of chemotherapy and surgery, a large retrospective series of operable patients [81] did not demonstrate any advantage in those patients undergoing resection as compared to those who received chemotherapy alone. There is evidence supporting the addition of radiotherapy to chemotherapy for patients with limited disease [82, 83]. Further trials are underway.

Multivariate analysis

The relative importance of clinical parameters at presentation has been evaluated in cooperative group studies. Performance status, disease extent and weight loss are the most significant prognostic factors in Cox regression analysis [14, 61, 68]. The relative ranking in 3 major studies is tabulated in Table 10. In the CALGB study [70], when the attainment of complete remission was entered into the model, it became most predictive of survival. Once again, of parameters available at presentation, performance status is of primary importance.

Acknowledgements

We gratefully acknowledge the help of Ms. Linda Godette for her technical and linguistic skills in the preparation of this manuscript.

References

1. Silverberg EA, Lubera J: Cancer Statistics, *CA* 36: 9–25, 1986
2. Karnofsky DA, Abelmann WH, Craver LF, Burchenal JH: The use of nitrogen mustard in the palliative treatment of carcinoma. *Cancer* 1: 634–656, 1948
3. Stanley KE: Prognostic factors for survival in patients with inoperable lung cancer. *J Nath Cancer Inst* 65: 25–32, 1980
4. Zelen M: Keynote address on biostatistics. *Cancer Chemother Rep* 4: 31–42, 1973
5. Ederer F, Mersheimer WL: Sex differences in the survival of lung cancer patients. *Cancer* 15: 425–532, 1962
6. Connelly RR, Cutler SJ, Baylis P: End results in cancer of the lung: comparison of male and female patients. *J Natl Cancer Inst* 36: 277–287, 1966
7. Higgins GA, Beebe GW: Bronchogenic carcinoma-factors in survival. *Arch Surg* 94: 539–549, 1966
8. Williams DE, Pairolero PC, Davis CS *et al.*: Survival of patients surgically treated for Stage I lung cancer. *J Thorax Cardiovasc Surg* 82: 70–76, 1981
9. Gail MH, Eagan RT, Mountain CF *et al.*: Prognostic factors in patients with resected Stage I non-small cell lung cancer. *Cancer* 54: 1802–1813, 1984
10. Lanzotti VJ, Thomas DR, Boyle LE, Smith TL, Gehan EA, Samuels ML: Survival with inoperable lung cancer. *Cancer* 39: 303–313, 1977
11. Axtell LM, Meyers MH, Shambaugh EM: Treatment survival patterns for black and white cancer patients diagnosed 1955 through 1964. *DHEW Publication* (NIH) 75–712, 1975
12. Page WF, Kuntz AJ: Racial and socioeconomic factors in cancer survival, a comparison of Veterans Administration results with selected studies. *Cancer* 45: 1029–1940, 1980
13. Dewys WD, Begg C, Larin PT *et al.*: Prognostic effect of weight loss prior to chemotherapy in cancer patients. *Am J Med* 69: 491–497, 1980
14. Ettinger DS, Lagakos S: Phase III study of CCNU, cyclophosphamide, adriamycin, vincristine and VP-16 in small cell carcinoma of the lung. *Cancer* 49: 1544–1554, 1982
15. Feinstein AR: Symptoms as an index of biological behavior and prognosis in human cancer. *Nature* 209: 241–245, 1966
16. Chahinian P: Relationship between tumor doubling time and anatomical features in 50 measurable pulmonary cancers. *Chest* 61: 340–345, 1972
17. Huhti E, Sutinen S, Saloheinio M: Survival among patients with lung cancer, an epidemiologic study. *Am Rev Respir Dis* 124: 13–16, 1981
18. Senior RM, Adamson JS: Survival in patients with lung cancer, an appraisal of Feinstein's symptom classification. *Arch Intern Med* 125: 975–980, 1970
19. Collins VP, Coeffler RK, Tivey H: Observations on growth rates of human tumors. *Am J Roent Rad Ther Nucl Med* 76: 988–1000, 1956
20. Chahinian AP, Israel L: Rates and patterns of growth of lung cancer. In: *Lung Cancer: Natural History, Prognosis and Therapy*. Israel L, Chahinian AP (eds). New York: Academic Press, 1976, pp 63–76
21. Geddes DM: The natural history of lung cancer: a review based on rates of tumor growth. *Br J Dis Chest* 73: 1–17, 1979
22. Mizuno T, Masaoka A, Ichimura H *et al.*: Comparison of actual survivorship after treatment with survivorship predicted by actual tumor volume doubling time from tumor diameter at first observation. *Cancer* 53: 2716–2720, 1984
23. Chahinian AP, Israel L: prognostic value of doubling time. In: *Lung Cancer: National History, Prognosis and Therapy*, Israel L, Chahinian AP (ed). New York: Academic Press, 1976, pp 95–106
24. Ali MK, Ewer MS, Atallah MR, Moutain CF *et al.*: Regional and overall pulmonary function

changes in lung cancer. Correlations with tumor stage, extent of pulmonary resection and patient survival. *J Thorax Cardiovasc Surg* 86: 1–8, 1983

25. Israel L, Mugica J, Chahinian P: Prognosis of early bronchogenic carcinoma, survival curves of 451 patients after resection of lung cancer in relation to the results of preoperative tuberculin skin test. *Biomedicine* 19: 68–72, 1973

26. Snell NJC: Tuberculin reactivity as a predictor of survival time in inoperable bronchial carcinoma. *Thorax* 34: 508–511, 1979

27. Wynder EL, Hoffman D: Tobacco and health. *N Eng J Med* 300: 894–903, 1979

28. Johnston-Early A, Cohen MH, Minna JD: Smoking abstinence and small cell lung cancer survival, an association. *JAMA* 244: 2175–2179, 1980

29. Markman M, Braine HG, Abeloff MD: Histocompatibility antigens in small cell carcinoma of the lung. *Cancer* 54: 2943–2945, 1984

30. Tongio MM, Kerschen C, Paul G *et al.*: HLA antigens and primary bronchial carcinoma. *Cancer* 49: 2485–2488, 1982

31. Ford CHJ, Newman CE, Mackintosh P: HLA frequency and prognosis in lung cancer. *Br J Cancer* 43: 610–614

32. Rogentine GN, Dellon AL, Chretien PB: Prolonged disease-free survival in bronchogenic carcinoma associated with HLA-AW19 and HLA-B5. *Cancer* 39: 2345–2347, 1977

33. Weiss GB, Nawrocki LB, Daniels JC: HLA type and survival in lung cancer. *Cancer* 46: 38–40, 1980

34. Svejgaard A, Jersild C, Nielsen LS, Bodmen WF: HLA antigens and disease: statistical and genetical considerations. *Tissue Antigens* 4: 95–105, 1974

35. Abe S, Makimura S, Itabahsi K *et al.*: Prognostic significance of nuclear DNA content in small cell carcinoma of the lung. *Cancer* 56: 2025–2030, 1985

36. Volm M, Drings P, Mattern J *et al.*: Prognostic significance of DNA patterns and resistance predictive tests in non-small cell lung carcinoma. *Cancer* 56: 1396–1403, 1985

37. Kreyberg L: Histologic typing of lung tumors. In: *International Histologic Classification of Tumors*, Kreyberg L (ed). Geneva: World Health Organization, 1967

38. Mountain CF, Carr DT, Anderson WAD: A system for the clinical staging of lung cancer. *Am J Roentgenol and Rad Ther Nucl Med* 120: 130–138, 1974

39. Feinstein AR, Gelfman NA, Yesner R: The diverse effects of histopathology on manifestations and outcome of lung cancer. *Chest* 66: 225–229, 1974

40. Williams DE, Pavoleno PC, Davis CS *et al.*: Survival of patients surgically treated for Stage I lung cancer. *J Thorac Cardiovasc Surg* 82: 70–76, 1981

41. Campobasso O, Invernizzi B, Musso M, Berrino F: Survival rates of lung cancer according to histological type. *Br J Cancer* 29: 240–246, 1974

42. Mountain CF: The relationship of prognosis to morphology and the anatomic extent of disease: Studies of a new clinical staging system. In: *Lung Cancer: Natural History, Prognosis and Therapy*. Irsael L, Chahinian AP (ed). New York: Academic Press, 1976, pp 107–140

43. Martini N: Preoperative staging and surgery for non-small cell lung cancer. In: *Lung Cancer*, Aisner J (ed). New York, Churchill, Livingstone, 1985, pp 101–130

44. Naruke T, Suemasu K, Ishikawa S: Lymph node mapping and curability at various levels of metastasis in resected lung cancer. *J Thorac Gardiovasc* Surg 76: 832–839, 1978

45. Bergh NP, Schersten T: Bronchogenic carcinoma: a follow-up study of a surgically treated series with a special reference to the prognostic significance of lymph node metastasis. *Acta Chir Scand* (Suppl) 341: 1–6, 1965

46. Vincent RG, Chu TM, Lane WW: The value of carcinoembryonic antigen in patients with carcinoma of the lung. *Cancer* 44: 685–691, 1979

47. Concannon JP, Dalbow MH, Hodgson SE *et al.*: Prognostic value of preoperative carcinoembryonic antigen (CEA) plasma levels in patients with bronchogenic carcinoma. *Cancer* 42: 1477–1483, 1978

48. Wolfsen AR, Odell WD: ProACTH: use for early detection of lung cancer. *Am J Med* 66: 765–771, 1979

49. Ariyoshi Y, Kato K, Ishiguro T *et al.*: Evaluation of serum neuron-specific enolase as a tumor marker of carcinoma of the lung. *Gann* 74: 219–225, 1983

50. Bignall JR, Moon AJ: Survival after lung resection for bronchial carcinoma. *Thorax* 10: 183–190, 1955

51. Martini N, Flehinger BJ, Nagasaki F *et al.*: Prognostic significance of N_1 disease in carcinoma of the lung. *J Thorac Cardiovasc Surg* 86: 646–653, 1983

52. Holmes EC, Gail M: Surgical adjuvant therapy for Stage II and Stage III adenocarcinoma and large cell undifferentiated carcinoma. *J Clin Oncol* 4: 710–715, 1986

53. Martini N, Flehinger BJ, Zaman MB, Beattie EJ: Prospective study of 445 lung carcinomas with mediastinal lymph node metastases. *J Thorac Cardiovasc Surg* 80: 390–399, 1980

54. Cormier Y, Bergeron D, LaForge J *et al.*: Benefits of polychemotherapy in advanced non-small cell bronchogenic cancer. *Cancer* 50: 845–849, 1982

55. Aisner J, Hansen HH: Commentary: Current status of chemotherapy for non-small cell lung cancer. *Cancer Treat Rep* 65: 979–985, 1981

56. Ruckdeschel JC, Finkelstein DM, Ettinger DS *et al.*: A randomized trial of the four most active regimens for metastatic non-small cell lung cancer. *J Clin Oncol* 4: 14–22, 1986

57. Coy P, Kennelly GM: The role of curative radiotherapy in the treatment of lung cancer. *Cancer* 45: 698–702, 1980

58. Sherman OM, Weichselbaum R, Hellman S: The characteristics of long-term survivors of lung cancer treated with radiation. *Cancer* 47: 2575–2580, 1981

59. Perez CA, Stanley K, Rubin P *et al.*: A prospective randomized study of various irradiation doses and fractionation schedules in the treatment of inoperable non-oat-cell carcinoma of the lung. *Cancer* 45: 2744–2753, 1980

60. Petrovich Z, Stanley K, Cox JD, Paig C: Radiotherapy in the management of locally advanced lung cancer of all cell types. *Cancer* 48: 1335–1340, 1981

61. Stanley KE: Prognostic factors in lung cancer. In: *Lung Cancer*. Aisner J (ed). New York, Churchill, Livingstone, 1985, pp 41–67

62. Radice PA, Matthews MJ, Ihde DC, Gazdar AF, *et al.*: The clinical behavior of 'mixed' small cell/large cell bronchogenic carcinoma compared to 'pure' small cell subtypes. *Cancer* 50: 2894–2902, 1982

63. Hirsch FR, Osterlind K, Hansen HH: The prognostic significance of histopathologic subtyping of small cell carcinoma of the lung according to the classification of the World Health Organization. *Cancer* 52: 2144–2150, 1983

64. Davis S, Stanley KE, Yesner R *et al.*: Small cell carcinoma of the lung – survival according to histologic subtype: a veteran's administration lung group study. *Cancer* 47: 1863–1866, 1981

65. Carney DN, Matthews MJ, Ihde DC *et al.*: Influence of histologic subtype of small cell carcinoma of the lung on clinical presentation, response to therapy and survival. *J Natl Cancer Inst* 65: 1225–1229, 1980

66. Souhami RL, Bradburg I, Geddes DM *et al.*: Prognostic significance of laboratory parameters measured at diagnosis in small cell carcinoma of the lung. *Cancer Res* 45: 2878–2882, 1985

67. Ihde DC, Makuch RW, Carney DM *et al*: Prognostic implications of stage of disease and sites of metastases in patients with small cell carcinoma of the lung treated with intensive combination chemotherapy. Am Rev Resp Dis 123: 500–507, 1981

68. Maurer LH, Pajak TF: Prognostic factors in small cell carcinoma of the lung: a cancer and leukemia group B study. *Cancer Treat Rep* 65: 767–774, 1981

69. Vogelsang GB, Abeloff MD, Ettinger DS, Booker SV: Long term survivers of small cell carcinoma of the lung. *Am J Med* 79: 49–55, 1985

70. Johnson BE, Ihde DC, Bunn PA *et al.*: Patients with small cell lung cancer treated with combination chemotherapy with or without irradiation. *Ann Intern Med* 103: 430–438, 1985

71. Meyer JA: Effect of histologically verified TNM stage on disease control in treated small cell carcinoma of the lund. *Cancer* 55: 1747–1752, 1985

72. Hirsch FR, Hansen HH: Bone marrow involvement in small cell anaplastic carcinoma of the lung. *Cancer* 46: 206–211, 1980

73. Carney DN, Marangos PJ, Ihde DC *et al.*: Serum neuron-specific enolase: a marker for disease extent and response to therapy of small cell lung cancer. *Lancet* i, 583–585, 1982

74. Goslin RH, Skarin AT, Zamcheck N: Carcinoembryonic antigen: a useful monitor of therapy of small cell lung cancer. *JAMA* 246: 2173–2176, 1981

75. Sorensen GD, Pettergill OS, Delprete SA, Carte CC: Biomarkers in small cell carcinoma of the lung. In: *Lung Cancer.* Aisner J (ed) New York, Churchill, Livingston, 1985, pp 203–239

76. Carney DN, Cuttita FC, Gazdar AF, Minna JD: Autocrine clonogenic factors are produced by cell lines of small cell lung cancer. *Proc Am Soc Clin Oncol* 2: C-55, 1983

77. Gazdar AF, Carney DM, Nan MN, Minna JD: Characterization of variant subclasses of cell lines derived from small cell lung cancer having distinct biochemical, morphological and growth properties. *Cancer Res* 45: 2924–2930, 1985

78. Johnson BE, Nan MN, Gazdar AF *et al.*: Oncogene amplification of c-myc in cell lines established from patients with small cell lung cancer as associated with shortened survival. *Proc ASCO* (Abstract) 4: 186, 1985

79. Aisner J, Alberto P, Bitran J *et al.*: Role of chemotherapy in small cell lung cancer: A consensus report of the International Association for the Study of Lung Cancer Workshop. *Cancer Treat Rep* 67: 37–43, 1983

80. Mountain CF: Clinical biology of small cell carcinoma: Relationship to surgical therapy. *Sem Oncol* 5: 272–279, 1978

81. Osterlind K, Hansen M, Hansen HH *et al.*: Treatment policy of surgery in small cell carcinoma of the lung: Retrospective analysis of a series of 84 consecutive patients. *Thorax* 40: 272–277, 1985

82. Perry MC, Eaton WL, Ware J *et al.*: Chemotherapy with or without radiation therapy in limited small cell cancer of the lung. *Proc Am Soc Clin Oncol* 3: 230, 1984

83. Catane R, Lichter A, Lee YJ, Brereton HD *et al.*: Small cell lung cancer: analyses of treatment factors contributing to prolonged survival. *Cancer* 48: 1936–1943, 1981

17. Prognostic indices in mouth and throat cancer

R.J. ZARBO and J.D. CRISSMAN

There are two types of prognostic variables in cancer– those that are important in epidemiologic evaluation and those more useful in patient management. The following discussion is on those that are of value in planning patient care and in predicting response to therapy and duration of survival in cancers of the oral cavity, pharynx and larynx. The tract is lined by squamous epithelium and the majority of malignant neoplasms arising in the mucosa are squamous cell carcinomas.

Host-related factors

While tumor staging usually represents the basis on which cancer therapy is selected, host-related factors may modify the choice.

Their possible influence depends on the mode of therapy selected for an individual. Thus, the general health of an individual patient may dictate the type and extent of therapy, so that patients with compromised renal function are not good candidates for aggressive chemotherapy. Head and neck cancer patients are commonly addicted to tobacco and alcohol abuse and these are not conducive to optimum health.

Age and Gender

Squamous cell carcinomas arising in younger age groups are sometimes said to be more aggressive and associated with a poorer prognosis than are tumors occurring in the elderly, but most reports do not confirm such differences. In a study of squamous cell carcinomas of the lip, patients under the age of 40 had a worse prognosis than those in the older age group [1], but in a Parge series of squamous cell carcinomas of the head and neck region, it was noted that *increasing* age was associated with a higher rater of recurrence at all sites [2].

Multivariate analysis of oral carcinomas in patients older than 70 years showed a poorer survival than in patients less than 70 years [3] but another extensive study of oral cavity carcinomas showed no consistent relationship between prognosis and age [4]. Nor was an association with age confirmed in the study of prognosis conducted by the Head and Neck Cancer Contracts Program of the National Cancer Institute [5].

Thus, there is little evidence that younger age is associated with a higher morbidity and mortality in squamous cell carcinomas of the head and neck, although there is evidence that carcinoma in older age groups usually compromises survival. This may be partly associated with a decreasing performance status in the aged, and the inherent restriction on the type and duration of therapies that may be administered without adverse morbidity. The natural survival of head and neck cancer patients not dying of their cancer is also decreased when compared to an age- and sexmatched control population [6]. It is clear that the population exposed to the risk factors for carcinoma of the head and neck (alcohol and tobacco) already have a compromised survival pattern due to associated diseases.

The majority of patients with cancer of the upper aerodigestive tract are male although the increasing use of cigarettes and alcohol by women has started to alter this male predominance. In one large series of squamous cell carcinomas of the oral cavity, females appeared to have a poorer survival rate compared to males [7], but in a second, more comprehensive, study of oral cavity tumors using multivariate analysis, no significant male/females differences were noted [3]. Yet, in some carefully controlled smaller studies, males were found to have a significantly poorer survival [8, 9].

Performance status

Patients with head and neck cancer often have histories of chronic tobacco and alcohol abuse which contribute to a compromised nutritional and performance status [10]. Nutritional deficiencies may in turn, result in altered host immune reactivities. Although deviations in immune parameters have been documented for head and neck cancer patients [11], correlations with prognosis have been inconsistent [12].

Initial performance status has been identified as an important prognostic factor for tumor response to chemotherapy (and for ultimate survival) in patients with advanced carcinoma of the head and neck [13]. The Radiation Therapy Oncology Group has similarly identified performance status as the most important factor in predicting initial complete response to radiation therapyin head and neck cancer patients [14], followed by staging and anatomical site of the primary tumor. In the Head and Neck Contracts Program, however, no significant association of performance status with tumor response rates was seen with more advanced head and neck cancers treated with pre-operative chemotherapy [5]. Selection of patients with a high performance status probably accounted for the lack of association with tumor response in this last group of patients. It requires a high level of performance status to allow for recovery from the surgical procedure and from the addition of chemotherapy.

Clinical staging

This is the most important criterion in planning therapy for head and neck squamous cell carcinoma. Tumor staging is based on the TNM system as defined by the American Joint Commission on Cancer Staging [15] and the International Union Against Cancer [16]. For the most part, the TNM staging is a clinical assessment of the extent and distribution of the neoplasm and takes into account not only the size, but in some instances also the anatomical distribution, of the primary tumor (T). Clinical assessment of regional lymph node metastases (N) and the presence or absence of distant metastases (M), complete the parameters required for clinical staging. The primary tumor staging classifications vary by site and are outlined in Table 1.

Staging of cervical lymph node involvement differs in the AJC and UICC staging classification in regard to the number, fixation, size and bilaterality of nodal assessment. These differences are outlined in Table 2. The determination and importance of distant metastases are the same in both systems. Because of the numerous potential combinations of TNM subgroups, four stages of disease have been defined and are outlined in Table 3. The purpose of grouping TNM combinations into four distinct stages is to assemble comparable groups of patients with similar clinical advancement of disease.

Determination of T category is modified by the anatomic distribution of the carcinoma in the case of the hypopharynx and larynx: it takes into account the invasion of contiguous anatomic structures which are known to influence the frequency of metastases and the likelihood of survival. In general, stages I and II tumors are more uniform in their behavior and response to therapy, while stages III and IV tumors are more heterogeneous. They include four and twelve TNM subcategories respectively, and encompass not only numerous tumor sizes but varying degrees of regional lymph node involvement (Table 3).

In the current staging system, stage IV disease may consist of tumors that are large but without palpable lymph node involvement, or small primary neoplasms with extensive regional lymph node metastases. Obviously, a tumor that has not demonstrated a tendency to metastasize would show a very different clinical behavior from that of a smaller tumor with extensive metastases. This inconsistency arises from surgical bias in the staging system because studies of chemotherapy and/or radiation therapy have demonstrated that the two subsets of tumors have a markedly different prognosis [17].

The major advantage of the TNM system and the subclassification into four stages of disease is that it reflects the natural history of head and neck squamous cell cancer. This is illustrated in Table 4 which summarizes selected large studies treated primarily by surgery with or without radiation and shows the average rates of survival [9, 18–35]. While it is agreed by most clinical investigators that the

Table 1. Primary tumor (T) classifications for head and neck sites.

Oral cavity	Larynx-supraglottis
TX Minimum requirements to assess the primary tumor cannot be met	Tis Carcinoma in situ
	T1 Tumor confined to region of origin with normal mobility
T0 No evidence of primary tumor	
Tis Carcinoma in situ	T2 Tumor involving adjacent supralottic site(s) or glottis without fixation
T1 Greatest diameter of primary tumor 2 cm or less	
	T3 Tumor limited to larynx with fixation or extension to involve postcricoid area, medial wall of pyriform sinus, or pre epiglottic space
T2 Greatest diameter of primary tumor more than 2 cm but not more than 4 cm	
T3 Greatest diameter of primary tumor more than 4 cm	
	T4 Massive tumor extending beyond the larynx to involve oropharynx, soft tissues of neck, or destruction of thyroid cartilage
T4 Massive tumor more than 4 cm in diameter with deep invasion to involve antrum, pterygoid muscles, base of tongue, skin of neck	

Oropharynx	Larynx-glottis
Tis Carcinoma in situ	Tis Carcinoma in situ
T1 Tumor 2 cm or less in greatest diameter	T1 Tumor confined to vocal cord(s) with normal mobility (includes involvement of anterior or posterior commissure)
T2 Tumor more than 2 cm but not more than 4 cm in greatest diameter	
	T2 Supralottic or suglottic extension with normal or impaired cord mobility, or both
T3 Tumor more than 4 cm in greatest diameter	
	T3 Tumor confined to the larynx with cord fixation
T4 Massive tumor more than 4 cm in diameter with invasion of bone, soft tissues of neck, or root (deep musculature) of tongue	T4 Massive Tumor with thyroid cartilage destruction or extension beyond the confines of the larynx, or both

Hypopharynx	Larynx-subglottis
Tis Carcinoma in situ	Tis Carcinoma in situ
T1 Tumor confined to one site	T1 Tumor confined to the sublottic region
T2 Extension of tumor to adjacent region or site without fixation of hemilarynx	T2 Tumor extension to vocal cords with normal or impaired cord mobility
T3 Extension of tumor to adjacent region or site with fixation of hemilarynx	T3 Tumor confined to larynx with cord fixation
T4 Massive tumor invading bone or soft tissues of neck	T4 Massive tumor with cartilage destruction or extension beyond the confines of the larynx, or both

staging system may lump together a heterogeneous collection of neoplasms, it remains a useful method for comparing a wide spectrum of tumors.

Site factors

Pathologists have been unable to identify distinct histological characteristics for the various primary sites, but it is clear that there are differences between sites in the biological aggressiveness of the tumors. This may be due in part to the clinical symptoms leading to diagnosis. Thus, squamous cell carcinomas developing on the glottis or the alveolar ridge will develop symptoms early so that voice change or ulceration with bleeding lead to diagnosis at an earlier stage in the disease progression, and a greater likelihood of cure.

Other factors, however, are also involved. In an analysis of 898 patients with squamous cell carcinoma of the oral cavity and oropharynx [36], equivalent-sized tumors of the lip, floor of the mouth, buccal mucosa, hard palate, and gingiva

Table 2. Comparison of AJC and UICC classifications of staging

AJC cervical node (N) classification

NX	Minimum requirements to assess the regional node cannot be met
N0	No clinically positive node.
N1	Single clinically positive homolateral node 3 cm or less in diameter
N2	Single clinically positive homolateral node more than 3 cm but not more than 6 cm in diameter or multiple clinically positive homolateral nodes, none more than 6 cm in diameter
N2a	Single clinically positive homolateral node more than 3 cm but not more than 6 cm in diameter
N2b	Multiple clinically positive homolateral nodes, none more than 6 cm in diameter
N3	Massive homolateral node(s), bilateral nodes, or contralateral node(s)
N3a	Clinically positive homolateral node(s), one more than 6 cm in diameter
N3b	Bilaterally clinically positive nodes (in this situation, each side of the neck should be staged separately; i.e., N3b: right, N2a; left N1)
N3c	Contralateral clinically positive node(s) only

UICC cervical node (N) classification

N0	No evidence of regional lymph node involvement
N1	Evidence of involvement of movable homolateral regional lymph nodes
N2	Evidence of involvement of movable contralateral or bilateral regional lymph nodes
N3	Evidence of involvement of fixed regional lymph nodes
NX	The minimum requirements to assess the regional lymph nodes cannot be met

Distant metastasis (M)

MX	Minimum requirements to assess the presence of distant metastasis cannot be met.
M0	No (known) distant metastasis.
M1	Distant metastasis present. Specify.

had approximately the same risk for metastasis to regional lymph nodes. In contrast, squamous cell carcinomas of the anterior two-thirds of the tongue had a much higher tendency to metastasize, while neoplasms arising in the posterior third of the tongue and oropharynx showed the most aggressive behavior.

It is not clear whether this aggressiveness reflects a true difference in the biological behavior of the primary neoplasm or the peculiarities of the host tissues infiltrated by tumor. It is possible that the anatomic site of involvement is of prognostic significance because of variations in local anatomy related to lymphatic drainage or to the size that tumors may attain without influencing function. It is also possible that neoplasms arising in some sites have an intrinsically more aggressive behavior which we cannot yet explain.

Laryngeal carcinomas are divided into several anatomical subgroups, (glottic, infraglottic, supraglottic and transglottic) and extensive data correlate the anatomic site with the frequency of lymph node metastasis. In one series, the frequency of metastasis was 0, 19%, 33% and 52% for glottic, infraglottic, supraglottic and transglottic carcinomas, respectively [37]. Contralateral metastases were most common in supraglottic and transglottic tumors [37, 38]. Transglottic tumors are usually larger than purely glottic tumors, and this confirms the association between tumor size and frequency of metastasis.

Carcinomas arising in other parts of the hypopharynx (pyriform sinus, posterolateral walls and post-cricoid areas) show almost twice the frequency of lymph node metastasis compared to those in the larynx [39]. In the case of carcinoma of the lip, the survival rate of patients with lesions of the upper lip is almost half that of those with carcinomas of the lower lip, and tumors of the oral commissures are even more lethal [40, 41].

Size of primary (T-Stage)

Larger tumors correlate with an increased frequency of metastasis [36]. While even small tumors are known to metastasize, the biological factors required for tumor invasion (infiltration of blood and lymph vessels, arrest and extravasation

Table 3. Stage grouping for head and neck cancer

Stage I	T1, N0, M0
Stage II	T2, N0, M0
Stage III	T3, N0, M0
	T1, T2, T3; N1, M0
Stage IV	T4, N0 or N1, M0
	Any T, N2 or N3, M0
	Any T, any N, M1

of tumor cells) seem to be features of larger tumors. In the oral cavity and oropharynx, tumors less than 3 cm generally share the same low percentage of metastasis, tumors measuring 3–4 cm are intermediate, and tumors over 4 cm have the highest rate of metastasis to regional lymph nodes [36].

In the case of carcinoma of the lip, tumors less than 2 cm in size have a 5% frequency of metastasis, tumors measuring 2–4 cm a 50% frequency, and tumors over 4 cm a 73% frequency of metastasis [42]. Glottic tumors also show a progressive increase in the frequency of lymph node metastasis – 1.9, 16.7, 25 and 65% in T1, T2, T3 and T4 tumors, respectively [43].

Lymph node metastasis (N-Stage)

Clinical assessment of lymph node metastasis is not absolute because obstructive submandibular gland enlargement, poor oral hygiene or ulceration of the primary neoplasm can elicit inflammatory and immunological responses within the draining lymph nodes. The frequency of false positive clinical assessments of palpable lymph nodes ranges from 24 to 56% for floor of the mouth carcinoma [44, 45]. On the other hand, clinically negative but histologically positive lymph nodes are found in 15% to 60% of patients [18, 46]. Histologic demonstration of metastases in radical neck dissections regarded as positive on clinical examination has varied from 44 to 88% [4].

Palpable and pathologically positive lymph node metastasis is the most important index of prognosis. The size of the primary neoplasm usually correlates with the frequency of lymph node metastasis, but some small tumors show the same frequency of metastases as do larger tumors [47, 48]. In a group of cases of oral carcinoma without palpable lymph nodes, the 5 year survival rate was 65%, without demonstrable effect of tumor size on survival [4]. Yet the finding of a

Table 4. 5 Year determinant survival by stage of disease for head and neck sites (includes studies with numerous treatment modalities)

Site	Overall (avg)	I	II	III	IV
Oral tongue [18, 19]	50–45	80–70	60–50	35–30	0
Floor of mouth [20, 21, 22]	50–35	85–70	60–50	40–25	15–0
Buccal mucosa [23]	42	77	65	27	18
Gingiva [24]	36	73	41	17	
Hard palate [9, 25, 26]	42	75	46	36	11
Soft palate [27, 28, 29]	50	68	44	31	3
Tonsil [30, 31, 32]	43	93	57	27	17
Supraglottis [33, 34]	65–50	90–80	70–60	55–40	0
Glottis [35]	82	89	85	59	0

single lymph node on the ipsilateral side decreased the survival rate to 52%, and when more than one lymph node was palpable, it decreased to 17%.

In a detailed study of oral cavity carcinomas, [49] the five year survival rate was 75% for patients without histological evidence of cervical lymph node metastasis, 49% for one positive node, 30% for two positive nodes and 13% for patients with three or more positive nodes. For cancer of the tongue, the finding of palpable lymph nodes decreases the 5 year survival rate by half [50]. For larynx and hypopharynx neoplasms, one pathologically proven lymph node metastasis reduces the five year survival rate from 70% to 29% [39]. The importance of lymph node metastases as a prognostic indicator may lie in the fact that many patients die from recurrent or uncontrolled regional disease in cervical lymph nodes, often associated with local recurrence in the primary site [49, 51].

Extranodal extension

Lymph node size and fixation to adjacent structures on clinical examination also influence prognosis. Lymph nodes become fixed by extranodal infiltration of tumor, especially in large metastases, so that multiple lymph nodes containing metastatic tumor may coalesce resulting in a large fixed mass of nodes. In a series of laryngeal and hypopharyngeal squamous cell carcinomas, patients with non-palpable, or non-fixed lymph nodes less than 2 cm in size, had similar five year survival rates of approximately 58%; those with fixed, or non-fixed lymph nodes greater than 2 cm, had similar survival rates of approximately 28%. [52]. In a large series of patients with carcinoma of the lip, oral cavity or oropharynx, clinically positive fixed lymph nodes were associated with a poorer prognosis than were clinically positive but mobile lymph nodes [3]. The number of lymph nodes found histologically positive had no statistical effect on survival in this study, but the presence of metastases at levels 3 and 4 of the lower neck resulted in a marked decrease in survival [3].

The histological finding of extracapsular spread of squamous cell carcinoma in lymph nodes removed at radical neck dissection is a significant prognostic indicator for survival [53]. In a study of supraglottic squamous cell carcinomas, patients without metastatic nodes or with positive cervical lymph nodes without capsular invasion, had a 71% and 79% three year disease free survival respectively, compared to 35% for those patients with extracapsular spread of tumor. Of the patients in this series who were clinically node-negative, 31% were demonstrated to have nodal metastasis, 20% of which showed extracapsular spread of tumor [54]. In a study of oral cavity carcinomas, it was shown that 33% of patients with intact lymph node capsules survived 5 years compared to only 11% of patients with infiltration of adjacent soft tissue [49].

Although some patients with extracapsular invasion into perivascular or adjacent soft tissue are still amenable to surgical extirpation, large metastases with extensive soft tissue infiltration (especially to the pre-vertebral fascia) are no longer resectable. Nevertheless, surgical resectability does not necessarily alter the prognostic importance of extranodal tumor invasion because lymph node metastases with an aggressive behavior pattern, as shown by invasion of adjacent tissues, are also likely to invade vascular structures.

Lymph node patterns of reaction

The recognition of histological subcompartments such as B-cell follicular centers, parafollicular or paracortical T-cell areas, and B-cell medullary areas has resulted in a number of studies on the histological response of lymph nodes in cancer patients. Reticuloendothelial compartments have been recognized for many years, and are known as indicators of host immune response. However, most studies of these compartments do not strongly correlate with either survival rate or frequency of lymph node metastasis [52, 55], despite an early report indicating increased survival rates in patients with lymph nodes displaying immunologic stimulation [56].

Distant metastases

Squamous cell carcinomas of the head and neck region usually metastasize to regional lymph nodes, and the majority of patients dying of head and neck squamous cell carcinoma show recurrence either at the primary site or in the neck [49, 57]. Systemic metastases were not considered a major clinical problem in the past and one report showed that only 1% of head and neck cancer patients had evidence of distant metastases at autopsy [58]. However, advances in the control of both primary and regional tumor have resulted in increased recognition of distant metastases. In 779 head and neck cancer patients treated between 1955 and 1967, 12.3% had evidence of distant metastases [59], and in 5,019 patients presenting from 1948 to 1973 without initial clinical evidence of distant metastases, 10.9% developed such metastases [60]. A more recent study (1968-1987) found distant metastases in 30.7% of 169 patients [61].

The incidence of distant metastasis ranges from 31% of patients dying of oral carcinoma who had initially negative neck dissections, to 59% of those with histologically positive nodes [49]. The autopsied population in this series demonstrated metastatic rates of 86% and 77%, respectively. In tumors of the larynx, the presence of cervical lymph node involvement and a persistent primary carcinoma are strongly correlated with the finding of distant metastases [58, 60]. No effect on the incidence of distant metastasis was noted from age, sex or other host variables [58]. Others have found that the incidence of distant metastasis for all head and neck sites increased with stage of disease, and that the correlation with N-stage was greater than with T-stage [60].

In the treatment of advanced cancer, it has been observed that chemotherapy may result in an increased frequency of distant metastases [62]. Although this was not a randomized study and the possibility of selection of more advanced disease for chemotherapy must be considered, improvements in local and regional tumor control must lead to longer survival and increased recognition of distant metastases. The presence of distant metastasis is usually the survival-limiting factor, as the metastases are often refractory to combined therapy [63].

Multiple primary cancers

The number of patients with multiple primary neoplasms of the upper aerodigestive tract and lung is increasing, possibly because of increased awareness of multicentric neoplasia and careful physical examination [64]. In a well controlled follow-up study, simultaneous primary tumors were found in over 10% of cases, and over 20% of the patients eventually developed second neoplasms [65]. In a similar study of oral cavity squamous cell carcinoma, 27% of 377 patients ultimately developed second primary tumors [66]. Evaluating the impact on treatment and survival is difficult, but in a community-based study, patients with a second tumor had an overall 5 year survival rate of 17% as compared to a 35% survival rate in patients with a single neoplasm [67].

The development of multiple primaries is thought to represent a field effect on the upper aerodigestive tract mucosa by carcinogens, and both alcohol abuse and smoking are causative factors for squamous cell carcinoma in these sites [10]. In patients developing one cancer, the rest of the mucosa is generally injured and is at increased risk to a second tumor. This appears to be particularly true in patients who continue to smoke and drink.

Histopathologic variables

Histological grade

The initial attempts at tumor cell grading were developed by Broders when he studied the relationship between histology and progression of carcinoma of the lip [68]. The value of histological differentiation in predicting the biologic behavior of squamous cell carcinomas of the upper aerodigestive tract has been disappointing in general, although individual parameters of grading may have prognostic importance.

The degree of differentiation has been found to be of value in predicting regional lymph node metastasis in squamous cell carcinomas of the larynx [37,

69, 70]. Most studies have found that poorly differentiated squamous cell carcinomas of the oral cavity and oropharynx have a higher metastatic rate than do better differentiated tumors [36], and a worse overall prognosis [3, 7]. An increased frequency of metastases has been shown for non-keratinizing squamous cell carcinomas of the pyriform sinus treated with pre-operative radiation [71].

Correlation between histological grade and the incidence of local recurrence has been looked for. In one study, poorly differentiated carcinomas of the larynx and hypopharynx were found more likely to recur locally after definitive surgery [52] but in another study highly keratinized carcinomas of the pyriform sinus were found more likely to recur [71]. These apparent contradictions have led to doubt as to the predictive value of histopathology in squamous cell carcinoma, especially as tumor grade does not appear to correlate well with tumor size and, therefore, appears to have limited prognostic value compared to clinical staging.

Jakobsson has suggested a multi-parametric grading system which leads to quantitative scoring for tumor grade of squamous cell carcinomas [12]. This grading scheme incorporates four tumor related parameters, including degree and pattern of keratinization, nuclear pleomorphism, number of mitoses and the structure and inter-relationships of the tumor cell population. It also includes four parameters related to tumor-host interface, including the mode or pattern of invasion, the stage of invasion, the presence or absence of vascular invasion and the cellular inflammatory response to the tumor.

In the original application of this quantitative assessment of tumor grade, the total score for laryngeal carcinomas correlated with survival better than did the current WHO grading format [72]. However, a more important contribution of the multi-parametric approach is that it uses multi-variate analysis to assess the contribution of each individual histological parameter either to recurrence, metastasis or ultimate survival. Thus, studies with laryngeal squamous cell carcinomas indicated that in T1 laryngeal tumors the pattern of invasion was prognostically most important while in larger T2–T4 neoplasms, nuclear pleomorphism was the most important predictor of tumor behavior. Studies applying these multiple histologic parameters have been used with varying degrees of success to assess prognosis for squamous cell carcinomas of the gingiva [73], lip [74], and the palate [75].

Observations on the structure of the tumor cells and the pattern in which the tumor invades normal host tissue were incorporated into a single observation in two studies on squamous cell carcinomas of the floor of the mouth [45] and oropharynx [8]. The stage of invasion does not appear to be pertinent, as microcarcinoma and early carcinoma represent different clinical problems and most squamous cell carcinomas fit into Jakobsson's group of 'massive involvement'. For this reason, this category was dropped in subsequent studies and the histological evaluation of multiple parameters was modified substantially (Table 5) [8].

Invasiveness

A study of uniformly treated squamous cell carcinomas of the oropharynx showed that the pattern of invasion was the histological feature of greatest prognostic importance [8]. In an evaluation of similar-sized tumors and excluding all clinical factors in the regression analysis, increased frequency of mitoses was also noted to show significant correlation with ultimate survival, but the infiltrating pattern of the tumor was found to be by far the most important factor.

In another study of squamous cell carcinomas of the oral cavity it was noted that an infiltrating pattern of invasion was associated with a high frequency of regional lymph node metastasis [76]. In this latter study, of the patients with cord-like or single cell patterns of infiltration, approximately two-thirds were noted to have regional metastasis, whereas only one-seventh of the patients with better organized or more cohesive infiltrating patterns of tumor invasion developed metastases. In the larynx, it has also been noted that nodal metastases from tumors with 'pushing' margins occur in approximately 5% of cases whereas the incidence of metastases from infiltrative tumors approaches 50% [70]. When squamous cell carcinomas are divided into those with pushing margins as compared to those with infiltrating patterns of invasion, the latter pattern achieves the

Table 5. Grading scheme for squamous cell carcinoma of the oropharynx [8]

Histologic parameter	Score			
	1	2	3	4
Cytoplasmic keratinization	High degree, well-formed pearls	Moderate, 20–50% of cells, attempts at pearl formation	Poor, 5–20% of cells with suggestion of keratinization	No evidence of keratinization
Nuclear differentiation	Few enlarged nuclei >75% mature appearing	50–75% mature appearing nuclei	considerable nuclear pleomorphism, 25% mature appearing	Anaplastic tumor
Mitoses, average number/HPF	0–1	2–3	4–5	>5
Inflammatory response	Continuous rim	Patchy rim	Occasional patch	None
Vascular/ lymphatic invasion	Not identified	Not identified	Not identified	Identified
Pattern of invasion	Pushing borders	Solid cords	Thin, irregular cords	Single cells

same degree of statistical significance in predicting regional lymph node metastasis as does tumor grade [37, 69].

Progression involves a propensity for the carcinoma to penetrate and release cells into lymph or blood vascular spaces. Although demonstration of vascular invasion has not been found an important prognostic factor except in isolated studies [8], its presence in initial biopsies from many head and neck sites is associated with regional lymph node metastases [11]. It has also been reported that lymph node metastasis is associated with nerve sheath invasion in carcinomas of the larynx [37], lip [78], and oral tongue [79].

Submucosal and soft tissue invasion by carcinomas of the floor of the mouth has been shown to be an important independent prognostic factor for T2 lesions of this region [45], predicting a high frequency of local recurrence and regional lymph node metastases. Depth of invasion is also indirectly assessed in the laryngeal TNM criterion of impaired vocal cord mobility or fixation which relates to vocalis muscle infiltration by tumor [80]. It may be concluded that in a comparison of tumor stage and histological features, the factors relating to stage have a much greater statistical power in predicting ultimate prognosis of squamous cell carcinomas of the upper aerodigestive tract [8].

Factors related to therapy

Tumor-free margins in the surgical resection are predictive of non-recurrence of carcinoma [2] but the criteria for such a margin differ between studies. A clinicopathologic study of hemi-laryngectomy specimens which defined positive margins as those with carcinoma and carcinoma *in situ* but not varying degrees of atypia, found that of 39 patients with positive margins, only 7 (18%) developed a local recurrence compared to 4 of 72 patients (6%) who had cancer-free margins [81].

In Looser's study of head and neck carcinomas, there was a significant increase in local recurrence and mortality for patients with tumor in the resection margins when compared to those with tumor-free margins [82]. In this study, the definition of a positive margin included tumor within 0.5 cm of a margin, epithelial atypia, *in situ* and invasive carcinoma. Overall, 71% of the patients with positive margins developed local recurrence, ranging from 62.5% for stage I to 90% for stage IV disease. In comparison, 31.7% of patients with negative margins developed local recurrence at the primary site, ranging from 14.5% for stage I neoplasms to 47.3% for stage IV tumors. The frequency of positive margins also appears to correlate with tumor size.

Both radiation and chemotherapy appear to have the greatest effect on rapidly dividing tumors but rapidly proliferating neoplasms are usually poorly differentiated and have the poorest survival rates. Higher response rates were reported in poorly differentiated carcinomas in patients treated with combination chemotherapy, radiation and surgery in one series [83], and confirmed in a multi-institutional RTOG study [84], but were not translated into improved survival rates. Improved survival rates were however observed in patients with differentiated tumors that responded to therapy [83].

Combination chemotherapy response rates vary greatly, with complete clinical responses rates as high as 54% reported from therapy with 5-FU infusion and cisplatin [17]. This report also noted an improved survival rate in patients achieving a complete clinical response and it is has also been observed in other studies [85]. It is noteworthy that no tumor recurrences have occurred at 36 months in patients with complete pathologic responses and patients with pathologically proven complete response appear to have the potential for cure [86]. Complete clinical responses are less likely to occur in patients with advanced regional lymph node metastases and the best responders are those reported as N0 on clinical examination [17]. The presence of node metastasis decreases the tumor sensitivity to chemotherapy, and distant metastases appear to be even more resistant [63].

Biological variables

It is possible to determine the percentage of cells within a tumor that are actively synthesizing DNA (S-phase fraction) by incubating viable tumor with tritiated thymidine. It has been demonstrated that well differentiated or verrucous carcinomas demonstrate S-phase incorporation of tritiated thymidine in the cells of the basal and parabasal zones, similar to that observed in normal squamous epithelium [87]. Infiltrating squamous cell carcinomas show tritiated thymidine uptake throughout the neoplasm, except in the maturing keratinized cells.

DNA histograms which reflect DNA content in neoplastic cells can be obtained either by Feulgen microspectrophotometry on thick tissue sections, or by use of flow cytometry on disaggregated single cell preparations of the tumor. Cytophotometrically-determined DNA indices, which for the most part reflect abnormally increased amounts of DNA within the neoplastic cell population, have been shown to correlate with survival in head and neck cancer [88]. Tumors with diploid or hypodiploid DNA values are associated with longer survival even in advanced stage disease [89].

Several studies have attempted to correlate stage of tumor, size of primary, degree of nodal involvement, and grade of tumor with abnormal or aneuploid DNA histograms [90, 91]. The incidence of aneuploidy in dissociated fresh tumor specimens [92] has been found to correlate well with retrospective study of nuclei retrieved from paraffin-embedded tissue specimens [93], where aneuploidy was demonstrated in 86% of squamous cell carcinomas from the head and neck region.

Using fixed sections for examining DNA histograms for the tumor S-phase fraction, it was noted that an aneuploid DNA index and high proliferative activity (as reflected by the S-phase fraction) were more commonly associated with nuclear pleomorphism, while well differentiated squamous cell carcinomas commonly displayed aneuploid DNA histograms but only a low S-phase fraction. In general, it appears that techniques measuring DNA ploidy and S-phase fractions within squamous cell carcinomas may be correlated with biological progression.

Conclusion

For squamous cell carcinoma of the head and neck region, the anatomic extent of disease, reflected in the clinical staging and confirmed by pathologic staging, is the most important factor in prognosis. In addition, the stage of disease is the major determinant in planning therapy. The site of the primary squamous cell carcinoma is the second most important parameter in determining prognosis, but stage and site are inter-related and cannot be evaluated separately. Squamous cell carcinomas occurring in sites such as floor of mouth and glottis lead to early diagnosis, whereas relatively 'silent' neoplasms occurring in maxillary sinus or hypopharynx often reach an advanced stage.

Histopathologic parameters are less well understood as factors in prognosis, but pattern of invasion and histologic grading may influence response to therapy. New biological indices may allow identification of other tumor characteristics with a clearer prognostic significance.

References

1. Boddie AWJr, Fischer EP, Byers M: Squamous carcinoma of the lower lip in patients under 40 years of age. *South Med J* 70: 711–712, 1977
2. Jacobs JR, Spitznagel EL, Sessions DG: Staging parameters for cancers of the head and neck: A multi-factorial analysis. *Laryngoscope* 95: 1378–1381, 1985
3. Platz H, Fries R, Hudec M, Tjoa AM, Wagner RR: The prognostic relevance of various factors at the time of the first admission of the patient. Retrospective DOSAK study on carcinoma of the oral cavity. *J Max-Fac Surg* 11: 3–12, 1983
4. Hibbert J, Marks NJ, Winter PJ, Shaheen OH: Prognostic factors in oral squamous carcinoma and their relation to clinical staging. *Clin Otolaryngol* 8: 197–203, 1983
5. Wolf GT, Makuch R, Baker S: Predictive factors for tumor response to preoperative chemotherapy in patients with head and neck squamous carcinoma. *Cancer* 54: 2869–2877, 1984
6. Niederer J, Hawkins NV, Rider WD, Till JE: Failure analysis of radical radiation therapy of supraglottic laryngeal carcinoma. *Int J Radiation Oncol Biol Phys* 2: 621–629, 1976
7. Shah JP, Cendon RA, Farr HW, Strong EW: Carcinoma of the oral cavity. Factors affecting treatment failure at the primary site and neck. *Am J Surg* 132: 504–507, 1976
8. Crissman JD, Liu WY, Gluckman JL, Cummings G: Prognostic value of histopathologic parameters in squamous cell carcinoma the oropharynx. *Cancer* 54: 2995–3001, 1984
9. Ratzer ER, Schweitzer RJ, Frazell EL: Epidermoid carcinoma of the palate. *Am J Surg* 119: 294–297, 1970

10. Cann CI, Fried MP, Rothman KJ: Epidemiology of squamous cell cancer of the head and neck. *Otolaryngol Clin N America* 18: 1–22, 1985

11. Saranath D, Mukhopadhyaya R, Rao R, Fakih AR, Naik SL, Gangal SG: Cell-mediated immune status in patients with squamous cell carcinoma of the oral cavity. *Cancer* 56: 1062–1070, 1985

12. Bier J, Ulrike N, Platz H: The doubtful relevance of nonspecific immune reactivity in patients with squamous cell carcinoma of the head and neck region. *Cancer* 52: 1165–1172, 1983

13. Amer MH, Al-Sarraf M, Vaitkevicius VK: Factors that affect response to chemotherapy and survival of patients with advanced head and neck cancer. *Cancer* 43: 2202–2206, 1979

14. Pajak T, Davis L, Faxekas J, Laramore G: Prognostic factors in head and neck tumors for patients initially treated with radiation therapy. *Proc Am Soc Clin Oncol* 3: 185, 1984

15. *Manual for Staging of Cancer,* American Joint Committee on Cancer (2nd edition) Beahrs OH, Meyers MH (eds), Philadelphia, Lippincott, 1983

16. Union Internationale Contre le Cancer. *TNM-Atlas, Illustrated Guide to the Classification of Malignant Tumors,* Spiessel B, Scheibe O, Wagner G (eds), Springer-Verlag, Berlin, 1982

17. Rooney M, Kish J, Jacobs J, Kinzie J, Weaver A, Crissman J, Al-Sarraf M.: Improved complete response rate and survival in advanced head and neck cancer after three-course induction therapy with 120–hour 5–FU infusion and cisplatin. *Cancer* 55: 1123–1128, 1985

18. Spiro RH, Strong EW: Surgical treatment of cancer of the tongue. *Surg Clin N America* 54: 759–765, 1974

19. Decroix Y, Ghoessein NA: Experience of the Curie Institute in treatment of cancer of the mobile tongue. I. Treatment policies and results. *Cancer* 47: 496–502, 1981

20. Harrold CC Jr: Management of cancer of the floor of the mouth. *Am J. Surg* 122: 487–493, 1971

21. Flynn MB, Mullias FX, Moore C: Selection of treatment in squamous cell carcinoma of the floor of the mouth. *Am J Surg* 126: 477–481, 1973

22. Ballard BR, Suess GR, Pickren IW, *et al*: Squamous cell carcinoma of the floot of the mouth. *Oral Surg* 45: 568–579, 1978

23. Bloom ND, Spiro RH: Carcinoma of the cheek mucosa. A retrospective analysis. *Am J Surg* 140: 556–559, 1980.

24. Nathanson A, Jakobsson PA, Wersall J: Prognosis of squamous cell carcinoma of the gums. *Acta Otolaryngol* 75: 301–303, 1973

25. Evans JF, Shah JP: Epidermoid carcinoma of the palate. *Am J Surg* 142: 451–455, 1981

26. Chung CK, Rahman SM, Lim ML, Constable WC: Squamous cell carcinoma of the hard palate. *Int J Radiat Oncol Biol Phys* 5: 191–196, 1979

27. Fee WE Jr, Schoeppel SL, Rubenstein R *et al*: Squamous cell carcinoma of the soft palate. *Arch Otolaryngol* 105: 710–718, 1979

28. Cheng VST, Shetty KS, Deutsch M: Carcinoma of the anterior tonsillar pillar and the soft palate-uvula: Treatment by radiation therapy. *Radiology* 134: 497–501, 1980

29. Chung CK, Constable WC: Squamous cell carcinoma of the soft palate and uvula. *Int J Radiat Oncol Biol Phys* 5: 845–850, 1979

30. Krause CJ, Lee JG, McCabe BF: Carcinoma of the oral cavity. A comparison of therapeutic modalities. *Arch Otolaryngol* 97: 354–358, 1973

31. Givens CD Jr, Johns ME, Cantrell RW: Carcinoma of the tonsil. Analysis of 162 cases. *Arch Otolaryngol* 107: 730–734, 1981

32. Barrs DM, DeSanto LW, O'Fallon WM: Squamous cell carcinoma of the tonsil and tongue-base region. *Arch Otolaryngol* 105: 479–485, 1979

33. Shah JP, Tollefsen HR: Epidermoid carcinoma of the supraglottic larynx. Role of neck dissection in initial treatment. *Am J Surg* 128: 494–499, 1974

34. Razack MS, Silapasvang S, Sako K, and Shedd DP: Significance of site and nodal metastases in squamous cell carcinoma of the epiglottis. *Am J Surg* 136: 520–524, 1978

35. Daly CJ, Strong EW: Carcinoma of the glottic larynx. *Am J Surg* 130: 489–492, 1975.

36. Shear M, Hawkins DM, Farr HW: The prediction of lymph node metastases from oral squamous carcinoma. *Cancer* 37: 1901–1907, 1976

37. McGavran MH, Bauer WC, Ogura JH: The incidence of cervical lymph node metastases from epidermoid carcinoma of the larynx and their relationship to certain characteristics of the primary tumor. A study based on the clinical and pathological findings for 96 patients treated by primary en bloc laryngectomy and radical neck dissection. *Cancer* 14: 55–66, 1961

38. Som ML: Conservation surgery for carcinoma of the supra-glottis. *J Laryngol Otol* 84: 655–678, 1970

39. Futrell JW, Bennett SH, Hoye RC, Roth JA, Ketcham AS: Predicting survival in cancer of the larynx or hypopharynx. *Am J Surg* 122: 451–457, 1971

40. Cross JE, Guralnick E, Daland EM: Carcinoma of the lip: A review of 563 case records of carcinoma of the lip at Pondville Hospital. *Surg Gynecol Obstet* 87: 153–162, 1948

41. Baker SR, Krause CJ: Cancer of the lip. In: *Cancer of the Head and Neck,* Suen JY, Myers EN (eds), Churchill Livingstone, New York, 1981, pp 280–300

42. Wurman LH, Adams GL, Myerhoff WL: Carcinoma of the lip. *Am J Surg* 130: 470–474, 1975

43. Skolnick EM, Yee KF, Wheatley MA, Martin LO: Panel discussion on glottic tumors. V Carcinoma of the laryngeal glottis therapy and end results. *Laryngoscope* 85: 1453–1466, 1975

44. Ballard BR, Suess GR, Pickren JW. *et al*: Squamous cell carcinoma of the floor of the mouth. *Oral Surg* 45: 568–579, 1978

45. Crissman JD, Gluckman J, Whiteley J, Quenelle D: Squamous cell carcinoma of the floor of the mouth. *Head Neck Surg* 3: 2–7, 1980

46. Lyall D, Shetlin CF: Cancer of the tongue. *Ann Surg* 135: 489, 1952

47. Lee JG, Litton WB: Symposium on malignancy. II. Occult regional metastasis: carcinoma of the oral tongue. *Laryngoscope* 82: 1273–1281, 1972

48. Stell PM. Tumors of the oropharynx. *Clin Otolaryngol* 1: 71–90, 1976

49. Kalnins IK, Leonard AG, Sako K, Razack MS, Shedd DP: Correlation between prognosis and degree of lymph node involvement in carcinoma of the oral cavity. *Am J Surg* 134: 450–454, 1977

50. Skolnick EM, Saberman MN: Cancer of the tongue. *Otolargyngol Clin N America* 2: 603, 1969

51. MacComb WS: Radical neck dissection. In: *Cancer of the Head and Neck,* MacComb, WS, Fletcher GH (eds), Williams and Wilkins Co, Baltimore, 1967, pp 488–506

52. Bennett SH, Futrell JW, Roth JA, Hoye RC, Ketcham AS: Prognostic significance of histologic host response in cancer of the larynx or hypopharynx. *Cancer* 28: 1255–1265, 1971

53. Johnson JT, Barnes EL, Myers EN, Schramm VL, Borochovitz D, Sigler BA: The extracapsular spread of tumors in cervical node metastasis. *Arch Otolaryngol* 107: 725–729, 1981

54. Snyderman NL, Johnson JT, Schramm VL Jr, Myers EN, Bedetti CD, Thearle P: Extracapsular spread of carcinoma in cervical lymph nodes. Impact upon survival in patients with carcinoma of the supraglottic larynx. *Cancer* 56: 1597–1599, 1985

55. Gilmore BB, Repola DA, Batsakis JG: Carcinoma of the larynx: lymph node reaction patterns. *Laryngoscope* 88: 1333–1338, 1978

56. Berlinger NT, Tsakraklides V, Pollak K, Adams GL, Yang M, Good RA: Prognostic significance of lymph node histology in patients with squamous cell carcinoma of the larynx, pharynx or oral cavity. *Laryngoscope* 86: 792–803, 1976

57. Batsakis JG, Hybels SR, Rice DH: Laryngeal carcinomas, stomal recurrences and distant metastases. In: *Centennial Conference on Laryngeal Cancer,* Alberti PW, Bryce DP (eds), Appleton-Century-Crofts, New York, 1976, pp 868–876

58. Crile GW: Carcinoma of the jaws, tongue, cheek and lips. *Surg Gyncol Obstet* 36: 159–184, 1923

59. Probert JC, Thompson RW, Bagshaw MA: Patterns of distant metastases in head and neck cancer. *Cancer* 33: 127–133, 1974

60. Merino OR, Lindberg RD, Fletcher GH: An analysis of distant metastases from squamous cell carcinoma of the upper respiratory and digestive tracts. *Cancer* 40: 145–151, 1977

61. Papac RJ. Distant metastases from head and neck cancer. *Cancer* 53: 342–345, 1984

304

62. Slotman GJ, Mohit T, Raina S, Swaminathan AP, Ohanian M, Rush BF: The incidence of metastases after multimodal therapy for cancer of the head and neck. *Cancer* 54: 2009–2014, 1984
63. Kish JA, Weaver A, Jacobs J, Cummings G, Al-Sarraf M: Cisplatin and 5–fluorouracil infusion in patients with recurrent and disseminated epidermoid cancer of the head and neck. *Cancer* 53: 1819–1824, 1984
64. Weaver A, Fleming SM, Knechtges TC, Smith D: Triple endoscopy: A neglected essential in head and neck cancer. *Surgery* 86: 493–496, 1979
65. Gluckman JL, Crissman JD, Donegan JO: Multicentric squamous cell carcinoma of the upper aerodigestive tract. *Head Neck Surg* 3: 90–96, 1980
66. Tepperman BS, Fitzpatrick PJ. Second respiratory and upper disgestive tract cancers after oral cancer. *Lancet* 2: 547–549, 1981
67. Gluckman JL, Crissman JD: Survival rates in 548 patients with multiple neoplasms of the upper aerodigestive tract. *Laryngoscope* 93: 71–74, 1983
68. Broders AC: Carcinoma. Grading and practical application. *Arch Pathol* 2: 376–381, 1926
60. Kashima HK: The characteristics of laryngeal cancer correlating with cervical lymph node metastasis (analysis based on 40 total organ sections). In: *Centennial Conference on Laryngeal Cancer,* Alberti PW and Bryce DP (eds), Appleton-Century-Crofts, New York, 1976, pp 855–864
70. Bauer WC, Edwards DL, McGavran MH: A critical analysis of laryngectomy in the treatment of epidermoid carcinoma of the larynx. *Cancer* 15: 263–270, 1962
71. Martin SA, Marks JE. Lee JY, Bauer WL, Ogura JH: Carcinoma of the pyriform sinus: predictors of TNM relapse and survival. *Cancer* 46: 1974–1981, 1980
72. Jakobsson PA: Histologic grading of malignancy and prognosis in glottic carcinoma of the larynx. In: *Centennial Conference on Laryngeal Cancer,* Alberti PW, Bryce DP (eds), Appleton-Century-Crofts, New York, 1976, pp 847–854
73. Willen R, Nathanson A: Squamous cell carcinoma of the gingiva. *Acta Otolaryngol* 75: 299–300, 1973
74. Lund C, Segaard H, Elbrond O, Jorgensen K, Anderson AP: Epidermoid carcinoma of the lip. *Acta Radiol Ther Phys Biol* 14: 465–474, 1975
75. Eneroth CM, Moberger G: Histological malignancy grading of squamous cell carcinoma of the palate. *Acta Otolaryngol* 75: 293–295, 1973
76. Yamamoto E, Miyakawa A, Kohama G: Mode of invasion and lymph node metastasis in squamous cell carcinoma of the oral cavity. *Head Neck Surg* 6: 938–947, 1984
77. Poleksic S, Kalwaic HJ: Prognostic value of vascular invasion in squamous cell carcinoma of the head and neck. *Plast Reconstr Surg* 61: 234–240, 1978
78. Byers RM, O'Brien J, Waxler J: The therapeutic and prognostic implications of nerve invasion in cancer of the lower lip. *Int J Radiat Oncol Biol Phys* 4: 215–217, 1978
79. Carter RL, Tanner HSB, Clifford P, Shaw HJ: Perineural spread in squamous cell carcinomas of the head and neck: a clinicopathologic study. *Clin Otolaryngol* 4: 271–281, 1979
80. Lesinski SG, Bauer WC, Ogura JH: Hemilaryngectomy for T3 (fixed cord) epidermoid carcinoma of the larynx. *Laryngoscope* 86: 1563–1571, 1976
81. Bauer WC, Lesinski SG, Ogura JH: The significance of positive margins in hemilaryngectomy specimens. *Laryngoscope* 85: 1–13, 1975
82. Looser KG, Shah JP, Strong EW: The significance of 'positive' margins in surgically resected epidermoid carcinomas. *Head Neck Surg* 1: 107–111, 1978
83. Ensley J, Crissman J, Kish J, Jacobs J, Weaver A, Kinzie J, Cummings G, Al-Sarraf M: The impact of conventional morphologic analysis on response rates and survival in patients with advanced head and neck cancers treated initially with cisplatin-containing combination chemotherapy. *Cancer* 57: 711–717, 1986
84. Crissman J, Pajak T, Al-Sarraf M, Marcial V: Prediction of response in advanced head and neck carcinomas by histologic parameters. An RTOG pathology study. *Proceedings AACR* abstract, Los Angeles, California, 1986

85. Kies MS, Gordon LI, Hauck WW, Krespi Y, Ossoff RH, Pecaro BC, Yuska c, Lamut CH, Brand WN, Chang SK, Shetty M, Sisson GA: Analysis of complete responders after initial treatment with chemotherapy in head and neck cancer. *Otolaryngol Head Neck Surg* 93: 199–205, 1985
86. Al-Kourainy K, Kish J, Ensley J, Tapazoglou E, Jacobs J, Weaver A, Crissman J, Cummings G, Al-Sarraf M: Improved survival in pathologic complete responders to cisplatinum combination in patients with locally advanced head and neck cancer. In press
87. Prioleau PG, Santa-Cruz DJ, Meyer JS, Bauer WC: Verrucous carcinoma. A light and electron microscopic, autoradiographic, and immunofluorescence study. *Cancer* 45: 2849–2857, 1980
88. Bocking A, Auffermann W, Vogel H, Schlondorff G, Goebbels R: Diagnosis and grading of malignancy in squamous epithelial lesions of the larynx with DNA cytophotometry. *Cancer* 56: 1600–1604, 1985
89. Holm LE: Cellular DNA amounts of squamous cell carcinomas of the head and neck region in relation to prognosis. *Laryngoscope* 92: 1064–1069, 1982
90. Crissman JD, Ensley J, Maciorowski Z: Flow cytometric analysis of DNA content in squamous cell carcinomas. *IAP abstract,* Toronto, Canada, 1985
91. Crissman JD, Ensley J: Histopathology as a prognostic factor in the treatment of squamous cell cancer of the head and neck. In: *Head and Neck Cancer,* Vol 1, Chretian P, Johns M, Shedd D, Strong E, Ward P (eds), BC Decker, Inc Philadelphia, 1985, pp 92–96
92. Grabel-Pietrusky R, Hornstein OP: Flow cytometric measurement of ploidy and proliferative activity of carcinomas of the oropharyngeal mucosa. *Arch Dermatol Res* 273: 121–128, 1982
93. Johnson TS, Williamson KD, Cramer MM, Peters LJ: Flow cytometric analysis of head and neck carcinoma DNA index and S-fraction from paraffin-embedded sections: Comparison with malignancy grading. *Cytometry* 6: 461–470, 1985

18. Prognostic indices in colorectal cancer

S.J. ARNOTT

Colorectal cancer shows considerable geographic variations in its incidence [1] and differences between the sexes in its age and site incidence [2]. Because the survival rates following surgery have remained static for many years [3, 4] it is now accepted that to determine the most appropriate management for each patient, we will need to recognise factors which determine the prognosis in that individual.

Clinical trials have been set up to evaluate the effectiveness of treatment in different subsets of patients and to evaluate the relative strengths of different prognostic factors [5, 6, 7]. Pointers to the possible outcome for any individual patient may come from the history and clinical findings at presentation, from information gained at the time of operation, from pathological examination of the resected specimen and from biological markers.

Symptomatology and prognosis

The vast majority of patients with colonic cancer present with vague symptoms and chronic ill-health. The remainder may have a variety of symptoms ranging from intestinal obstruction or perforation to altered bowel habit and, especially in rectal tumours, the passage of blood and mucus.

Bleeding

Patients who present with rectal bleeding have a better than average prognosis [8]. This symptom causes patients concern and expedites their seeking medical advice. They are predominantly cases with rectal tumours, and their better prognosis suggests that bleeding from rectal cancers may occur at an earlier pathological stage than bleeding from more proximal tumours. However, it should be noted that those patients with right sided tumours who present with haemorrhage also have a better prognosis [9].

Obstruction

Colorectal cancer presenting with obstruction is said to be associated with a poor prognosis [8, 9, 10, 11, 12]. Obstruction is seen particularly with tumours of the transverse and descending colon and rectosigmoid junction and the survival rates of patients with obstructing cancers is said to be half of that of those who do not have evidence of obstruction [8, 21].

Several reasons may combine to explain this poor survival. First, only about 50% of patients presenting in this way are suitable for curative surgery [10, 12]. Second, surgery is associated with much higher operative morbidity and mortality rates [12]. Even in those patients who do have a potentially curative operation, survival rates are still poor and as a general rule, patients presenting with obstruction have tumours of a more advanced stage. Finally, experiments on dogs in whom the intraluminal pressure of the bowel was increased, show that lymph flow may be increased by a factor of four to six [13]. Thus patients with obstructing carcinomas are more likely to have lymph node metastases and a correspondingly poorer survival [14]. While the majority view is that intestinal obstruction is associated with a poor prognosis, there have been reports to the contrary [11, 15].

Perforation

As might be expected, patients presenting with perforation of the bowel due to tumour have a dismal prognosis, probably related to the implantation of tumour cells within the abdomen. When obstruction and perforation are both present, the prognosis is even worse [16].

Duration of symptoms

Convincing evidence that early detection of colorectal cancer in asymptomatic patients leads to improved survival comes from a long-term clinical study in Minnesota [17]. Over a 28 year period 21,150 men and women were examined by annual proctosigmoidoscopy. At the first examination 27 tumours were found. Subsequently at each annual examination all adenomatous polyps were removed. The subsequent incidence of developing cancers was only 15% of that expected from epidemiological data. The five year survival of the 27 patients detected at the first examination was 64%, twice that reported for symptomatic cancer [18]. The prognosis for patients whose tumours were detected subsequently was even better, with an 85% five year survival.

The disadvantages of annual proctosigmoidoscopy are that it is time-consuming and expensive and the return is low [19]. These problems have stimulated the introduction of faecal occult blood testing [20] and patients with a positive test are then subjected to proctocolonoscopy.

A paradoxical finding is that patients who present with symptoms of long duration have an improved prognosis [8], whereas for those with a short history the outlook is poorer [21]. This is, at least in part, explained by the fact that those tumours which cause patients to seek early advice are often biologically aggressive [10]. A higher proportion of patients in this category have obstructing cancers [22] of high grade [21, 22]. Thus, any potential benefit which might result from the seeking of early attention is offset by the virulent nature of the tumour. On the other hand, in those with less acute symptoms which may be of long duration, there is a tendency for the tumour to be less aggressive, and therefore associated with a better prognosis.

This does not imply that delay in dealing with symptomatic patients is to be encouraged, since it may mean that emergency surgery becomes necessary in a greater proportion with a correspondingly greater related hospital mortality. Earlier diagnosis may place a higher proportion of patients in the elective surgical group [23]. However, for most patients with colorectal cancer with histories of intermediate length, there is no clear correlation between prognosis and length of history.

Age and gender

In patients over the age of 70 the prognosis is worse [24], but it is likely that the effect on survival is through a higher operative mortality [25, 26], and a higher rate of death from diseases other than colorectal cancer [26]. Some have suggested that patients under the age of thirty who develop colorectal cancer fare badly, with survival nearly half that of older patients [10], while improved survival in young patients has been reported from other centres [27]. When the reports of several series are pooled, it seems that patients under the age of 30 have a greater proportion of poorly differentiated and mucinous tumours, both of which carry a poorer prognosis [10].

Most reports do not describe any influence of gender on prognosis in colorectal cancer, although a more favourable outlook has been reported in female patients [8, 27]. The latter reports come from single centres and there may be a selection bias producing such an effect.

Clinical findings and prognosis

Size of the primary tumour

There is a close relationship between the size of a tumour and its potential to spread for nearly every type of human cancer. However, in the case of colorectal cancer, the size of the tumour as determined by the clinicial is frequently not an accurate assessment ot its true size, and it is therefore difficult to correlate tumour size with prognosis [10].

Configuration of the primary tumour

Colorectal tumours which are exophytic and of a polypoid nature tend to have a better prognosis than those which are sessile and ulcerated [10]. Although different clinicians may use different descriptive terms for the same lesion [28], a correlation between the configuration of the primary tumour, incidence of lymph node metastases, venous invasion and survival has been made. Coller *et al.* [29] noted a 54% incidence of lymph node metastases in polypoid tumours and an 81% incidence in sessile lesions.

In a review of 1592 patients from St. Mark's Hospital in London [30], fungating tumours were found to have a 23% incidence of venous invasion, ulcerating tumours a 31% incidence and stenosing tumours a 45% incidence. Therefore, while there are differences between clinicians in their assessment of the configuration of the primary tumour, it provides useful guidance to prognosis.

Anatomical site of the primary tumour

There is some controversy concerning the influence of tumour site on prognosis. While some reports indicate that long-term survival is not influenced by whether the tumour arises in the colon or the rectum [31, 8], differences in survival rates between patients with colonic and rectal tumours have been described, particularly in the USA [32].

Site does however clearly affect survival in rectal cancer with tumours of the lower rectum faring significantly worse. The height of the tumour within the rectum, as assessed preoperatively was found to be one of the most important prognostic indices [24]. When the tumour arose in the lower 5 cm of the rectum the five-year survival was 42% and this increased to 64% when the carcinoma was found above 9 cm. Similar findings have been demonstrated by other investigators [33].

Tumours lying below the level of the peritoneal reflection are covered by one less protective tissue layer, and in addition are more diffucult to remove surgically because of their anatomical position [34]. A further factor which may be of importance is the lymphatic drainage pathways for low lying tumours. Carcinomas of the upper rectum metastasize via the superior haemorrhoidal lymphatics whereas lower tumours would also spread via the middle and inferior haemorrhoidal lymphatic vessels.

Number of quadrants involved

The number of quadrants of the bowel wall involved by tumour has prognostic importance in rectal cancer [24, 28, 35]. This is probably true for colonic tumours as well, because as noted above, colonic tumours presenting with obstruction carry a particularly poor prognosis [8, 12]. In a group of patients with rectal cancer, curative resection was possible in 72% of cases when only one quadrant was involved, compared with 55% if two or more quadrants were involved [24]. A relationship has been postulated between the number of quadrants involved and the incidence of lymph node involvement [29] and venous invasion [36].

Mobility

A significant prognostic factor in patients with rectal cancer is the degree of 'tethering' of the tumour as discerned clinically. Although this may be due to inflammatory changes rather than malignant extension [4], the surgeon is capable of detecting this feature with accuracy, and it does have a close relationship to survival rates [24, 28, 35]. When there is obvious invasion of adjacent organs or structures, survival is poor [10], but even when less extensive spread has occurred, it may be the single most important factor determining the outlook for patients [11, 35]. In one trial, the survival rate for patients with mobile tumours was 48% compared to only 29% when tethering was present. No clear difference could be demonstrated between patients with partially fixed and those with completely fixed cancers [24].

Dukes and Bussey [37] in a large review, found that the age-corrected survival rate for patients with only slight extra-rectal invasion was 89.7%, but 57% in those with extensive spread. They also demonstrated that the greater the degree of extra-rectal spread, the more likely was the tumour to be of high grade malignancy, to be associated with lymphatic metastases and to have venous spread. Nevertheless, controversy continues on the ability of the clinician to differentiate on clinical grounds between malignant and inflammatory tethering. Newer imaging techniques such as computerised tomography (CT) are capable of identifying the cause of tethering with a great deal of accuracy [4], and are of particular value in patients with high rectal and colonic tumours where clinical assessment is more difficult.

Pathological features and prognosis

Tumour grading

One of the earliest efforts by pathologists to predict the outcome for individual cancer patients was by the use of histopathological grading [38]. Grinnell introduced a widely used modification specifically applicable to colorectal cancer, which attempts to evaluate the behaviour of the tumour according to invasiveness, glandular arrangement, loss of polarity and number of mitoses [39]. Another widely employed system is that of Dukes [40], which graded the tumour according to the cell type, but was later modified to incorporate also the differentiation of the cells [37].

Whilst there is general agreement that poorly differentiated tumours carry a worse prognosis in the case of colorectal cancer, there are few reproducible criteria for the classification of degree of malignancy. New gradings have been developed [41] and are becoming more widely used, but except at the extremes of grade, tumour differentiation and survival are not closely correlated. Most tumours are heterogeneneous, and different degrees of differentiation may be found in different areas of the lesion [42, 43, 44]. However, if multiple biopsies are performed, especially of the deep margins of the tumour, then the discrepancies are reduced [4, 39]. The deep margins of the tumour are likely to contain the areas of poorest differentiation and the behaviour of the cancer is most closely related to these cells.

Tumours of high grade carry a poor prognosis because such cancers have a higher incidence of local invasion [11, 39], an increased frequency of venous invasion [30, 36, 44] and metastases to lymph nodes [37,39, 40]. There is some controversy as to whether poorly differentiated lesions have an increased frequency of distant metastases [11] but the increased incidence of lymphatic and venous invasion seen with such tumours make this likely.

Flow cytometry

Biopsies used for histological assessment may be analysed for DNA content using flow cytometry. It has been demonstrated that patients with non-diploid cancers of the colon and rectum have a significantly worse prognosis than those with diploid tumours [4, 45]. Various staining techniques may be used, but perhaps the most useful is that employing acridine orange and ethidium bromide which allows scattergrams to be made of DNA/RNA concentrations rather than DNA histograms [42]. When over 10% of cells in a tumour contain more than twice the normal DNA content, they are defined as non-diploid [4].

Cell type

Adenocarcinomas of the colon and rectum of certain cell types are considered to carry a particularly poor prognosis. For example, tumours which secrete large amounts of mucus are said to fare particularly badly [43] and in a study carried out by Symonds and Vickery [46], the five year survival in patients with mucoid adenocarcinoma was found to be only 34% compared to 53% in those with non-mucoid tumours. The outlook for patients with mucoid rectal cancers was particularly bad, only 18% surviving for five years compared with non-mucoid lesions. This poor prognosis exists even if the tumour is well differentiated and the lymph nodes are uninvolved by tumour [39], but if nodes are clearly involved, there are few long term survivors [10].

When mucus production is large, but intracellular, the tumour cells have a signet-ring appearance. This variant also has a particularly poor outlook. Mucoid tumours as a whole, tend to occur with greater frequency in young people, and this may contribute to the poor outlook seen in patients below the age of 30 [10].

Local tumour invasion

The factor most clearly influencing whether a curative resection can be performed is the local invasiveness of the tumour, and pre-operative assessment of mobility will decide the likelihood of such an operation being possible. Loco-regional recurrence increases when tumours extend completely through the bowel wall, and prognosis is closely correlated with the degree of extra-rectal spread [34]. In one study [47], local tumour invasion appeared as important as lymph node involvement in influencing survival but these two factors are closely interrelated. Lymph node metastases only rarely occur before the primary tumour has penetrated through the bowel wall, yet at the same time the extent of penetration is associated with a poorer prognosis independent of lymph node status.

Lymph node metastases

It is difficult to assess the significance of lymph node metastases as an independent factor, since other features which adversely influence prognosis are closely related to the involvement of lymph nodes. For example, in the MRC1 trial of rectal cancer [24] those patients found to have lymph node metastases also had a higher proportion of poorly differentiated tumours, cancers of larger size, and a greater proportion of tethered tumours. In addition, a smaller proportion of curative resections were performed when nodal metastases were present [26].

However, one series has shown that the presence of lymph node metastases can adversely affect survival irrespective of the degree of extramural infiltration [48].

When the degree of infiltration was slight and the nodes were negative the five-year survival rate was 73%, but when positive nodes were found the survival rate was only 43%. When extensive infiltration was present, the five-year survival was 45% when the nodes were negative, but only 15% when the nodes were positive.

There is evidence that when the nodes are not involved by tumour, but are instead demonstrating reactive changes such as histiocytosis and paracortical immunoblastic activity, the prognosis is improved [49].

Venous invasion

The majority of patients dying from colorectal cancer do so as a result of vascular spread [30, 48]. While invasion of intramural veins is not of prognostic significance and is not correlated with the development of metastases, invasion of extramural veins is strongly related to survival. This is particularly so when thick-walled extramural veins are involved [48]. Many reported series have not differentiated between intra- and extramural venous invasion. It has been suggested that venous invasion may be demonstrated histologically in as many as 52% of cases [50]. That it is directly related to the development of distant metastases is suggested by the observation that in patients in whom venous invasion was found the five-year survival rate was 43%, compared to 13% when venous spread was not present [50].

Venous invasion may occur in the absence of lymphatic metastases but its incidence increases along with the finding of other features which adversely affect prognosis. For example, invasion of veins is seen in about 70% of excavated, invasive tumours, but in only 36% of exophytic lesions [48]. The greater the depth of penetration of the bowel wall by tumour, the greater are the chances of developing distant metastases [50, 51]. The combination of venous invasion and local invasion has an additive unfavourable effect on prognosis [48]. Venous invasion is also found with increasing frequency in poorly differentiated tumours [51].

Metastases

Metastatic disease is found at the time of presentation in approximately one third of patients with large bowel cancer. The most common site of metastasis is the liver but lung secondaries may also occur. Metastatic disease in other situations is uncommon especially in the absence of liver or lung deposits. The site of the primary tumour is related to the site of metastases. Thus, pulmonary metastases in patients with rectal cancer may have arisen via the middle haemorrhoidal system and have by-passed the liver, but pulmonary metastases from a colonic primary will almost certainly have been derived from hepatic metastases. Therefore, while the presence of either pulmonary or hepatic metastases suggests a poor prognosis, liver deposits are by far the more serious [10].

The overall prognosis for patients with hepatic metastases is dismal but for patients with truly solitary metastatic disease, the median one-year survival is of the order of 80% and the three year survival 55%, following surgical resection [52]. On the other hand, all patients with localised or widespread multiple metastases are usually dead at four years and most die within two or three years [55].

Biological markers and prognosis

Since the first description of carcinoembryonic antigen (CEA) by Gold and Freedman [54], it has been found to be of value as a prognostic indicator, both at the pre-treatment stage of assessment and following surgical removal of colorectal cancer [11]. It was clearly shown that elevation of CEA could predict tumour recurrence in a large proportion of patients, often with a considerable lead time over clinical detection [55, 56].

The detection of elevated CEA levels following surgery frequently indicates the presence of recurrence [51] but in addition, the *pattern* of rise of the CEA titre following operation may differentiate between local recurrence and distant metastatic disease. A rapidly rising CEA level was said to be typically associated with metastatic spread, whereas slowly increasing titres were more frequently seen in patients with local recurrence [58]. Pre-operative CEA levels could also be of prognostic value, and there was a positive correlation between the level of pre-operative CEA and disease recurrence [58]. This was greatest when the CEA level was high [59].

More recently, it has been suggested that a combination of tumour-associated factors (such as CEA) together with various non-specific reactions to the presence of tumour will provide a better prognostic index than the use of any of these factors alone [4, 59, 60, 61]. A number of non-specific markers of malignancy have been studied including the acute phase reactant proteins (APRP's) c-reactive protein (CRP), α_1-acid glycoprotein (AGP) and α_1 antichymotrypsin (ACT). APRP's are primarily produced by the liver and increase as a non-specific response to a variety of stimuli, including malignancy. Other factors investigated are phosphohexose isomerase (PHI), gamma-glutamyl transpeptidase (γGT), serum pseudouridine (SPU), albumin and pre-albumin levels and transferrin.

Cooper and O'Quigley [60] have investigated the relationship of pre- and post-surgical levels of CEA and γGT to survival. They found that serial measurement of both these factors and any change in the levels which had occurred two months after surgery had a much greater prognostic significance than the estimation of either alone. Other studies have confirmed that a combination of CEA and APRP levels can be related to the fixity of tumours [61], especially fixation due to tumour extension rather than inflammation [4].

To summarise this section. Whilst measurement of CEA levels may provide information regarding prognosis, the accuracy of this information is limited when the levels are only slightly raised. The incorporation of measurements of APRP's into the equation significantly improves the accuracy of such information and in particular, seems capable of identifying those patients with locally invasive tumours which carry an especially poor prognosis. A rise often occurs in the serum level of acute phase proteins and in general, the tendency is for serum total proteins to fall with advancing disease, reflecting the patient's nutritional state.

Clinical staging and prognosis

Clinical staging of colorectal cancer allows clinicians to make treatment decisions based on knowledge of tumour extent, and also permits a comparison of different treatments in patients with similar stage disease. The system of Lockhart-Mummery [62] divided cases into three classes A, B and C, according to the extent of local tumour invasion and involvement of lymph nodes. Dukes refined and modified this staging classification, defining prognostic groups of patients according to the level at which lymphatic metastases were found [44, 63].

Most widely employed in the USA is the staging system of Astler and Coller [64]. Whilst tumours are still classified as A, B and C, the C categories in the Astler-Coller system refer to different depths of penetration of tumour in the bowel wall when lymph nodes are involved by tumour, and does not refer to different levels of lymph node metastases. The controversy surrounding staging persists and has mainly centred on the relative importance of local invasion and lymph node metastases in determining prognosis [47, 48].

With the introduction of adjuvant therapies into the management of patients with colorectal cancer, the importance of making therapeutic decisions *before* surgery has become apparent and this has led to increased enthusiasm for pre-operative staging systems [4, 28, 35]. The majority of these approaches are appropriate only for rectal cancers, although new technology, biochemistry and histopathological techniques may allow a clinical staging system to be used for colon cancers also.

Multivariate analysis of prognostic factors

Multivariate analyses of patients with colorectal cancer have been reported [8, 26]. These are based on a method of analysis using non-parametric data [65], which allows for the simultaneous evaluation of the relative effect on survival of each of a number of variables. Analysis of data from the MRC1 trial [24] revealed a number of factors of prognostic significance in patients considered to have operable tumours [26]. Pre-operative and post-operative classifications were devised. Curative resection was used as the end-point for the pre-operative classification, as it was considered that this was the factor most strongly related to the future prognosis of the patient.

The factor of greatest importance in determining whether a curative resection could be performed was the pre-operative mobility of the tumour. The only other factor having influence was the number of quadrants of the bowel wall involved. If more than one quadrant was involved, the curative resection rate was reduced for both mobile and fixed tumours. Following surgery the factor most closely influencing length of survival was a curative radical resection. When patients having a curative resection were examined, age and the height of the tumour appeared most strongly to influence survival but factors having an overall influence, such as mobility and number of quadrants involved, had little effect. It was therefore in the prediction of the possibility of a curative resection that these latter factors were important.

Pathological factors found to be important in influencing prognosis were Dukes' classification, tumour grade and venous spread. Using multivariate analysis, a scoring system was devised based on Dukes' classification, histological grade, height of tumor and venous spread. This classified patients into five groups. Group I, consisting of 20% of the patients, had a good prognosis with an 80% five-year survival rate. Group V patients, forming 14% of the total, had a poor outlook with a 19% five-year survival. There were three intermediate groups.

Patients who did not have a curative resection had a particularly poor prognosis. When a radical non-curative operation was performed, 83% of patients were dead within five years. Prognostic factors of importance in this group were Dukes' classification, venous spread and local invasion. A similar scoring system was constructed for these patients. However, in the non-radical resection groups, the median survival time was only 7,5 months and no prognostic factors were identified.

This investigation clearly identified pre- and post-operative factors of prognostic importance which could be incorporated into a scoring system of great accuracy, and which therefore would be of value in making pre-operative as well as post-operative management decisions. A large Australian study has provided similar answers [8].

Prognostic criteria at relapse

In a study of patients with large bowel cancer who died following apparently curative surgery [66], autopsies were carried out on 267 patients. A total of 207 patients had recurrent disease of whom 110 had local recurrence, but local recurrence as an isolated phenomenon was found in only 12 of the 110 patients. However, the incidence of local recurrence reported by different series depends upon whether planned reoperation was performed [34] or whether autopsy data are being examined [37], and local recurrence rates in various surgical series vary from 15-50% [1].

Only 10–15% of local recurrences are resectable and of these patients about 10% will survive more than three years [3]. Showing that even local recurrence of colorectal cancer (the form of recurrence most amenable to subsequent treatment) carries a poor prognosis. Thus, attempts to identify local recurrence at a stage when it would be resectable have included routine 'second-look' procedures [67] and the use of CEA-mediated 'second-look' operations [68]. Routine 'second-look' procedures have been advocated largely in the USA [67], and have not been generally accepted because of the associated operative morbidity and mortality [3]. Poor histological differentiation of tumour and extensive local spread are the characteristics most likely to be associated with local recurrence.

Alternatives to surgical removal of recurrence are few, although there have been reports of success using radiotherapy [69]. Again, the survival rate is low and only about 3–4% of patients receiving radical radiotherapy are alive at five years. Interestingly, one of the best predictors of a response to radiotherapy was found to be the pre-treatment CEA level [70], and only patients with CEA levels less than 75 ng/ml showed worthwhile survival rates. For patients with levels greater than this palliative radiotherapy was advised.

The response of colorectal cancer to chemotherapy is poor [71]. The best single agent response rates are only of the order of 15–20%, and there is no evidence that their use prolongs survival [72]. Although higher response rates are quoted when combinations of drugs are used, again no survival advantage has been demonstrated [12].

Careful follow up of patients following surgical resection of colorectal tumours is important for reasons other than detecting recurrence. A second primary large bowel cancer will develop in 3–15% of patients and must be differentiated from recurrent disease. Surveillance and detection of adenomata before frank malignant change has occurred has the advantage of early detection of second primary tumours. Finally, patients who develop large bowel cancer are at high risk of developing a second primary tumour in other organs [10].

Conclusion

A number of factors which influence prognosis in patients with colorectal cancer have been clearly identified. Information may come from clinical examination of patients at the time of presentation, from features found at operation, and from examination of the operative specimen. Additional information may be provided by the use of biological markers. Multivariate analysis is being increasingly employed to provide scoring systems to predict prognosis more accurately than is possible by current staging systems.

Recurrent colorectal cancer carries a particularly poor prognosis since there is no effective treatment except in a minority of cases. Increasingly, adjuvant treatments are being incorporated into the management of high risk patients in order to improve survival. These regimens must be based on a knowledge of those indices known to affect prognosis.

References

1. Fraser P, Adelstein AM: Recent trends in colorectal cancer epidemiology. In: *Recent Results in Cancer Research – Colorectal Cancer*. Duncan W (ed). Heidelberg. Springer-Verlag, 1982, pp 1–10
2. Giles GR, Moosa AR: The colon, rectum and anal canal. In: *Essential Surgical Practice*. Cuschieri A, Giles GR, Moosa AR (eds). Bristol, Wright, 1982, pp 980–1015
3. Nicholls RJ: Surgery for colorectal cancer. In: *Recent Results in Cancer Research – Colorectal cancer*. Duncan W (ed). Heidelberg. Springer-Verlag, 1982, pp 101–112
4. Williams NS, Durdey P, Quirke P, Robinson PJ, Dyson JED, Dixon MF, Bird CC: Pre-operative staging of rectal neoplasm and its impact on clinical management . *Br J Surg* 72: 868–874, 1985
5. Higgins GA: Adjuvant radiation therapy in colon cancer. *Int Advances in Surg Oncol* 2: 1–24, 1979
6. First report of an MRC working party: A trial of pre-operative radiotherapy in the management of operable rectal cancer. *Br J Surg* 69: 513–519, 1982
7. Porter NH, Nicholls RJ: Pre-operative radiotherapy in operable rectal cancer; interim report of a trial carried out by the Rectal Cancer Group. *Br J Surg* 72 (suppl): 62–64, 1985
8. Chapuis PH, Dent OF, Fisher R, Newland RC, Pheils MT, Smyth E, Colquhoun K: A multivariate analysis of clinical and pathological variables in prognosis after resection of large bowel cancer. *Br J Surg* 72: 698–702, 1985
9. Thomas WH, Larson RA, Wright HK, Cleveland JC: An analysis of patients with carcinoma of the right colon. *Surg Gynecol Obstet* 127: 313–318, 1968
10. Sugarbaker PH, MacDonald JS, Gunderson LL: Colorectal cancer. In: *Cancer Principles and Practice of Oncology*. DeVita VT, Hellman S, Rosenberg SA (eds). Philadelphia. Lippincott, 1982, pp 643–723
11. Wood CB: Prognostic factors in colorectal cancer. In: *Recent Advances in Surgery*, no 10. Taylor S (ed). Edinburgh. Churchill Livingstone, 1980, pp 259–280
12. Öhman V: Prognosis in patients with abstructing colorectal carcinoma. *Am J Surg* 143: 742–747, 1982
13. Ragland JJ, Londe AM, Spratt JS: Correlation of the prognosis of obstructing colorectal carcinoma with clinical and pathologic variables. *Am J Surg* 121: 552–556, 1971
14. Ackerman NB: The influence of mechanical factors on intestinal lymph flow and their relationship to operations for carcinoma of the intestine. *Surg Gynecol Obstet* 138: 766–682, 1974
15. Dutton JW, Hreno A, Hampson LG: Mortality and prognosis of obstrucing carcinoma of the large bowel. *Am J Surg* 131: 36–41, 1976
16. Glenn F, McSherry CK: Obstruction and perforation in colorectal cancer. *Am Surg.* 173: 983–992, 1971
17. Gilbertsen VA, Nelms JM: The presentation of invasive cancer of the rectum. *Cancer.* 41: 1137–1139, 1978

18. Gill PG, Morris PJ: The survival of patients with colorectal cancer treated at a regional hospital. *Br J Surg* 65: 17–20, 1978

19. Sherlock S, Winawer SJ: The role of early diagnosis in controlling large bowel cancer. *Cancer* (suppl 5) 40: 2609–2615, 1977

20. Hardcastle JD, Vellacott KD: Early diagnosis and detection of colorectal cancer. In: *Recent Results in Cancer Research. – Colorectal cancer.* Duncan W (ed). Heidelberg. Springer-Verlag, 1982, pp 86–100

21. McDermott FT, Hughes ESR, Pihl E, Milne BJ, Price AB: Prognosis in relation to symptom duration in colon cancer. *B J Surg* 68: 846–849, 1981

22. Devlin HB, Plant JA, Morris D: The significance of the symptoms of carcinoma of the rectum. *Surg Gynecol Obstet* 137: 399–402, 1973

23. Holliday HW, Hardcastle JD: Delay in diagnosis and treatment of symptomatic colorectal cancer. *Lancet* 1: 309–311, 1979

24. Third report of an MRC working party: Clinico-pathological features of prognostic significance in operable rectal cancer in 17 centres in the UK. *Br J Cancer* 50: 435–442, 1984

25. Block GE, Enker WE: Survival after operation for rectal carcinoma in patients over 70 years of age. *Am Surg* 174: 521–527, 1971

26. Freedman LS, Macaskill P, Smith AN: Multivariate analysis of prognostic factors for operable rectal cancer. *Lancet* 2: 733–736, 1984

27. McDermott FT, Hughes ESR, Pihl E, Milne BJ, Price AB: Comparative results of surgical management of single carcinomas of the colon and rectum: a series of 1939 patients managed by one surgeon. *Br J Surg* 68: 850–855, 1981

28. Zorzitto M, Germanson T, Cummings B, Boyd NF: A method of clinical prognostic staging for patients with rectal cancer. *Dis Colon Rectum* 25: 759–765, 1982

29. Coller FA, Kay EB, MacIntyre RS: Regional lymphatic metastasis in carcinoma of the colon. *Am Surg* 114: 56–63, 1941

30. Dionne L: The pattern of blood borne metastasis from carcinoma of the rectum. *Cancer* 18: 775–781, 1965

31. Slaney G: Results of the treatment of carcinoma in the colon and rectum. In: *Modern Trends in Surgery.* Irwine WT (ed). London. Butterworths 3rd Edn, 1971, pp 69–78

32. Dwight RW, Higgins GA, Keehn RJ: Factors influencing survival after resection in cancer of the colon and rectum. *Am J Surg* 117: 512–522, 1969

33. Morson BC, Vaughan EG, Bussey HJR: Pelvic recurrence after excision of rectum for carcinoma. *Br Med J* 2: 13–18, 1963

34. Gunderson LL, Sosin H: Areas of failure found at reoperation (second or symptomatic look) following 'curative surgery' for adenocarcinoma of the rectum. *Cancer* 34: 1278–1292, 1974

35. Nicholls RJ, Galloway DJ, Mason AY, Boyle P: Clinical local staging of rectal cancer. *Br J Surg* 72 (suppl): pp 51–52, 1985

36. Grinnell RS: The lymphatic and venous spread of carcinoma of the rectum. *Am Surg* 112: 138–149, 1940

37. Dukes CE, Bussey HJR: The spread of rectal cancer and its effect on prognosis. *Br J Cancer* 12: 309–320

38. Broders AC: Carcinoma: Grading and practical application. *Arch Pathol* 2: 376–381, 1926

39. Grinnell RS: The grading and prognosis of carcinoma of the colon and rectum. *Am Surg* 109: 500–533, 1939

40. Dukes CE: Cancer of the rectum; an analysis of 1000 cases. *J Pathol Bacteriol* 50: 527–539, 1940

41. Blenkingsopp WK, Stewart-Brown S, Blesovsky L, Kearny G, Fielding LP: Histopathology reporting in large bowel cancer. *J Clin Pathol* 34: 509–513, 1981

42. Quirke P, Dyson JED, Dixon MF, Bird CC, Joslin CAF: Heterogeneity of colorectal adenocarcinomas evaluated by flow cytometry and histopathology. *Br J Cancer* 51: 99–106, 1985

43. Qualheim RE, Gall EA: Is histopathologic grading of colon cancer a valid procedure? *Arch Pathol* 56: 466–472, 1953
44. Dukes CE: The classification of cancer of the rectum. *J Pathol Bacteriol* 35: 323–332, 1932
45. Wolley RC, Schreiber K, Koss LG, Karas M, Sherman A: DNA distribution in human colon carcinoma and its relation to clinical behaviour. *J Nat Cancer Inst* 69: 15–22, 1982
46. Symonds DA, Vickery AL: Mucinous carcinoma of the colon and rectum. *Cancer* 37: 1891–1900, 1976
47. Wood CB, Gillis CR, Hole D, Malcolm AJH, Blumgart LH: Local tumour invasion as a prognostic factor in colorectal cancer. *Br J Surg* 68: 326–328, 1981
48. Talbot IC: The pathology of colorectal cancer and its natural history. In: *Recent Results in Cancer Reserach – Colorectal cancer*. Duncan W (ed). Heidelberg. Springer-Verlag, 1982, pp 59–66
49. Pihl E, Malahy MA, Khankhanian N *et al.*: Immunomorphological features of prognostic significance in Dukes' class B colorectal carcinoma. *Cancer Res* 37: 4145, 1977
50. Talbot IC, Ritchie S, Leighton MH, Hughes AO, Bussey HJR, Morson BC: The clinical significance of invasion of veins by rectal cancer. *Br J Surg* 67: 439–442, 1980
51. Brown CE, Warren S: Visceral metastasis from rectal carcinoma. *Surg Gynecol Obstet* 66: 611–621, 1938
52. Taylor I: Colorectal liver metastases – to treat or not to treat. *Br J Surg* 72: 511–516, 1985
53. Wood CB: Natural history of liver metastases. In: *Liver Metastases*. Van de Velde CJH, Sugarbaker PH (eds). Amsterdam. Martinus Nijhoff, 1984, pp 47–54
54. Gold P, Freedman SO: Demonstration of tumour specific antigens in human colonic carcinomata by immunological tolerance and absorption techniques. *J Exp Med* 121: 439–462, 1965
55. Minton JP, James KK, Hurturbise PE, Rinker L, Joyce S, Martin EW Jr: The use of serial carcinoembryonic antigen determination to predict recurrence of carcinoma of the colon and the time for second-look operation. *Surg Gynecol Obstet* 147: 208–210, 1978
56. MacCay AM, Patel S, Carter V, Lawrence DJR, Cooper EH, Neville AM: Role of serial plasma CEA assays in detection of recurrent and metastatic colorectal carcinomas. *Br Med J* 4: 382–385, 1974
57. Moertel CG, Schutt AJ, Go VLW: Carcinoembryonic antigen test for recurrent colorectal carcinoma. Inadequacy for early detection. *JAMA* 239: 1065–1066, 1978
58. Staab HJ, Anderer FA, Brümmendorf T, Stumpf E, Fischer R: Prognostic value of pre-operative serum CEA level compared to clinical staging. I Colorectal cancer. *Br J Cancer* 44: 652–662, 1981
59. deMello J, Struthers L, Turner R, Cooper EH, Giles GR and the Yorkshire Regional Gastrointestinal Cancer Research Group: Multivariate analysis as aids to diagnosis and assessment of prognosis in gastrointestinal cancer. *Br J Cancer* 48: 341–348, 1983
60. Cooper EH, O'Quigley J: Biochemical markers in colorectal cancer. In: Recent Results in Cancer Research – Colorectal Cancer. Duncan W (ed). Heidelberg. Springer-Verlag, 1982, 67–76
61. Durdey P, Williams NS, Brown DA: Serum carcinoembryonic antigen and acute phase reactant proteins in the pre-operative detection of fixation of colorectal tumours. *Br J Surg* 71: 881–884, 1984
62. Lockhart-Mummery JP: Two hundred cases of cancer of the rectum treated by perineal excision. *Br J Surg* 14: 110–124, 1926–1927
63. Gabriel WB, Dukes C, Bussey HJR: Lymphatic spread in cancer of the rectum. *Br J Surg* 23: 395–413, 1935
64. Astler VB, Coller FA: The prognostic significance of direct extension of carcinoma of the colon and rectum. *Am. Surg* 139: 846–852, 1954
65. Cox DR: Regression models and life tables. *J Stat Soc Br* 34: 187–220, 1972
66. Berge T, Ekeland G, Mellner C, Wenckert P: Carcinoma of the colon and rectum in a defined population. *Acta Chir Scand* (suppl) 438, 1972
67. Gilbertsen VA, Wangensteen OH: A survey of thirteen years experience with the second look program. *Surg Gynecol Obstet* 114: 438–442, 1962

68. Northover J: Carcinoembryonic antigen and recurrent colorectal cancer. *GUT* 27: 117–122, 1986
69. Arnott SJ: Radiotherapy of colorectal cancer. In: *Recent Results in Cancer Research*. Duncan W (ed). Heidelberg. Springer-Verlag, 1982, 83: 113–125
70. Arnott SJ: Plasma carcinoembryonic antigen (CEA) as an indicator for radical or palliative radiotherapy in patients with rectal cancer. *Cancer det Prev* 6: 155–160, 1983
71. Whitehouse JMA: Chemotherapy in colorectal cancer. In: *Recent Results in Cancer Research*. Duncan W (ed). Heidelberg. Springer-Verlag, 1982, 83: 126–134
72. Moertel CG: Current concepts in cancer: Chemotherapy of gastrointestinal cancer. *N Engl J Med* 299: 1049–2052, 1978

19. Prognostic indices in stomach cancer

J.L. CRAVEN

The prognosis of a patient with stomach cancer is determined above all else by the completeness of its surgical resection; few, if any, patients will survive 5 years unless the cancer has been removed. The use of prognostic criteria either preoperatively or after resection, is to help predict the outcome of apparently curative surgery. These include the site of the primary tumour, duration of symptoms, histological features, staging and lymph node metastases, and monitoring of tumour products. Neither age nor sex has been shown to influence prognosis, and race is considered later when comparing Japanese and Western survival data.

Site of primary tumour

Most reports, whether from the West or Japan, agree that there is a significantly worse outcome after treatment of tumours arising in the cardia or proximal third of the stomach. Fundal cancer often presents at an advanced stage due to symptoms being unnoticed in its early stages. It is frequently polypoidal rather than ulcerative, and is situated in a more distensible part of the stomach where its growth may proceed undetected [1]. Its prognostic disadvantage is significant and persists even if allowance is made for the increased operative mortality that follows total gastrectomy.

From Japan, Miwa [1] records a 50% 5 year survival rate after resection of distal tumours, but only 19% for proximal tumours. In Europe similarly, Gennari and colleagues [2] have reported that only 11% of patients with tumours of the cardia who survived postoperatively lived for 5 years after resection, whilst the survival rates for cancers of the body and antrum were 53% and 49% respectively.

Duration of symptoms

It has been suggested that length of symptoms is a useful guide to prognosis –

the longer the history the better the prognosis [3, 4] – but some surveys have not found such a relationship. Most surveys are retrospective and in these circumstances, assessment of the length of symptoms is difficult and frequently unreliable. However, in a few cases of gastric cancer that have been followed prospectively, reports suggest that tumour growth, particularly of the ulcerating type of early gastric cancer, may be very slow, and that mucosal cancers of this form may exist for several years without progression to advanced cancer [6, 7]. In this subset of gastric cancer, slow growth and good cure rates are related.

It has to be emphasised that these reports largely comprise ulcerating (and therefore symptomatic) cancers; polypoid cancers rarely ulcerate, and because they are usually asymptomatic, rarely present early. As their presentation tends to be delayed until they produce noticeable distant effects, surgical cure is unlikely. In this group, short length of symptoms and poor cure rates are likely to be related.

Okabe's investigation of the natural history of gastric cancer verified these findings [8]. It was based partly on a retrospective study of advanced gastric cancers (collating symptoms and histological staging with previously misinterpreted radiographic and gastrocamera data) and partly on a prospective study of 27 gastric cancers found by annual mass survey. He demonstrated that there is a wide variation in the growth and invasion patterns of gastric cancers and constructed a hypothetical graph which summarised the varying relationship of growth to symptoms.

He suggest that at one extreme is the incurable cancer which grows and invades insidiously without symptoms, so that diagnosis is not made until it is markedly advances with remote metastases (see Fig. 1, Line CH). Early diagnosis would, in these cases, only be made by serendipity or a screening programma. At the other extreme (lowest line in figure) are the very slowly growing tumours, which Okabe thinks may represent 10% of all stomach cancers and are all ulcerating. (Eckhardt [7] documents the very benign course of one such tumour which was followed over more than 10 years). They may stay within the mucosa for many years.

The two lines embrace the range of biological behaviour of gastric cancer. It is likely that up to 70% of cancers have the insidious pattern of growth and they are usually unlikely to be diagnosed before remote metastasis has occurred, even if the patient submits himself to investigation at the first appearance of symptoms. The fact that 'early gastric cancer' accounts for almost 40% of new cases is not in conflict with these views, for only a small minority of these early cases are not ulcerated.

Thus, duration of symptoms prior to diagnosis provides substantial prognostic information. The slowly growing types are ulcerative in type and symptomatic at an early stage, so that treatment tends to be offered when the tumour may be cured by resection. In addition, ulcerative forms of gastric cancer (particularly the early forms) metastasize less commonly via the blood stream than do polypoid forms [9].

324

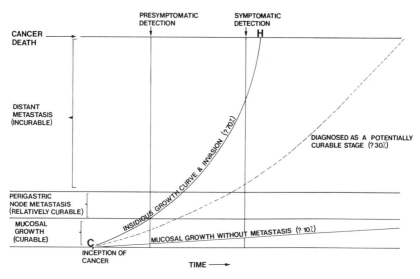

Figure 1. Hypothetical history of gastric cancer (after Okabe [8] and McDonald [45]. The vertical axis is divided into the stages of growth (and of curability) of the cancer and the horizontal axis, which is of time, is divided by vertical lines to define the hypothetical times at which the cancer first becomes detectable (presymptomatic detection) and later when the cancer first produces symptoms. Extremes of growth and invasion of gastric cancer are represented by two lines; a) insidious growth and invasion in which only presymptomatic screening offers any chance of diagnosis at a stage amenable to cure; b) mucosal growth without metastasis representing the 'early gastric cancers' which never progress to advanced cancers. All gastric cancers can be accomodated between these lines.

Histological features

Gastric cancers show marked variation in their microscopic structure, not only between different tumours, but often between different areas of the same tumour. The early attempts at pathological classification were too complicated, each attempting to describe cellular types and patterns and the surrounding stroma. The lack of correlation between macroscopic and microscopic features led Stout to state tha the histological classification of gastric cancer was valueless and that gross appearances were more relevant as prognostic indicators [10]. However, this view is no longer shared by the majority of pathologists, and the several classifications currently employed are briefly summarised as follows:

WHO Classification. This divides gastric cancer into papillary, tubular, mucinous, signet ring and undifferentiated types based on its predominant component [11]. Each tumour type may be graded as either well-, moderately-, or poorly-differentiated. Apart from the well known relationship between papillary adenocarcinoma and polypoid tumours, there is little association between this microscopic classification and macroscopic features.

Lauren Classification [12]. This allocates the cancer into two main groups – intestinal and diffuse types – which differ not only in general and cellular structure, but in secretion, mode of growth and clinical correlation. Intestinal types have a glandular structure, whereas diffuse types comprise single cells or small clusters without glandular formation. Only a loose association with macroscopic structure exists; most of the intestinal types are polypoid, and infiltrating carcinomata form the largest fraction of the diffuse type. Some 15 to 20 per cent of carcinomas, however, cannot be classified because of their poor differentiation. The three year survival rate reported after curative resection was 43% in intestinal types and 35% in diffuse type tumours.

Ming Classification [13]. This grouping emphasises the growth pattern of a gastric cancer rather than its architecture. It divides the cancers into expanding (67%) and infiltrative types, the former growing by expansion and forming nodules, the latter by penetration and diffuse involvement. Though glandular formation tends to be commoner in the expansive type, degrees of differentiation are divided equally between the two types. There is some relationship to macroscopic type; the majority of infiltrative type cancers form diffuse or ulcerated tumours while polypoid cancers are most commonly formed by expanding tumours.

Relationship of histology to prognosis

While the WHO classification is the easiest to apply and most widely used, it does not best aid the assessment of prognosis. The Lauren classification does provide some prognostic determinants [12, 14], but has not been used widely enough in surveys of treatment results for its potential to be firmly defined. The Ming classification has not yet been tested for prognostic value.

The relationship of the histology of gastric cancer to prognosis has largely been judged from surgically resected cases. On this basis, highly differentiated carcinoma [1], intestinal type carcinoma [15] and differentiated carcinoma [16] are thought to carry the better prognosis while diffuse type carcinoma [17] and poorly differentiated tumours [18] are said to spread more frequently to regional lymph nodes.

Ishii *et al.* [19] in an autopsy study of 294 cases, carefully assessed the extent of metastases and concluded that tumours could be divided by histological type into two groups – those of limited invasiveness and those of generalised invasiveness. While there might be considerable histological variation within the primary tumour, they found an unfavourable biological behaviour even when a histological type with the potential for generalised invasiveness formed only a minor part of the tumour. Poorly differentiated adenocarcinoma, poorly differentiated mucoid carcinoma and all three types of diffuse carcinoma were the histological types which showed generalised invasiveness. It suggests that the prognostic features of the primary tumour's histology *depend on its invasive behaviour*.

Circumscribed growths with no evidence of infiltration appear to have the best prognosis; they were found in 25 of 30 five year survivors and, in another review of 105 patients, those with a noninfiltrative tumour margin had a 52.6% five year survival rate, whereas those with an infiltrative margin had only a 13% five year survival rate [21]. The prognosis seems to be improved in those tumours surrounded by a marked inflammatory and plasma cell infiltration [11–24]. Even with invasion of the serosa the prognosis of this type of tumour was said to be good [25], and an immunological basis was suggested as the reason for this favourable prognostic influence.

These findings could not be confirmed in a subsequent Finnish study [26], but these workers did find that paracortical activity (PCA) within the regional lymph nodes was positively related to improved patient survival and that where PCA was most marked, no tumour metastases could be found. They suggested that thymus-dependant lymphocytes are an integral part of host resistance against gastric carcinoma, and may be less well recognised in the stromal reactions around a tumour than in the paracortical region of the lymph node. More clinical data is required to confirm the role of paracortical lymphocytes in host resistance to gastric cancer.

Clinical staging

Gastric cancer spreads directly, both horizontally and vertically through the gastric wall, and metastasizes to regional lymph nodes. It also shows a tendency to vascular invasion which is not strongly related either to to lymph node involvement or to depth of spread in the gastric wall. Transcoelomic spread across the peritoneum frequently follows full thickness penetration of the stomach wall by the cancer.

The extent of spread, whether direct, by lymphatics or blood stream, is clearly a most important prognostic determinant. Distant metastases (whether blood borne or carried by the lymphatics) define incurability and few, if any, of the patients with distant metastases survive five years after tumour resection. Attempted curative resections, in which the surgeon believes (by macroscopic of microscopic staging) that he has probably removed the whole of the tumour and its metastases, result in five year survival rates ranging from 21% [27] to 37% [28] in the Western World and 28% [29] to 54% [30] in Japan. The commonest cause of death after resection of a gastric cancer is recurrent tumour and retrospective analysis of operative series reveals that the two most important prognostic determinants are the depth of spread of the cancer through the gastric wall and the extent of involvement of regional lymph nodes.

Depth of spread

Outside of Japan, few series of resected gastric cancers contain more than 5% of 'early gastric cancers' (i.e. confined to the mucosa and submucosa) and at least 75% will have infiltrated the serosa. Paile [24] showed the five year survival rate to be 50% when the tumour was confined to the mucosa, yet only 20% when the muscle coat has been penetrated. Miwa [30], reporting the collaborative data of 113 Hospitals in a survey of 5706 patients who had undergone gastrectomy, was able to show a graded relationship of prognosis to depth of invasion (Table 1). It is likely that this relationship is in part due to the increasing likelihood of nodal and distant metastases with deeper penetration of the gastric wall by the tumour notwithstanding that supposed relationship, the five year survival rate declines sharply from 40% when the infiltration, though extending to serosa is confined by it, to 22% when the infiltration extends to invade the serosa.

Nakajima and colleagues [31] examined exfoliative cytology after peritoneal lavage at the time of laparotomy in 458 patients with gastric cancer. Positive cytological specimens were found in 21% of patients who had no visible dissemination in the peritoneal cavity, and all but 2 of the positive results were found in patients with microscopic serosal involvement. No patient with positive cytology in their peritoneal washings survived five years (Table 2).

Peritoneal dissemination is the most common type of recurrent disease after attempted curative surgery. Peritoneal lavage is a good prognostic indicator because serosal involvement seriously diminished the potential benefits of attempted curative resection.

Table 1. Relationship of 5 year survival rate to depth of invasion, judged microscopically

Depth of penetration	Relative 5-year survival rate %*
Mucosa	101.6
Submucosa	90.3
Muscularis propria	70.2
Subserosal	49.8
Serosal	
S_1 (covered by intact connective tissue)	39.6
S_2 (extending through all layers of serosa)	22.1
S_3 (invading into adjacent organs)	7.3

* Relative 5 year survival rate excludes operative deaths occurring 30 days or less after surgical operation (after Miwa [30])

Lymph node metastases

A major factor in the assessment of prognosis is the presence and extent of involvement of the regional lymph nodes. The presence of lymph node metastases points to a poor prognosis, so that Hawley and colleagues [22] found a five year survival rate of 40% when no lymph node metastases were present, but 12% when they are present. Hoerr [28] similarly found that lymph node involvement reduced the five year survival rate from 62% to 21%.

In addition, patients with few nodal metastases fare better than those with many [22, 32] and lymph node deposits more than 2.5 cm from the tumour point to a poor prognosis [33].

The most convincing report on the prognostic significance of lymph node deposits and the extent of nodal involvement was provided by the Japanese collaborative study of 5706 operated cases [30] (see Table 3).

Tumour products

So far no tumour-specific antigen has been detected in human gastric cancer, but a relationship has been claimed with neofoetal antigens – α foetoprotein (AFP), carcinoembryonic antigen (CEA) and foetal sialo-glycoprotein antigen (FSA). Their estimation for diagnostic or follow-up studies has not been widespread because elevated levels in the serum are rarely present other than in advanced (and differentiated) tumours, or in patients with hepatic metastases. Postoperative monitoring of serum levels of these, so called, tumour-associated antigens has not been found of value in stomach cancer patients.

Both CEA and FSA have been found in gastric juice. The level of CEA is raised in the gastric aspirates from gastric cancer patients, as it is also in those from patients with benign gastric ulcers, and according to one report it does not provide a sensitive tool for the diagnosis of gastric cancer [34]. However, Hakkinen and his colleagues have stressed the estimation of FSA in gastric juice in the diagnosis of gastric cancer [35], and in a large screening survey in Finland which was based on this technique, he appears to have used it successfully. His laboratory methods though are complex and qualitative and, as yet, lack reproducibility.

Table 2. Correlation of survival after attempted curative surgery with serosal involvement and peritoneal washings examined cytologically (after Nakajima *et al.* [31])

	5-Year survival rate %
Intact serosa, negative peritoneal cytology	86%
Involved serosa, negative peritoneal cytology	52%
Involved serosa, positive peritoneal cytology	0%

There are no reports available on the prognostic significance of these tumour-associated antigens, nor on other biological markers that have been reported to be associated with gastric cancer, such as lactic acid dehydrogenase [36], neutrophil acid phosphatase [37] or urinary polyamines [38].

Multivariate analysis

It has long been suggested that the extent of the disease, in terms of mural invasion and lymph node metastasis may determine the outcome more precisely than either a histological or a macroscopic classification [34] and a similar proposal came from the Japanese Research Society for Gastric Cancer [40, 41]. It represents a combination of prognostic indices that can be both macroscopically and micro-scopically defined, but until recently, multivariate analysis was not applied to the particular parameters used.

None of the variables shown to have prognostic importance in gastric cancer act in isolation; they act always in the presence of other factors aiding or hindering the progression of the disease. Multivariate analysis of all known prognostic factors is required in order to establish their relative importance. The statistical methods employed in this type of analysis are complex and debatable.

Curtis *et al.* [42] analysed data from 4,784 cases documented by the Surveillance, Epidemiology and End Results Program of US National Cancer Institute (SEER-USA) and studies eleven variables; age, sex, race, depth of invasion, lymph node metastasis, distant metastasis, location, histological type, grade of differentiation, localised or diffuse growth and degree of extension to adjacent

Table 3. Correlation of survival with extent of lymph node deposits (after Miwa [30])

Extent of lymph node involvement*	5 Year survival rate %
Node (n_0)	79
Perigastric nodes (n_1)	38
Nodes around gastric, hepatic and splenic arteries, coeliac axis and hilum of spleen (n_2)	22
Distant nodes; porta hepatis, retropancreatic, para-oesophageal, root of mesentery (n_3)	11
More distant nodes (n_4)	8

*The General Rules of the Japanese Research Society for gastric cancer (33) have designated four groups of nodes ($n_1 - n_4$) whose involvement by metastases represents, they say, an advancement of the cancer. Their survival data would tend to support this view.

tissue. Multivariate analysis revealed that the three most important variables were depth of invasion, lymph node metastases and distant metastasis and they suggested that a staging system be based on these three factors.

Similar conclusions had been reached by Japanese workers (personal communication) who reported on a multivariate analyses of 10 variables; age, sex total or partial resection, location of primary, postoperative complication, size of tumour, lymph node metastasis, serosal invasion, cancer type, and use of adjuvant chemotherapy. Serosal involvement (which is equivalent to Curtis' depth of invasion), lymph node metastasis, and distant metastasis were found to be the most important. In a smaller study Bedikian et al. [43] reported from Texas that serosal invasion, histological type and lymph node metastasis were the three most important prognostic factors. The signet ring type of cancer was, they found, associated with a significantly worse prognosis than any other type.

All reports agree that serosal invasion and lymph node involvement are pointers to a poor prognosis, and such findings reinforce the basis of present staging systems for both the TNM [44], American Joint Committee on Cancer [42] and the Japanese Research Society for Gastric Cancer [40]. Each employs these two factors as major components in their staging systems. However, their staging systems are not identical; size of tumour is given weight by the TNM, but extent of lymph node involvement by the Japanese and the American groups.

These three groups (the UICC, AJC and the Japanese) are attempting to produce a staging system acceptable to all. Since each group has been using their staging system for several years, multivariate analysis will be used to reveal the strengths and weaknesses of each. Their report is not yet out, but it is likely that neither size of tumour nor histological type will play any part in the new staging system which has been agreed.

Conclusion

The adoption of an internationally accepted staging system will do much to promote international comparison, not only of treatment results but of treatment techniques. It may be a most important advance in the understandign of this disease whose treatment results show such a great variation between one country and another.

References

1. Miwa K: Treatment results of stomach carcinoma WHO-CC Monograph No 2. Published by WHO-CC Stomach Cancer, Tokyo, 1979
2. Gennari L, Bonfanti G, Salvadori B: Prognostic factors in gastric cancer. In: Diagnosis and Treatment of Upper Gastro-intestinal Tumours. Friedman M (ed), published by Excerpta Medica, Oxford, pp 173–184

3. Swynnerton BF, Truelove SC: Carcinoma of the stomach. *Brit Med J* 1: 287, 1952
4. Waterhouse JAH: Regional Variations and established prognostic factors in gastric cancer. In: *Gastric Cancer*. Fielding J (ed). Pergamon Press, Oxford, 1981, pp 17–34
5. ReMine WH, Games MMR, Dockerty MB: Longterm survival (10–56 years) after surgery for carcinoma in the stomach. *Amer J Surg*: 117–177, 1969
6. Tsukuma H, Mishuma T, Oshima A: Prospective Study of 'early' gastric cancer. *Int J Cancer* 31: 421–426, 1983
7. Eckhardt VF, Willems D, Kanzler G *et al*,: 80 months persistence of poorly differentiated early gastric cancer. *Gastroenterology* 87: 719–724, 1984
8. Okabe H: Clinical ctudy of growth and invasion patterns of early gastric cancer: its position in the natural history of gastric cancer. In: *Gann Monograph on Cancer Research*. Murukami T (ed). University of Tokyo Press, 1971, pp 67–79
9. Kidokoro T: Frequence of resection, metastasis and five-year survival rate of early gastric carcinoma in a surgical clinic. *Gann Monograph on Cancer Research* 11. Murukami T (ed). University of Tolyo Press, 1971, pp 45–49
10. Stout AP: Tumours of the stomach. *Atlas of Tumour Pathology*, Fascicle 21, US Armed Forces Institute of Pathology, Washington, 1953, p 65
11. Oota K: Histological typing of gastric and oesophageal tumours. *WHO Monograph*, Geneva, 1927
12. Lauren P: The two histological main types of gastric carcinoma: diffuse and so-called intestinal type carcinoma. An attempt at a histo-clinical classification. *Acta Path Microbiol Scand* 64: 31–49, 1965
13. Ming SC: Gastric carcinoma. A pathological classification. *Cancer* 39: 2475–2485, 1977
14. Correa P, Cuello PC, Dugue E: Carcinoma and intestinal metaplasia of the stomach in Colombian migrants. *Journal of the National Cancer Institute* 44: 297–306, 1970
15. Stemmerman GN, Brown C: A survival study of intestinal and diffuse forms of carcinoma. *Cancer* 33: 1190, 1974
16. Morimura Y: Prognosis of gastric carcinoma in the autopsy result. A Statistical Survey. *Saishini-gaku* 14: 21, 1959
17. Stalsberg H: Histological typing of gastric carcinoma. A comparison of surgical and autopsy materials and of primary tumours and metastases. *Acta Path Microbiol Scand* Section A 80, 509, 1972
18. Ohman V, Wellerfars J, Maberg A: Histological grading of gastric cancer. *Acta Chir Scand* 138: 384, 1972
19. Ishii T, Ikegami N, Hosoda Y *et al*.: The biological behaviour of gastric cancer. *J Pathology* 134: 97–117, 1981
20. Steiner PD, Maimon SN, Palmer WL and Kirsner JB: Gastric cancer: morphologic factors in five-year survival after gastrectomy. *American Journal of Pathology* 24: 947–969, 1948
21. Martin C, Kay S: The prognosis of gastric carcinoma as related to its morphologic characteristics. *Surgery, Gynecology and Obstetrics* 119: 319–322, 1964
22. Hawley PR, Westerholm P, Morson BC: Pathology and prognosis or carcinoma in the stomach. *British Journal of Surgery* 57: 877–883, 1970
23. Inberg MV, Lauren P, Vuori J, Viikari SJ: Prognosis in intestinal-type and diffuse gastric carcinoma with special reference to the effect of the stromal reaction. *Acta chirurg Scandin* 139: 273–278, 1973
24. Paile A: Morphology and prognosis of carcinoma of the stomach. *Ann Chirurg et gyneacolog. (fenniae)* 60, Suppl. 175: 1–56, 1977
25. Wanotabe HM, Enjoji M, Imai T: Gastric carcinoma with lymphoid stroma. Its morphological characteristics and prognostic correlations. *Cancer* 38: 232–243, 1976
26. Syrjamen KJ, Hjelt LH: Paracortical activity of the regional lymph nodes as a prognostic determinant in gastric carcinoma. *Scand J Gastroenterol* 12: 897–902, 1977

27. Inberg MV, Heinonen R, Rantakokklo V, Viikari SJ: Surgical treatment of gastric carcinoma. *Arch Surg* 110: 703–707, 1975

28. Hoerr SO: Prognosis for carcinoma of the stomach. *Surg, Gynec and Obst* 137: 204–209, 1973

29. Mine M, Majima S, Harada M, Etani S: End results of gastrectomy for gastric cancer. *Surgery* 68: 753–758, 1970

30. Miwa K: Cancer of the stomach in Japan. *Gann Monograph* 22: 61–75, 1979

31. Nakajima T, Harashima S, Hirate M, Kajitani T: Prognostic and Therapeutic Values of Peritoneal Cytology in Gastric Cancer. *Acta Cytologica* 22: 225–229, 1978

32. Cantrell E: The importance of lymph nodes in the assessment of gastric carcinoma at operation. *Brit J Surg* 58: 384–386, 1971

33. ReMine W, Dockerty M, Priestly J: Some factors which influence prognosis in surgical treatment of gastric carcinoma. *Ann Surg* 138: 311–317, 1953

34. Micali B, Florio MG, Venuti A, Artemisia A, Caputo G, Broncato U: Usefulness of CEA measurement in gastric juice of patients with gastric disorders. *J Clin Gastroenterol* 5: 411–415, 1983

35. Hakkinen I: Serum and gastric juice tumour markers. In *Advances in the Biosciences Vol. 32, Gastric Cancer* Fielding J, Newman C, Ford C, Jones B (ed). Pergamn Press. Oxford, 1981, pp 85–94

36. Piper D, Griffith E, Macoun M, Broderick F, Fenton B: Relationship of activities of lactic dehydrogenase, beta glucuronidase and glutamic oxaloacetic transaminase in gastric carcinoma to that in fundic and pyloric mucosa. *Cancer* 8: 1055–1058, 1965

37. Sulowicz W: Activity of some lysosomal enzymes in neutrophils. A cytochemical study. *Rev Esp Oncol* 28: 509–514, 1981

38. Takeda Y, Tommaga T, Kitamura M, Taguchi T, Takeda T, Miwatani T: Urinary polyamines in Patients with Gastric Cancer and their change after gastrectomy. *Gann* 66: 445–447, 1975

39. Hoerr SO: A Surgeon's Classification of Carcinoma of the Stomach. *Surg, Gynec and Obst* 99: 281–286, 1954

40. Japanese Research Society for Gastric Cancer. General rules for the gastric cancer study in surgery and pathology. Kanehara Shuppari, Tokyo, 1962 (quotes in 41).

41. Japanese Research Society for Gastric Cancer. The general rules for the gastric cancer study in surgery. *Japan J Surg* 3: 61–71, 1973

42. Curtis RE, Kennedy BJ, Myers MH, Honkey BF: Evaluation of AJC stomach cancer staging using the SEER population. *Seminars in Oncology* 12: 21–31, 1985

43. Bedikian AY, Chen TT, Khankhanian N, Heilbrun LK, McBride CM, McMurtrey MJ and Bodey GP: The Natural History of Gastric Cancer and Prognostic Factors Influencing Survival. *J Clin Oncol* 2: 305–310, 1984

44. UICC: TNM, Classification of malignant tumours. Stomach. Livre de Poche 1974, Second edition. *Livre de Poche* 1978, Third edition. Geneve

20. Prognostic factors in lymphoma

M.A. RICHARDS, W.M. GREGORY and T.A. LISTER

A significant proportion of patients with malignant lymphoma, especially Hodg-kin's disease, live many years following treatment with current 'conventional' radiotherapy, cytotoxic chemotherapy or combined modality therapy. A larger proportion, however, die either because of treatment failure or from treatment-related causes. The identification of those groups of patients who are at high risk of failure for either of the above reasons is of considerable importance, in order to permit application of alternative strategies. This chapter reviews reports on the major prognostic factor analyses in lymphoma, concentrating on those based on large numbers of patients and those which have employed multivariate analysis.

Methods of analysis

Most reports of clinical trials of treatment for lymphoma record the results in terms of achievement of complete remission, duration of remission and survival, and provide univariate analysis of prognostic factors for these three parameters. Many of the factors thus identified are, however, interrelated, and the relative importance and independence of factors identified by univariate analysis can be assessed by multivariate analysis as proposed by Cox [1]. At the outset, however, certain cautions are necessary about the practice of multivariate analysis for prognostic factors.

First, the precise methods of analysis must be recorded in order that results from different centres may be compared. Second, all variables examined should be listed (whether positive or negative) and, as far as possible, any factor which has previously been shown to be of major significance should be included. Third for continuous variables, such as age or serum albumin, any subdivisions used need to be defined, as the use of different subsets may yield significantly different results. Finally, the greater the number of variables examined, the greater the likelihood of finding a chance factor which is significant at the $p = 0.05$ level, and thus, stricter criteria may be necessary.

The importance of a particular factor may become apparent only if its effects on achievement of remission, duration of remission and survival after relapse are assessed separately, because it may affect survival in those who fail to achieve remission. For example, a recent study of advanced Hodgkin's disease (HD) at St. Bartholomew's Hospital [M.S. Dorreen, personal communication] has shown that increasing age is correlated with short survival of patients failing to respond to initial therapy, and short survival after relapse for those who do achieve remission. Advanced age, however, had relatively little effect on the achievement of remission itself.

One limitation of multivariate analysis needs special mention. A profound effect of a characteristic which is found in only a small proportion of patients may appear to be of lesser importance than a minor effect which is seen in a large number of patients. For example, the prognostic importance of localized disease in non Hodgkin's lymphoma may be overlooked, as such presentations occur in less than twenty per cent of patients.

The significance of prognostic factors may depend on treatment strategy used and the relative strengths of different indices may need to be reviewed frequently. Hoppe et al. [2], for example, found that for stage III HD treated by radiotherapy alone, patients with constitutional ('B') symptoms had a significantly worse prognosis than those who were asymptomatic. This difference was not observed when combined modality treatment (ie radiotherapy and chemotherapy) was given.

The relative importance of different pretreatment characteristics also depends on the methods of investigation used. For example, studies of patients with clinical stages I and II HD have identified mixed cellularity as an adverse feature [3, 4, 5]. However, when laparotomy is used in the pretreatment evaluation, such a relationship may not be apparent [6], possibly due to a higher incidence of clinically occult infradiaphragmatic disease in patients with mixed cellular histology.

Hodgkin's Disease (Table 1)

As noted above, the prognostic relevance of pretreatment characteristics depends on the treatment strategy and this is illustrated by the changing pattern of survival in patients with Hodgkin's disease (HD). Histology and clinical stage were of enormous significance when the natural history of the disease was allowed to run its course, but are now much less important with the introduction of extended field megavoltage radiotherapy and cyclical combination chemotherapy. These treatments have introduced their own influence on prognosis, so that choice of treatment now depends upon the relative risk of the disease, the relative chance of cure with one of the treatment options, and also their relative risks.

The Ann Arbor staging classification [7] has been used for the past 15 years as the basis for treatment decisions; broadly speaking, those patients with 'localised' disease (stages I and II) receive irradiation, those in stages IIIB to IVB receive chemotherapy and those in stage IIIA receive either or both. Radiotherapy is highly effective for patients with stage I disease, but recurrence is frequent after the achievement of remission in stage II cases, although survival following radiotherapy 'failure' may be excellent because of successful 'salvage' chemotherapy. It is important to identify those patients whose likelihood of failure following radiotherapy is arbitrarily high enough to recommend that they receive chemotherapy or combined modality therapy at presentation, in spite of the considerable morbidity (and especially the risk of infertility).

Histology

The Rye modification of the Lukes and Butler classification [8] divides HD into four histological subgroups – lymphocyte predominant (LP), nodular sclerosis (NS), mixed cellularity (MC) and lymphocyte depleted (LD). Histological subtype is regarded as having a strong influence on the tempo at which the disease evolves [9], with LP the most indolent and LD the most aggressive. However, the prognostic significance of histological subtype is complicated by the fact that it correlates with age, constitutional symptoms and stage.

Table 1. Factors reported to be of prognostic significance in Hodgkin's Disease

Age	
Sex	
Histological subtype	
Constitutional ('B') symptoms	
Extent of Disease:	Clinical stage
	Pathological stage
	Number of involved sites
	Presence of mediastinal mass/hilar mass
	Anatomic substage
	Extensive splenic involvement
	Extranodal involvement: pulmonary
	pleural
	liver
	bone marrow
	Number of extranodal sites
Laboratory tests:	ESR
	serum copper
	Lymphocyte count
Immunological tests:	DNCB sensitivity
	HLA AW19 phenotype
	In vitro lymphocyte function tests
Pre-existing atopy	

Thus, a Swedish study [10] of patients with all stages of HD, showed by univariate analysis that patients with LP and NS histology had a significantly better overall survival than those with MC and LD histology, but this difference was not significant for patients under fifty years of age. By multivariate analysis, histopathological subtype did not correlate significantly with prognosis, whereas age, stage and symptoms did so.

In localised HD confirmed by laparotomy (ie pathologically staged I and II), histological subtype was not of prognostic importance in three major studies [11, 12, 13]. (LD histology is very uncommon in this setting [6] and it more usually presents with advanced disease [14]). However, in three studies of clinically staged I and II patients [3–5], histology was prognostically significant, with MC and LD types carrying an adverse prognosis, confirmed in each case by multivariate analysis (Table 2). This difference may reflect the increased incidence of occult dissemination of disease in MC and LD Hodgkin's Disease.

Several recent studies of advanced HD (stages III & IV) have failed to show an independent impact on prognosis by histology [15–17]. DeVita et al [18] using MOPP chemotherapy found that patients with NS Hodgkin's Disease had significantly shorter disease-free intervals than did patients with MC or LD histology ($p < 0.02$). They suggest that as these effects are opposite to those generally found in studies where radiotherapy is employed, these patients might benefit from combined modality therapy.

Table 2. Prognostic factors for overall survival in 'localised' Hodgkin's Disease: Results of multivariate analysis

Study (ref)	EORTC (3)	Toronto (4)	BNLI (5)
No. of Pts	1139	252	753
Stages	CS I + II	CS I + II	CS I + IIA
Age	+ + +	+ + +	+ +
Sex	+		+
ESR	} + +		+ +
Symptoms			(all 'A')
Stage	−	} + +	
No. of Sites	+		
Mediastinum	−		+
Bulk		−	
Histology	+ +	+ +	+ +

+ = independent significance (no. of + gives approximation of relative importance of a factor)
− = not significant
blank spaces = not mentioned by authors
{ + denotes that the two factors were combined in that study

Age and sex

Many studies have identified increasing age as a major adverse prognostic factor both in localized [3–5] and advanced HD [15, 19, 20]. The study from Sweden [10] which examined the prognosis of patients with all stages of HD showed that age was the most significant prognostic factor for survival. (The mean age of the patients in that study was forty-seven years, which is considerably higher than in most other series, and probably reflects the referral pattern for that region). The adverse effect of age was most pronounced for patients over fifty years and Surcliffe *et al.* [4] similarly reports a marked adverse effect for age greater than fifty years. Many series are biased towards younger patients, and this may explain why age is not a prognostic factor in these analyses.

In localized HD, age was found to be an independent factor for survival in each of the three studies which used multivariate analysis (Table 2) and it also has a lesser but definite impact on disease-free survival (Table 3). These results presumably arise from poor survival after relapse in elderly patients, perhaps reflecting poor tolerance to salvage chemotherapy. In the case of patients with advanced HD, the impact of age on survival may be due to a lower rate of achievement

Table 3. Prognostic factors for disease-free survival in 'localised' Hodgkin's Disease: Results of multivariate analysis

Study (ref) No. of Pts Stages	EORTC (3) 1139 CS I + II	Toronto (4) 252 CS I + II	BNLI (5) 743 CS I + IIA	Stanford (11) 109 PS I + II	MD Anderson (13) 155 PS I + II
Age	+ +	+ +	–		–
Sex	+		–		–
ESR	} + + +		+ + +		
Symptoms			(All 'A')	–	+ + +
Stage	–	} + +	+ +		
No. of Sites	+ +			–	
Mediastinum	–	{ +	–	+ + +	–
Bulk					
Histology	–	+ + +	+ +		–
Hilar involvement					–
E disease				–	
Treatment				+ +	

+ = independent significance (no. of + gives approximation of relative importance of a factor)
− = not significant
blank spaces = not mentioned by authors
{ + denotes that the two factors were combined in that study

of complete remission [19, 20] as well as lower freedom from relapse [20], although this was not found at St. Bartholomew's Hospital [M.S. Dorreen, personal communication].

The effect of sex in HD is at most a minor one. However, both the EORTC [3] and the BNLI [5] have found that sex is a small but independent factor for survival in localized HD, with females faring better than males. This effect has not been shown in any of the recent major studies of advanced HD.

Extent of disease

The Ann Arbor conference [7] classified patients with HD into four stages according to extent of disease (Table 4). Patients were classified by clinical stage (CS) according to the results of physical examination and investigations (including x-rays and lymphography) and by 'pathological' stage (PS) following bone marrow biopsy and/or staging laparotomy (including splenectomy, biopsy of potential nodal sites of involvement and liver biopsy). Thus, following laparotomy, patients with CS I or II disease may be reallocated to PS III (or occasionally IV). The reverse may also occur, when a patient with CS III (e.g. because of splenomegaly or a positive lymphogram) is found after laparotomy to have no infradiaphragmatic disease and is therefore downgraded to PS I or II.

Patients with localized disease (stages I and II) mantain their prognostic advantage over those with advanced disease, despite the great improvements in therapy of the past twenty years [9]. However, the question is whether stage itself is a prognostic indicator, the difficulty being to separate the influence of stage from that of related factors, such as constitutional symptoms, the presence of a mediastinal mass or raised ESR level.

The actual number of involved sites is probably a better discriminator than the Ann Arbor category of stage I or II. For CS I and II patients, Tubiana *et al.* [21]

Table 4. Ann Arbor staging classification for Hodgkin's Disease

Stage I	Involvement of a single lymph node region (I) or of a single extralymphatic organ or site (I_E).
Stage II	Involvement of 2 or more lymph node regions on the same side of the diaphragm (II) or localized involvement of extralymphatic organ or site and of 1 or more lymph node regions on the same side of the diaphragm (II_E).
Stage III	Involvement of lymph node regions on both sides of the diaphragm (III), which may also be accompagnied by localized involvement of extralymphatic organ or site (III_E) or by involvement of the spleen (III_S), or both (III_{SE}).
Stage IV	Diffuse or disseminated involvement of 1 or more extralymphatic organs or tissues with or without associated lymph node enlargement.

found a highly significant difference in prognosis between patients with one or two involved sites and those with three or more involved sites. Similarly, Peckham et al. [22] reported that disease – free survival was dependent on the number of sites involved, with a poor prognosis for patients with four or more involved lymph node chains. Supradiaphragmatic relapse correlated with the number of sites involved in the studies by Carmel and Kaplan [23] and Thar et al. [24].

Kaplan has stressed that the normal pattern of spread in HD is by contiguous involvement of lymph node chains [9]. Tubiana et al. [3] confirmed that for patients with two sites of disease, contiguous territories were involved in over ninety per cent of cases. However, for patients with three or four involved sites, the proportion falls to sixty-seven per cent, which may imply haematogenous spread in some of these cases (and in turn, could be the cause of the adverse effect of multiple sites of involvement). The number of involved sites, has also been shown by Hoppe et al. [2] to be significant in patients with stage IIIA disease, where patients with five or more sites of disease (supra or infradiaphragmatic) had a worse disease-free survival.

The effect of substaging within stage III has yielded varying results in different trials. Desser et al. [25] found that patients with involvement of para-aortic, iliac or inguinal nodes (substage III_2) with or without upper abdominal involvement (spleen, splenic hilar, coeliac or porta hepatis nodes) had a worse prognosis than those with upper abdominal involvement alone (substage III_1). This finding was subsequently confirmed by Stein et al [16] in a collaborative study of one hundred and thirty PS IIIA patients treated with radiotherapy with or without chemotherapy. The adverse prognosis for substage $IIIA_2$ was statistically significant only in those treated with radiotherapy alone.

Hoppe et al. [26] reported a conflicting result in one hundred and seventy-one patients treated at Stanford for PS IIIA disease. For patients treated with total lymphoid irradiation, the five year freedom from relapse for $IIIA_1$ and $IIIA_2$ was nearly identical. For patients treated with combined modality treatment, those with $IIIA_1$ disease had significantly better freedom from relapse (but not overall survival) than did those with $IIIA_2$ disease. Stein et al. [16] suggested that the apparent discrepancy between their results and those from Stanford might be due to differences in radiotherapy technique, as patients at Stanford frequently receive radiotherapy to the liver and lung as well as to lymph nodes, as part of total lymphoid irradiation. However, at St. Bartholomew's Hospital [27] no difference in the rate of relapse was demonstrated between the two substages of stage IIIA regardless of the initial therapy used. In that study patients were treated either with chemotherapy or with total node irradiation without radiation to the liver or lung.

In the Stanford study [26], a new prognostic factor was identified for patients within PS IIIA treated with radiotherapy. The presence of extensive spleen involvement (defined as 5 or more nodules visible in the sectioned spleen) had a significant adverse effect on freedom from relapse (p = 0.007) but not on survival. The authors suggested a possible correlation of extensive splenic involvement with occult extralymphatic disease, particularly as subsequent bone marrow relapse appeared to be related to previous extensive splenic involvement.

For patients with stage IV disease no particular site of extranodal disease has consistently been shown to be an adverse prognostic factor (Table 5), although CALGB [19] found that patients with pulmonary disease had a lower complete remission rate than others. Pleural involvement has been identified as an adverse site of disease [18, 28] as is also liver involvement [18]. On the other hand, Pillai et al. [17] found no difference in survival between patients with hepatic, pulmonary or bone marrow involvement, but patients with more than one site of extranodal involvement had a significantly worse complete remission rate and survival than those with only one site of extranodal disease. Prosnitz et al. [15] also found this to be a significant factor.

Table 5. Prognostic factors for survival in patients with advanced Hodgkin's Disease: Results of multivariate analysis

Institution (Ref)	CALGB (19)	Yale (20)	NCI (18)	Stanford (28)	MDA (17)
Stages	III + IV	IIIB + IV	(II) III, IV	Predominantly III + IV	IV
Therapy	CT	CT + RT	CT	CT	CT
Previous RT		−		−	
Age	+ +	+		+	−
Sex	(−)	−			
Constitutional symptoms	(−)	+	+ +	+	−
Mediastinal mass					−
Number of 'E' sites		+			+ +
Pulmonary inv.	(+)				−
Pleural inv.			+	+ +	
Hepatic inv.	(−)		+		−
Bone marrow inv.					−
Histology	(−)	−	+ (subtype)		−
Response	+ +		+ +	+ + +	+
Drug dosage			+	+	+

In the CALGB study response was included in the multivariate analysis for survival. The factors which did or did not predict for response are therefore shown in brackets.
+ = independent significance (no. of + gives approximation of relative importance of factor)
− = not significant
blank spaces = not mentioned by authors

Mediastinum and bulk

The significance of mediastinal involvement is controversial. Early reports before current staging techniques were introduced, suggested a favourable influence of mediastinal involvement [29–31], but more recently the adverse effect of large mediastinal masses has been stressed [4, 11, 12, 32–35], particularly for patients treated with radiotherapy alone. At St. Bartholomew's Hospital, for example, no patient with PSIIA with a normal chest radiograph had relapsed, whereas, with bulky mediastinal masses the actuarial risk of relapse following RT alone was one hundred per cent [33].

The problem is that mediastinal masses frequently occur in the context of disease involving several sites, and are often associated with constitutional symptoms. This has been examined by Tubiana *et al.* [3] by multivariate analysis. They noted a high correlation between mediastinal involvement and sex (female), age (less than 40 years) and nodular sclerosis histological type, which were all favourable indicators, and between mediastinal involvement and number of areas of involvement which were unfavourable prognostically. However, mediastinal involvement itself was not correlated with significant increase in the relative risk of relapse or death. Another study from the Institut Gustave Roussy [36] has also shown that neither the presence nor the size of a mediastinal mass were of adverse significance, and the authors suggested that this could perhaps be linked to their use of a 'split course' radiotherapy technique.

Mauch *et al.* [37] reported that those patients with disease limited to the mediastinum had a favourable prognosis and that relapse-free survival and overall survival rates at 8 years were 85% and 100% respectively. Most of these patients had small masses and only two out of twenty-two had 'B' symptoms. However, in keeping with the majority of recent publications, the authors noted a high relapse rate for patients with large mediastinal masses (greater than one third thoracic diameter). More recently, a further report from Harvard [12] showed that patients with large mediastinal adenopathy treated with radiotherapy alone had a significantly worse overall survival, as well as poorer disease-free survival, than did patients with lesser or no mediastinal adenopathy. The combination of a large mediastinal mass with hilar lymphadenopathy was found to be prognostically worse than a large mediastinal mass alone by Hagemeister *et al.* [13].

Wiernik and Slawson [38] noted a marked adverse effect on prognosis from local pulmonary extension in patients treated with radiotherapy alone. The high relapse rate for large mediastinal masses treated with radiotherapy alone may have several causes. Firstly the mass may be poorly vascularized and therefore less radiosensitive. Secondly, local extension may occur because of inadequate initial assessment of the extent of mediastinal disease. (Accurate assessment with CT scanning may be of assistance for this). Thirdly, the biological behaviour of the disease may theoretically be more aggressive in patients with large mediastinal masses.

Constitutional symptoms

The Ann Arbor staging classification recognises the importance of constitutional symptoms by classifying asymptomatic patients as 'A' and those with fever, sweats and/or weight loss (greater than 10% of body weight) as 'B'. Pruritus is not included in this classification as it is thought to have little, if any, prognostic significance [9]. The presence of 'B' symptoms does not appear to be age-related. The Swedish study [10] showed that for patients aged less than fifty, 'B' symptoms were second only to clinical stage in their importance while for those over fifty years, age was more important.

In localized HD, the importance of 'B' symptoms is seen both in clinically- and pathologically-staged patients [3, 13]. This difference was not observed in the Stanford series [11] where generally, more extensive radiotherapy was used. In advanced HD, the importance of 'B' symptoms may depend on the mode of treatment used. At Stanford [26] the prognosis for stage IIIB patients was significantly worse than for stage IIIA when patients were treated with total lymphoid irradiation, but not when combined modality therapy was used. The study from the MD Anderson Hospital [6] also observed no significant difference between 'A' and 'B' patients when treated with combined modality therapy. However, at the National Cancer Institute [18] where chemotherapy was used, a difference was observed in both disease-free survival and overall survival. A difference in disease-free survival alone was noted at Yale [15] using chemotherapy and low dose radiotherapy.

ESR and biochemical tests

The value of the erythrocyte sedimentation rate (ESR) in HD tends to be overlooked, despite being simple and cheap to measure. Tubiana *et al.* [39] found that ESR level was the most important single prognostic factor in their study of localized HD. Although closely correlated with the presence of systemic symptoms, the ESR gave independent prognostic information. They have therefore combined ESR and 'B' symptoms to give a new indicator, which has a stronger influence than either alone. The good prognostic group is made up of patients who are either 'A' with an ESR of less than 50, or 'B' with an ESR of less than 30. Conversely, the poor prognostic group consists of 'A' patients with an ESR greater than 50, and 'B' patients with an ESR greater than 30.

The British National Lymphoma Investigation (BNLI) studies [5] have independently confirmed the significance of ESR level in CS I and II patients. In their multivariate analysis of 743 patients, it was found to be the most significant factor. However, the role of ESR in advanced disease does not appear to have been adequately assessed recently.

Serum copper level has in the past been used as a marker for activity in HD.

Elevated levels are correlated with stage of disease and, to a lesser extent, with 'B' symptoms and histology [40]. However, large fluctuations in serum copper level can be induced by changes in oestrogen levels (for instance with the contraceptive pill) and it is therefore no longer routinely measured by most centres specializing in HD management. Other biochemical tests such as LDH and albumin assays probably do not add prognostic information in HD beyond that given by clinical stage [10].

Lymphocyte count and immunological factors

In 1973 Young *et al.* [41] found that lymphopenia (lymphocyte count less than $1 \times 10^9/1$) at presentation was a significant adverse factor for survival in patients with advanced (stages III and IV) HD, but not in patients with localized disease. A recent study of advanced HD at St. Bartholomew's Hospital [M.S. Dorreen, personal communication] has again identified lymphopenia (lyphocyte count less than $0.75 \times 10^9/1$) as a strongly adverse prognostic factor, second only to age in its effect. Contrary to this, Bjorkholm *et al.* [42] found that the peripheral lymphocyte count had no relation to survival either in stage I/II or in stage III/IV disease.

Impaired delayed hypersensitivity to skin testing and defective *in vitro* lympho-cyte function are recognised features of HD. Young *et al.* [41] have shown that impaired hypersensitivity correlates with advanced stage, presence of 'B' symp-toms and MC or LD histology. Furthermore, skin anergy was associated with low peripheral blood lymphocyte counts. Low levels of lymphocyte transformation by phytohaemoagglutinin correlated with stage IV disease. Bjorkholm *et al.* [42] found that increased spontaneous lymphocyte DNA synthesis and decreased activity in response to concanavalin and pokeweed mitogen were poor prognostic features for stages I and II patients.

A personal or family history of atopy prior to the diagnosis of HD has been demonstrated to be a favourable factor for survival even after allowance has been made for age, symptoms and histology [43]. Conversely patients with AW19 HLA phenotype apparently have a significantly worse prognosis than others with HD [44].

Response to treatment

Achievement of complete remission is of paramount importance for prolonged survival in HD [18, 19, 28] but the possible importance of rate of regression of tumour with treatment has been less thoroughly examined. In localized HD treated with radiotherapy the speed of resolution of a mass may not be important. Carmel and Kaplan [23] found an almost identical incidence of relapse for patients who still had radiographic evidence of intrathoracic HD after completion of mantle radiotherapy as for those whose chest x-rays returned to normal. However, with initial chemotherapy for early stage HD, Zittoun *et al.* [45] found that achievement of remission with the first three cycles of chemotherapy (which was followed by radiotherapy with or without subsequent chemotherapy) was the most significant prognostic factor in their study for overall survival. Kuentz *et al.* [46] demonstrated that chemotherapy-induced complete remission after three cycles of MOPP was a favourable prognostic indicator for both localized and extensive HD. Use of this would allow early discrimination between high risk and low risk patients and help determine appropriate subsequent therapy.

The total dose of drugs administered and their rate of delivery may also be important. Carde *et al.* [28] demonstrated a dose response effect for achievement of remission with MOPP. A factor which combined the dose of drugs administered (as a percentage of the planned dose) with the rate of delivery, was highly significant by multivariate analysis for achievement of remission, particularly for patients with 'B' symptoms. The effect of drug dose on survival was less pronounced, but patients who received more than sixty-five per cent of the planned dose of nitrogen mustard for six cycles did better than those who received smaller doses. Pillai *et al.* [17] found that dosage and therapeutic intensity were important for disease-free survival and overall survival, but not for achievement of remission.

Hodgkin's Disease – Summary

Increasing age is a major adverse factor in most large series of patients with HD whether the disease is localized or extensive. Sex is, if anything, only a minor factor. Histological subtype has proved important in trials of HD which have employed clinical staging for localized disease, but otherwise appears to have little independent effect once age and extent of disease have been accounted for.

In localized disease, ESR level, 'B' symptoms and the number of sites involved probably all give independent information regarding prognosis. The majority of authors have found a large mediastinal mass to be an adverse factor requiring special attention either by the use of specialized radiotherapy techniques or the use of chemotherapy.

Advanced HD undoubtedly still carries a worse prognosis than localized disease. However, the relative importance of symptoms, anatomical substage and different extranodal sites remains unclear, probably reflecting differences in patient populations, treatment methods and, to an extent, methods of statistical analysis.

Non Hodgkin's lymphoma

The term 'non Hodgkin's lymphoma' (NHL) encompasses a heterogenous group of diseases with varied natural histories, patterns of spread and outcome following treatment. If all histological subtypes of NHL are considered together, important prognostic factors may be submerged because of opposing influences in different subgroups.

Histology

Several histological classifications of NHL have been introduced in the past twenty years. The most widely used are those of Rappaport [47], Lukes and Collins [48] and Lennert [49]. Each lays emphasis on the presence or absence of a follicular (or nodular) architectural pattern and on the predominant cell type present. Recently these classifications have been compared in detail and the clinical relevance in terms of prognostic significance of each classification has been confirmed [50]. The NHL Pathological Classification Project created a working formulation (Table 6) which separates the group into ten major subtypes based on morphological criteria alone, in order to facilitate comparison between centres using different classifications. The working formulation also identified three major subgroups of NHL namely low grade, intermediate grade and high grade.

The significance of the terms 'low grade' and 'high grade' can best be appreciated by reference to actuarial survival curves (Fig. 1). Low grade lymphomas typically pursue an indolent course with a steady decline in survival, and hence a relatively steady gradient on a survival curve with a median survival of between seven and ten years, and with little evidence of a plateau. Conversely, high grade lymphomas

Table 6. Working formulation classification of non Hodgkin's lymphoma

---

1. Low Grade
A. small lymphocytic
B. follicular, predominantly small cleaved cell
C. follicular mixed small cleaved and large cell
2. Intermediate Grade
D. follicular, predominantly large cell
E. diffuse, small cleaved cell
F. diffuse mixed small and large cell
G. diffuse large cell (cleaved + non cleaved)
3. High Grade
H. large cell, immunoblastic
I. lymphoblastic
J. small non cleaved (Burkitts)

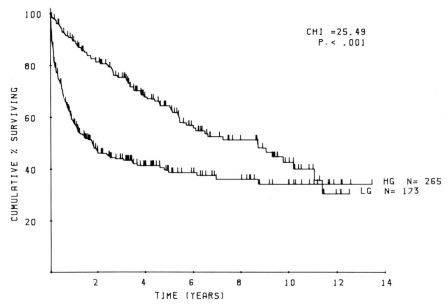

Figure 1. Actuarial survival curves in non Hodgkin's lymphoma, comparing low grade with high grade tumour patients. (St. Bartholomew's Hospital series).

show a steep initial slope reflecting a high early death rate, but thereafter the curve flattens reflecting prolonged disease free survival for many of those who have achieved a complete remission with treatment.

The clinical significance of follicularity, independent of cell type, has been observed in several studies comprising all histological subtypes of NHL [51–55]. This was confirmed by the NHL Pathological Classification Project [50]. Furthermore, in that project there was agreement between pathologists concerning the presence or absence of follicularity in almost ninety per cent of cases. The prognostic favourability of a follicular pattern is maintained whether or not the pattern is totally follicular or partially diffuse [50–52, 56].

Cell type is also of major independent prognostic significance [50, 51]. Within the follicular lymphomas the relatively rare subtype of 'follicular – predominantly large cell' (the nodular histiocytic category of Rappaport) may behave more like its 'diffuse' counterpart both in its aggressive natural history and in its response to intensive chemotherapy, rather than pursuing the typical course of a follicular lymphoma [57]. A further caveat to the prognostic advantage of follicularity has been made by Stein *et al.* [58]. They found that within the 'small cleaved cell' subtype of the Lukes and Collins classification, there was no significant difference in survival between those with follicular and those with diffuse patterns.

For lymphomas of diffuse architectural pattern there is a marked variation in survival according to cell type. At one end of the spectrum is diffuse 'small lymphocytic' lymphoma which is the lymphomatous counterpart of chronic lymphocytic leukaemia (the 'diffuse well differentiated lymphocytic' category of Rappaport). This conforms to the pattern of a low grade lymphoma, whereas all other diffuse lymphomas are of intermediate or high grade.

The diffuse large cell lymphomas (the diffuse 'histiocytic' category of Rappaport) can also be subdivided morphologically – as is done in both the Keil and Lukes and Collins classifications. However, the prognostic significance of such subclassification has been disputed. This may in part reflect the difficulty in achieving reproducibility between pathologists. The NHL Pathological Classification Project examined this problem in detail, and found a statistically significant survival difference in favour of the group of patients whose lymphomas were classified as follicular centre cell type (large cleaved and large non cleaved) over those with immunoblastic lymphomas. Armitage et al. [59] also found a survival advantage for 'large non-cleaved cell' lymphoma. The Manchester group [60] identified the 'centroblastic' histological type within the Kiel classification as a favourable group in terms of relapse-free survival and survival of remitters, but response and overall survival were not affected by histological subtype. Both the South West Oncology Group [61] and the National Cancer Institute [62] found that morphological subdivision of diffuse histiocytic lymphoma did not identify a subgroup of patients with longer survival despite earlier results to the contrary [63].

It should be noted that most current classifications are made on morphological criteria, rather than on the basis of immunological tests of B cell or T cell origin of the different lymphomas. As there is such a marked difference in natural history between histologically low grade and high grade lymphomas, and as most of the literature on prognostic factors in NHL concerns either follicular lymphomas or high grade lymphomas or high grade lymphomas, these two categories will be considered separately.

Follicular lymphoma (Table 7)

Relatively few centres have reported the results of analysis of prognostic factors in follicular lymphoma. However, there is a large degree of agreement between four centres that have done this [51, 56, 64, 65].

Age
Anderson et al. [51] found that age over forty-six years (the median age at presentation for all lymphomas at the National Cancer Institute) was associated with poorer survival (p = 0.002). Gospodarowicz et al [64] found a gradual decline in the cause-specific survival with increasing age above forty years but the greatest difference was observed by comparing those below and above seventy years of

age. Rudders *et al.* [56] found a similar effect of age, with patients over seventy years faring very poorly. However, age was not a significant factor in the study from St. Bartholomew's Hospital [65].

Stage and extent of disease

A high proportion of patients with truly localized follicular lymphoma can achieve long term disease free survival with radiotherapy, with or without adjuvant chemotherapy [66]. In the study by Rudders *et al.* [56], all eight stage I patients remain alive, and in Gallagher's study [65], each of the eleven stage I patients treated with radiotherapy achieved complete remission and only two have relapsed. The Toronto study [64] also found excellent results for patients with either stage I disease or contiguous and non-bulky stage II disease.

All four studies confirmed the marked difference in survival pattern between stages I and IV, with stages II and III having an intermediate position. However, Rudders *et al* found no significant difference in overall survival between stages II and III despite a more radical therapeutic approach being adopted for stage II patients. Gallagher *et al*'s study showed very similar relapse-free survival patterns for patients in stages II and III. This lack of separation between stages II and III, together with the fact that only a small minority of patients with follicular lymphoma present with truly localized disease, limits the clinical usefulness of the Ann Arbor classification for these patients. In addition, a proportion of stage II patients have disease for which radical radiotherapy is not feasible.

Within stage IV the influence of different sites of extranodal involvement is

Table 7. Factors reported to be of prognostic significance in non Hodgkin's lymphoma

---

Age
Sex
Histology – follicularity + cell type
Constitutional ('B') symptoms
Extent of Disease
Stage
Bulk of disease
Extranodal involvement – gastrointestinal
                        bone marrow
                        liver
Number of extranodal sites
Mediastinal involvement
Laboratory Tests
Haemoglobin
L.D.H.
Albumin
Lymphocyte count
ESR
C reactive protein

---

difficult to assess at present. Bone marrow biopsy was not performed on all patients in some studies of prognostic factors in follicular lymphoma. Liver involvement is difficult to assess clinically but hepatomegaly and abnormal liver function tests were significant adverse factors in Gallagher *et al.*'s study, whereas bone marrow involvement was not.

The Toronto group identified bulk as a major independent adverse prognostic factor (p = 0.00005). They therefore divide patients with stage II disease into a favourable group with non bulky and contiguous groups of involved lymph nodes, and an unfavourable group with bulky or non contiguous nodes.

Constitutional symptoms

Relatively little attention has been given to the significance of constitutional symptoms in NHL. Even though there is a strong correlation between constitutional symptoms and advanced stage, all three studies which used multivariate analysis found that the presence of constitutional symptoms had an independent adverse effect on survival. The fourth study (that of Rudders *et al*) also found that constitutional symptoms were a very strong negative prognostic determinant even after stratification for stage.

Haemoglobin and other laboratory tests

Gallagher *et al* found that anaemia (haemoglobin less than 11.5 g/dl) was an independent pretreatment factor of equivalent importance to that of B symptoms. Abnormal biochemical tests of liver function (alkaline phosphatase and aspartate transaminase) were also significant, but neither lymphocyte count nor levels of serum immunoglobulins were found to be important. Leonard *et al.* [67] also found haemoglobin levels to be important prognostically for all low grade lymphomas, as did Ciampi *et al.* [53] for 'lymphocytic' lymphomas: both of these studies included patients with follicular and diffuse histology.

Follicular lymphoma – Summary

Assessment of the extent of disease in follicular lymphoma by the Ann Arbor staging system gives useful information, but as about eighty per cent of patients fall within stages III and IV, this is of limited value. Additional significant information regarding prognosis can be gained by taking other factors into account, particularly age, 'B' symptoms, bulk of disease, haemoglobin level and histological subtype. As these factors affect prognosis independently, they should be combined to identify groups with different prognoses. This gives a better separation of groups than the use of stage alone [64], and should help to identify patients who might benefit from new treatment strategies.

After treatment has commenced, by far the most significant factor in determining overall survival is the response to treatment [65]. The intensity of therapy, however, may not be important in this group of patients [68]. Failure to respond may in some cases be associated with the early appearance of a high grade lymphoma, which may have been present but undetected prior to treatment. Histological transformation is usually associated with very poor prognosis.

High grade lymphomas

Several centres have published data concerning prognostic factors in high grade lymphoma within the past five years. The results of seven studies [59, 61, 62, 69–72] which give data on univariate analysis are shown in Table 8. Four of these have also used multivariate analysis as has also the study from Manchester [60] and the results are shown in Table 9. Only the reports from the National Cancer Institute and Iowa include patients with localized (stage I) disease. Various combination chemotherapy regimens, with or without radiotherapy to sites of bulky disease, have been used. The median age in the eight different studies ranged from forty-nine to sixty-four years, with six between fifty-three and fifty-six years.

Table 8. Prognostic factors for survival in patients with high grade non Hodgkin's lymphoma: results of univariate analysis

Study (ref)	NCI (62)	MSK (69)	MDA (70)	MDA (71)	SWOG (61)	SBH (72)	Iowa (59)
Histology	DM, DH, DU	DH	DLc	DLc	DH	HG	DH
Stages	All	III + IV	III + IIIE	IV	Adv	Adv	All
No. of pts	151	65	47	61	162	103	75
Age			−	+	−	+	
Sex	+			−	−		
Histological subtype	−				−		+
'B' symptoms	+			+	+	+	
Stage	+				+	+	
Bulk ⎫	+		+	−			
GI involvement ⎭							
Bone marrow	+			+			+
Liver	+					+	
No. of E sites				+			
Mediastinum			+	+			
Haemoglobin	+			−		+	
LDH·	+	+		+			
Albumin						+	
Previous CT		+				+	+
Response	+	+	+				

+ = significant factor
− = not significant
blank spaces = not specifically mentioned in report
{ + denotes that the two factors were combined in that study

A large number of factors have been found to have prognostic significance both by univariate and multivariate methods, with apparently little agreement between centres. This may be due to differences in the populations being treated, or differences in the treatments given, or differences in the methods of analysis used. If factors which reflect extent of disease are considered jointly, the apparent discrepancies between centres become less incomprehensible. When all the multivariate analyses in high grade NHL are examined together, greater importance should probably be attributed to factors which have either been shown to be highly significant ($p < .001$) by a single institution, or have been found to be significant at the $p < 0.05$ level in more than one study.

Age and sex

At both the MD Anderson Hospital and St. Bartholomew's Hospital advanced age has been shown to be a major adverse factor for survival (Table 8), whereas

Table 9. Prognostic factors for survival in patients with high grade non Hodgkin's lymphoma: results of multivariate analysis

Study (ref) Stages	NCI (62) All	MDA (71) IV	Manchester (60) Adv	SBH (72) Adv	Iowa (59) All
Age	−	+ < .01	−	+ .0005	−
Sex	+	−	−	−	−
Histological subtypes	−		−	−	+ .01
Symptoms	+	−	−	−	+ .043
Bulk	} +	−	−	−	
GI involvement			−	−	−
Bone marrow	+	−	−	−	+ .002
Liver	−		+ .001	−	−
No. of E sites		+ < .01			
Haemoglobin	−	−	−	−	−
LDH	−	+ < .05	+ .001		−
Albumin			−	+ .00001	
Previous CT	None	None	None	+ .05	−
Response	(+)	(+)	+ .001	(+)	(+)

+ = significant factor
(+) = significant factor but not included in analysis of factors for survival
− = not significant
blank spaces = not assessed or not mentioned in report
Numbers relate to p values by regression analysis where reported.
+ denotes that the two factors were combined in that study

other studies have not shown age to be important. Interestingly the two reports from the MD Anderson Hospital, one evaluating stage III and the other evaluating stage IV patients, differed regarding the importance of age.

The adverse effect of male sex which was noted by Cabanillas *et al.* [52] in their study of patients with advanced lymphoma of all histological types, was not found in the two recent studies of high grade lymphoma from the same institution. Indeed, amongst the studies outlined in Table 8 only the National Cancer Institute found sex to be important for survival, with male sex being an adverse factor.

Constitutional symptoms and extent of disease

Constitutional symptoms, stage, bulk of disease, liver involvement, and low serum albumin are all interrelated as is also high serum lactic dehydrogenase level (LDH). Each study has identified at least one of these factors as significant, and no study using multivariate analysis has shown that more than two of these factors give independent information. Although for follicular lymphomas a consistent independent effect of constitutional symptoms has been found, this does not appear to be the case for high grade NHL.

As with follicular lymphoma, truly localized disease, although rare, carries a favourable prognosis [62]. Amongst the studies of 'advanced' high grade NHL (ie stages III and IV with some stage II patients) Ann Arbor stage itself has not emerged as an independent prognostic indicator although each of the commoner sites of extranodal involvement (namely bone marrow, liver and gastrointestinal tract) in association with bulk have been shown to be significant factors in different studies. The study by Jagannath *et al.* [71] found that the number of extranodal sites was more important than any single site.

Lactic dehydrogenase level has been shown to be a useful prognostic indicator in NHL [73] and, its significance for survival in high grade lymphoma was confirmed both by the Manchester and the MD Anderson group. It probably reflects both tumour bulk and growth rate, and has the great merit of objectivity and being simple to measure (unlike bulk of disease). Recently, serum albumin level was shown to have very strong prognostic significance in the St. Bartholomew's Hospital study, and the Manchester group had also found this to be significant for achievement of remission. Whether these two simple biochemical tests yield different information deserves further investigation.

Haemoglobin level does not appear to be a good prognostic indicator in high grade lymphoma. The ESR has been little evaluated in these patients, but Leonard et al [67] found that neither ESR nor immunoglobulin levels were significant in their study of all patients with NHL, whereas elevated levels of acute phase proteins (particularly C reactive protein) were important, especially in asymptomatic patients.

Response to treatment

Achievement of complete remission with treatment has consistently been shown to be of paramount importance for prolonged survival, and is the only factor on which all studies appear to agree. This underlines the importance of assessing factors which predict achievement of remission separately from those which predict disease-free survival and overall survival. In this way, patients who need a different initial treatment strategy can be identified. Equally, it may be possible to select those who need consolidation therapy after the achievement of remission. For instance the Manchester group found that histological subtyping could identify patients at high risk of relapse following their initial treatment programme. At St. Bartholomew's Hospital, patients who had received prior chemotherapy were not at a disadvantage in terms of achieving remission, but had a high subsequent relapse rate. At the MD Anderson Hospital, relapse was highest in patients who had a high LDH level, constitutional symptoms or mediastinal involvement at presentation.

High grade NHL – Summary
The outlook for patients with high grade NHL has changed considerably in the past decade. Multivariate analysis of prognostic factors for these patients has only recently been undertaken by more than a very few centres, but, it does appear that better prognostic groupings can be identified than that given by the Ann Arbor staging classification alone. It is still uncertain as to what weight should be attributed to individual factors such as age, bulk of disease, sites of involvement and biochemical tests as LDH and albumin levels.

References

1. Cox DR: Regression models and life tables. *J R Stat Soc* 34: 187–220, 1972
2. Hoppe RT, Rosenberg SA, Kaplan HS, Cox RS: Prognostic factors in pathological stage IIIA Hodgkin's disease. *Cancer* 46: 1240–1246, 1980
3. Tubiana M, Henry-Amar M, Van der Werf-Messing B, Henry J, Abbatucci J, Burgers M, Hayat M, Somers R, Laugier A, Carde P: A multivariate analysis of prognostic factors in early stage Hodgkin's disease. *Int J Radiation Oncology Biol Phys* 11: 23–30, 1985
4. Sutcliffe SB, Gospodarowicz MK, Bergsagel DE, Bush RS, Alison RE, Bean HA, Brown TC, Chua T, Clark RM, Curtis JE, Dembo AJ, Fitzpatrick PJ, Hasselback RH, Rideout DF, Sturgeon JFG, Quirt I, Yeoh L, Peters MV: Prognostic groups for management of localized Hodgkin's disease. *J Clin Oncol* 3: 393–401, 1985
5. Haybittle JL, Easterling MJ, Bennett MH, Vaughan Hudson B, Hayhoe FGJ, Jelliffe AM, Vaughan Hudson G, MacLennan KA: Review of British National Lymphoma Investigation studies of Hodgkin's disease and development of prognostic index. Lancet i: 967–972, 1985
6. Fuller LM, Madoc-Jones H, Gamble JF, Butler JJ, Sullivan MP, Fernandez CH, Gehan EA: New assessment of the prognostic significance of histopathology in Hodgkin's disease for laparotomy-negative stage I and II patients. *Cancer* 39: 2174–2182, 1977
7. Carbone PP, Kaplan HS, Mushoff K, Smithers DW, Tubiana M: Report of the committee on Hodgkin's disease staging classification. *Cancer Res* 31: 1860–1861
8. Lukes RJ, Butler JJ: The pathology and nomenclature of Hodgkin's disease. *Cancer, Red* 26: 1063–1081, 1966

9. Kaplan HS: Hodgkin's disease: Unfolding concepts concerning its nature, management and prognosis. *Cancer* 45: 2439–2474, 1980

10. Wedelin G, Bjorkholm M, Biberfeld P, Holm G, Johansson B, Mellstedt H: Prognostic factors in Hodgkin's disease with special reference to age. *Cancer* 53: 1202–1208, 1984

11. Hoppe RT, Coleman CN, Cox RS, Rosenberg SA, Kaplan HS: The management of stage I-II Hodgkin's disease with irradiation alone or combined modality therapy: The Stanford experience. *Blood* 59 (3): 455–465, 1982

12. Leslie NT, Mauch PM, Hellman S: Stage IA to IIB supradiaphragmatic Hodgkin's disease: Long term survival and relapse frequency. *Cancer* 55: 2072–2078, 1985

13. Hagemeister FB, Fuller LM, Velasquez WS, Sullivan JA, North L, Butler JJ, Johnston DA, Shullenberger CC: Stage I and II Hodgkin's disease: Involved field radiotherapy versus extended field radiotherapy versus involded field radiotherapy followed by six cycles of MOPP. *Cancer Treat Rep* 66: 789–798, 1982

14. Bearman RM, Pangalis GA, Rappaport H: Hodgkin's disease, lymphocyte depletion type. A clinicopathologic study of 39 patients. *Cancer* 41: 293–302, 1978

15. Prosnitz LR, Farber LR, Kapp DS, Bertino JR, Nordlund M, Lawrence R: Combined modality therapy for advanced Hodgkin's disease: Long term follow up data. *Cancer Treat Rep* 66: 871–879, 1982

16. Stein RS, Golomb HM, Diggs CH, Mauch P, Hellman S, Wiernik PH, Ultmann JE, Rosenthal DS: Anatomic substages of stage IIIA Hodgkin's disease. *Ann Int Med* 92: 159–165, 1980

17. Pillai GN, Hagemeister FB, Velasquez WS, Sullivan JA, Johnston DA, Butler JJ, Shullenberger CC: Prognostic factors for stage IV Hodgkin's disease treated with MOPP with or without Bleomycin. *Cancer* 55: 691–697, 1985

18. DeVita VT, Simon RM, Hubbard SM, Young RC, Berard CW, Moxley JH, Frei E, Carbone PP, Canellos GP: Curability of advanced Hodgkin's disease with chemotherapy. Long term follow up of MOPP treated patients at the National Cancer Institute. *Ann Int Med* 92: 587–595, 1980

19. Rodgers RW, Fuller LM, Hagemeister FB, Johnston DA, Sullivan JA, North LB, Butler JJ, Velasquez WS, Conrad FG, Shullenberger CC: Reassessment of prognostic factors in stage IIIA and IIIB Hodgkin's disease treated with MOPP and radiotherapy. *Cancer* 47: 2196–2203, 1981

20. Peterson BA, Pajak TF, Cooper MR, Nissen NI, Glidewell OJ, Holland JF, Bloomfield CD, Gottlieb AJ: Effect of age on therapeutic response and survival in advanced Hodgkin's disease. *Cancer Treat Rep* 66: 889–898, 1982

21. Tubiana M, Henry-Amar M, Hayat M, Burgers M, Qasim M, Somers R, Sizoo W, Van der Schueren E: Prognostic significance of the number of involved areas in the early stages of Hodgkin's disease. *Cancer* 54: 885–894, 1984

22. Peckham MJ, Ford HT, McElwain TJ, Harmer CL, Atkinson K, Austin DE: The results of radiotherapy for Hodgkin's disease. *Br J Cancer* 32: 391–400, 1975

23. Carmel RJ, Kaplan HS: Mantle irradiation in Hodgkin's disease: An analysis of technique, tumor eradication and complications. *Cancer* 37: 2813–2825, 1976

24. Thar TL, Million RR, Hausner RJ, McKetty MHB: Hodgkin's disease stages I and II. Relationship of recurrence to size of disease, radiation dose and number of sites involved. *Cancer* 43: 1101–1105, 1979

25. Desser RK, Golomb HM, Ultmann JE, Ferguson DJ, Moran EM, Griem ML, Wardiman J, Miller B, Oetzel N, Sweet D, Lester EP, Kinzie JJ, Blough R: Prognostic classification of Hodgkin's disease in pathologic stage III, based on anatomic considerations. *Blood* 49: 883–893, 1977

26. Hoppe RT, Cox RS, Rosenberg SA, Kaplan HS: Prognostic factors in pathologic stage III Hodgkin's disease. *Cancer Treat Rep* 66: 743–749, 1982

27. Lister TA, Dorreen MS, Faux M, Jones AE, Wrigley PFM: The treatment of stage IIIA Hodgkin's disease. *J Clin Oncol* 1: 745–749, 1983

28. Carde P, MacKintosh FR, Rosenberg SA: A dose and time response analysis of the treatment of Hodgkin's disease with MOPP chemotherapy. *J Clin Oncol* 1: 146–153, 1983

29. Peters MV: A study of survival in Hodgkin's disease treated radiologically. *Am J Roentgenol* 63: 299–311, 1950
30. Papillon J: The curability of Hodgkin's disease. In: Diagnosis and Therapy of Malignant Lymphoma, Musshoff K (ed). Berlin: Springer Verlag 1974, pp 195–200
31. Fuller LM, Gamble JF, Ibrahim E, Jing B-S, Butler JJ, Shullenberger CC: Stage II Hodgkin's disease (significance of mediastinal and non mediastinal presentations). *Radiology* 109: 429–435, 1973
32. Fuller LM, Hutchison GB: Collaborative clinical trial for stage I and II Hodgkin's disease: Significance of mediastinal and non mediastinal disease in laparotomy and non-laparotomy staged patients. *Cancer Treat Rep* 66: 775–787, 1982
33. Dorreen MS, Wrigley PFM, Laidlow JM, Plowman PN, Neudachin L, Tucker AK, Malpas JS, Stansfeld AG, Faux MMML, Jones AE, Lister TA: The management of stage II supradiaphragmatic Hodgkin's disease at St. Bartholomew's Hospital, *Cancer* 54: 2882–2888, 1984
34. Ferrant A, Hamoir V, Binon J, Michaux J-L, Sokal G: Combined modality therapy for mediastinal Hodgkin's disease: Prognostic significance of constitutional symptoms and size of disease. *Cancer* 55: 317–322, 1985
35. Lee CKK, Bloomfield CD, Goldman AI, Levitt SH: Prognostic significance of mediastinal involvement in Hodgkin's disease treated with curative radiotherapy. *Cancer* 46: 2403–2409, 1980
36. Cosset JM, Henry-Amar M, Carde P, Clarke D, Le Bourgeois JP, Tubiana M: The prognostic significance of large mediastinal masses in the treatment of Hodgkin's disease. The experience of the Institut Gustave-Roussy. *Haemat Oncol* 2: 33–43, 1984
37. Mauch P, Gorshein D, Cunningham J, Hellman S: Influence of mediastinal adenopathy on site and frequency of relapse in patients with Hodgkin's disease. *Cancer Treat Rep* 66: 809–817, 1982
38. Wiernik PH, Slawson RG: Hodgkin's disease with direct extension into pulmonary parenchyma from a mediastinal mass; A presentation requiring special therapeutic considerations. *Cancer Treat Rep* 66: 711–716, 1982
39. Tubiana M, Henry-Amar M, Burgers MV, Van der Werf-Messing B, Hayat M: Prognostic significance of erythrocyte sedimentation rate in clinical stages I and II of Hodgkin's disease. *J Clin Oncol* 2: 194–200, 1984
40. Thorling EB, Thorling K: The clinical usefulness of serum copper determinations in Hodgkin's disease. *Cancer* 38: 225–231, 1976
41. Young RC, Corder MP, Benard CW, DeVita VT: Immune alterations in Hodgkin's disease. *Arch Intern Med* 131: 446–454, 1973
42. Bjorkholm M, Wedelin C, Holm G, Ogenstad S, Johansson B, Mellstedt H: Immune status of untreated patients with Hodgkin's disease and prognosis. *Cancer Treat Rep* 66: 701–709, 1982
43. Amlot PL, Slaney J, Brown R: Atopy – a favourable prognostic factor for survival in Hodgkin's disease. *Br J Cancer* 48: 209–215, 1983
44. Osoba D, Falk JA, Sousan P, Ciampi A, Till JE: The prognostic value of HLA phenotypes in Hodgkin's disease. *Cancer* 46: 1825–1832, 1980
45. Zittoun R, Audebert A, Hoerni B, Bernadou A, Krulik M, Rojouan J, Eghbali H, Merle-Beral H, Parlier Y, Diebold J, Grellet J, Laugier A, Debray J: Extended versus involved fields irradiation combined with MOPP chemotherapy in early clinical stages of Hodgkin's disease. *J Clin Oncol* 3: 207–214, 1985
46. Kuentz M, Reyes F, Brun B, Le-Bourgeois JP, Bierling P, Farcet JP, Vernant JP, Imbert M, Le Bezu M, Rochant H, Dreyfus B: Early response to chemotherapy as a prognostic factor in Hodgkin's disease. *Cancer* 52: 780–785, 1983
47. Rappaport H: Tumors of the haematopoietic system. In: *Atlas of Tumour Pathology,* section 3, fascicle 8. Washington DC, US Armed Forces Institute of Pathology 1966
48. Lukes RJ, Collins RD: Immunological characterization of human malignant lymphomas. *Cancer* 34: 1488–1503, 1974

356

49. Lennert K: *Malignant lymphomas other than Hodgkin's disease.* Springer-Verlag, New York, Heidelberg, Berlin 1978

50. The Non Hodgkin's Lymphoma Pathologic Classification Project: National Cancer Institute sponsored study of classifications of non-Hodgkin's lymphomas. Summary and description of a working formulation for clinical usage. *Cancer* 49: 2112–2135, 1982

51. Anderson T, DeVita VT, Simon RM, Berard CW, Canellos GP, Garvin AJ, Young RC. Malignant lymphoma. II Prognostic factors and response to treatment of 473 patients at the National Cancer Institute. *Cancer* 50: 2708–2721, 1982

52. Cabanillas F, Burke JS, Smith TL, Moon TE, Butler JJ, Rodriguez V: Factors predicting for response and survival in adults with advanced non-Hodgkin's lymphoma. *Arch Intern Med* 138: 413–418, 1978

53. Ciampi A, Bush RS, Gospodarowicz M, Till JE: An approach to classifying prognostic factors related to survival experience for non Hodgkin's lymphoma patients (based on a series of 982 patients 1967–1975). *Cancer* 47: 621–627, 1981

54. Bloomfield CD, Goldman A, Dick F, Brunning RD, Kennedy BJ: Multivariate analysis of prognostic factors in the non Hodgkin's malignant lymphomas. *Cancer* 33: 870–879, 1974

55. Jones SE, Fuks Z, Bull M, Kadin ME, Dorfman RF, Kaplan HS, Rosenberg SA, Kim H: Non Hodgkin's lymphomas IV. Clinicopathologic correlation in 405 cases. *Cancer* 31: 806–823, 1973

56. Rudders RA, Kaddis M, DeLellis RA, Casey H: Nodular non Hodgkin's lymphoma (NHL) – factors influencing prognosis and indications for aggressive treatment. *Cancer* 43: 1643–1651, 1979

57. Osborne CK, Norton L, Young RC, Garvin AJ, Simon RM, Berard CW, Hubbard S, DeVita VT: Nodular histocytic lymphoma; An aggressive nodular lymphoma with potential for prolonged disease free survival. *Blood* 56: 98–103, 1980

58. Stein RS, Cousar J, Flexner JM, Graber SF, McKee LC, Krantz S, Collins RD: Malignant lymphomas of follicular center cell origin in man. III prognostic features. *Cancer* 44: 2236–2243, 1979

59. Armitage JO, Dick FR, Corder MP, Garneau SC, Platz CE, Slymen DJ: Predicting therapeutic outcome in patients with diffuse histiocytic lymphoma treated with cyclophosphamide, adriamycin, vincristine and prednisolone (CHOP). *Cancer* 50: 1695–1702, 1982

60. Steward WP, Todd IDH, Harris M, Jones JM, Blackledge G, Wagstaff J, Anderson H, Wilkinson PM, Crowther D: A multivariate analysis of factors affecting survival in patients with high grade histology non Hodgkin's lymphoma. *Eur J Cancer Clin Oncol* 20: 881–889, 1984

61. Nathwani BN, Dixon DO, Jones SE, Hartsock RJ, Rebuck JW, Byrne GE, Sheehan WW, Kim H, Coltman CA, Rappaport H: The clinical significance of the morphological subdivision of diffuse 'histiocytic' lymphoma: A study of 162 patients treated by the Southwest Oncology Group. *Blood* 60: 1068–1074, 1982

62. Fisher RI, Hubbard SM, DeVita VT, Berard CW, Wesley R, Cossman J, Young RC: Factors predicting long term survival in diffuse mixed, histiocytic, or undifferentiated lymphoma. *Blood* 58: 45–51, 1981

63. Strauchen JA, Young RC, DeVita VT, Anderson T, Fantone JC, Berard CW: Clinical relevance of the histopathological subclassification of diffuse histiocytic lymphoma. *N. Engl J Med* 299: 1382–1387, 1978

64. Gospodarowicz MK, Bush RS, Brown TC, Chua T: Prognostic factors in nodular lymphomas: A multivariate analysis based on the Princess Margaret Hospital experience. *Int J Radiation Oncology Biol phys* 10: 489–497, 1984

65. Gallagher CJ, Gregory WM, Jones AE, Stansfeld AG, Richards MA, Dhaliwal HS, Malpas JS, Lister TA: Follicular lymphoma. Prognostic factors for response and survival. *J clin Oncol* 1986. In press

66. Chen MG, Prosnitz LR, Gonzalez-Serva A, Fischer DB: Results of radiotherapy in control of stage I and II non Hodgkin's lymphoma. *Cancer* 43: 1245–1254, 1979

67. Leonard RCF, Cuzick J, MacLennan ICM, Vanhegan RI, MacKie PH, McCormick CV and the Oxford Lymphoma Group: Prognostic factors in non Hodgkin's lymphoma: The importance of symptomatic stage as an adjunct to the Kiel histopathological classification. *Br J Cancer* 47: 91–102, 1983

68. Lister TA, Cullen MH, Beard MEJ, Brearley RL, Whitehouse JMA, Wrigley PFM, Stansfeld AG, Sutcliffe SBJ, Malpas JS, Crowther D. Comparison of combined and single-agent chemotherapy in non-Hodgkin's lymphoma of favourable histological type. *Br Med J* 1: 533–537, 1978

69. Koziner B, Little C, Passe S, Thaler HT, Sklaroff R, Straus DJ, Lee BJ, Clarkson BD: Treatment of advanced diffuse histiocytic lymphoma: An analysis of prognostic variables. *Cancer* 49: 1571–1579, 1982

70. Velasquez W, Fuller LM, Oh KK, Hagemeister FB, Sullivan JA, Manning JT, Shullenberger CC: Combined modality therapy in stage III and stage IIIE diffuse large cell lymphomas. *Cancer* 53: 1478–1483, 1984

71. Jagannath S, Velasquez WS, Tucker SL, Manning JT, McLaughlin P, Fuller LM: Stage IV diffuse large-cell lymphoma: A long term analysis. *J Clin Oncol* 3: 39–47, 1985

72. Dhaliwal HS, Richards MA, Gallagher CJ, Ash CM, Gregory W, Barnett MJ, Ganesan TS, Rohatiner AZS, Stansfeld AG, Malpas JS, Wrigley PFM, Lister TA: MACOP therapy of advanced high grade non Hodgkin's lymphoma with moderate dose mid-cycle methotrexate and CHOP-type chemotherapy. In preparation

73. Ferraris AM, Giuntini P, Gaetani GF. Serum lactic dehydrogenase as a prognostic tool for non Hodgkin's lymphomas. *Blood* 54: 928–932, 1979

Index